Pathophysiology and Management
of
THROMBOEMBOLIC DISORDERS

Edited by
Kenneth K. Wu

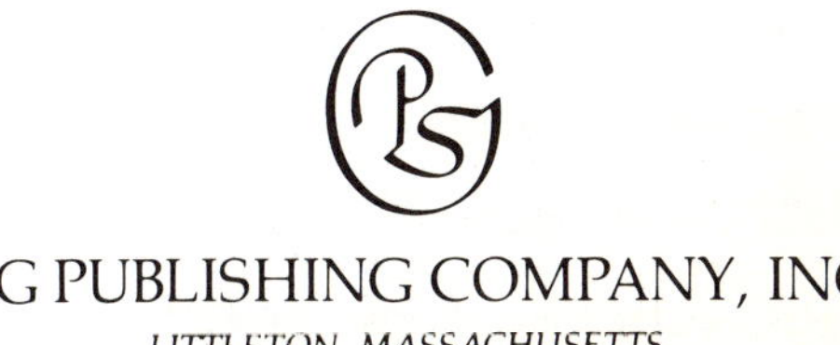

PSG PUBLISHING COMPANY, INC.
LITTLETON, MASSACHUSETTS

Library of Congress in Publication Data
Main entry under title:

Pathophysiology and management of thromboembolic
   disorders.

   Bibliography: p.
   Includes index.
   1. Thromboembolism.   I. Wu, Kenneth K. [DNLM:
1. Thromboembolism—Physiopathology.   2. Thromboembolism—
Therapy.   3. Arterial occlusive diseases—Physiopathology.
4. Arterial occlusive diseases—Therapy.   QZ 170 P297]
RC694.3.P34   1984   616.1′45   84-4292
ISBN 0-88416-460-8

Published by
PSG Publishing Company, Inc.
545 Great Road
Littleton, Massachusetts 01460

Medicine is an ever-changing science. As new research and clinical experience broaden our knowledge, changes in treatment and drug therapy are required. The author and the publisher of this work have made every effort to ensure that the treatment and drug dosage schedules herein are accurate and in accord with the standards accepted at the time of publication. Readers are advised, however, to check the product information sheet included in the package of each drug they plan to administer to be certain that changes have not been made in the recommended dose or in the indications and contraindications for administration. This recommendation is of particular importance in regard to new or infrequently used drugs.

Printed in the United States of America.

International Standard Book Number: 0–88416–460–8

Library of Congress Catalog Card Number: 84-4292

To my wife
Lung-Chin

Contributors

Edmond Cole, PhD
Associate Professor
Departments of Medicine and
  Biochemistry
Rush Medical College
Chicago, Illinois

L. Henry Edmunds, Jr, MD
W. M. Measey Professor
Chief Cardiothoracic Surgery
University of Pennsylvania
Philadelphia, Pennsylvania

Elizabeth R. Hall, PhD
Assistant Professor
Department of Internal Medicine
University of Texas Medical
  School
Houston, Texas

Paul D. Hirsh, MD
Assistant Professor
Department of Medicine
Medical College of Virginia
Virginia Commonwealth
  University
Richmond, Virginia

Jack Hirsh, MD
Professor and Chairman
Department of Medicine
McMaster University
Hamilton, Ontario
CANADA

Russell D. Hull, MD, FRCP(C)
Associate Professor
Department of Medicine
McMaster University
Hamilton, Ontario
CANADA

Richard Jay, MD, FRCP(C)
Clinical Research Fellow
Department of Medicine
McMaster University
Hamilton, Ontario
CANADA

Jacques Leclerc, MD, FRCP(C)
Clinical Research Fellow
Department of Medicine
McMaster University
Hamilton, Ontario
CANADA

Bruce J. Pardy, ChM, FRCS
Consultant Surgeon
St. Andrew's Hospital and
  Newham Hospital
London
UNITED KINGDOM

John A. Payne, MD
Associate Professor
Department of Medicine
Rush Medical College
Chicago, Illinois

Max E. Rafelson, PhD
Professor
Department of Biochemistry
Rush Medical College
Chicago, Illinois

Ennio C. Rossi, MD
Professor and Chief
Section of Hematology
Department of Medicine
Northwestern University Medical
  School
Chicago, Illinois

Richard J. Sassetti, MD
Assistant Professor
Department of Medicine
Rush Medical College
Chicago, Illinois

Robert W. Stein, MD
Fellow
Department of Neurology
Michael Reese Hospital and
    Medical Center
Chicago, Illinois

William J. Weiner, MD
Professor
Department of Neurology
University of Miami Medical
    School
Miami, Florida

James W. West, MD
Assistant Professor
Department of Medicine
Rush Medical College
Chicago, Illinois

Michael J. Weston, MD, FRCP
Consultant Physician
Dulwich Hospital
London
UNITED KINGDOM

James T. Willerson, MD
Professor and Director
Division of Cardiology
Department of Medicine
University of Texas Southwest
    Medical School
Dallas, Texas

Kenneth K. Wu, MD
Professor and Co-Director
Division of Hematology–Oncology
Department of Internal Medicine
University of Texas Medical
    School
Houston, Texas

Contents

Preface

In the past decade, there has been a rapid advance in the basic and the clinical understanding of thrombosis. It is recognized as one of the most important pathologic processes in causing human diseases. This book represents our attempt to provide practicing physicians, house officers and students with an updated overview of the basic principles of thrombogenic mechanisms and their involvement in the pathogenesis of various vascular thromboembolic disorders.

For the sake of convenience, the book is divided into five major sections. The first section deals with the basic subjects that are directly related to thrombogenesis. Certain subjects, such as atherosclerosis which is obviously important in arterial occlusive disorders, are described only in brief fashion because they have been widely covered in numerous books and review articles. Readers interested in pursuing further knowledge of these subjects are advised to consult the relevant publications. Sections II through V are arbitrarily divided into arterial venous-, microvascular- and artificial surface-related thromboembolic diseases. Emphasis is placed on the thromboembolic nature of these disorders. Detailed information with respect to the grave consequences of thromboembolism such as myocardial infarction and its complications is beyond the scope of this book and readers are referred to standard textbooks in the field of cardiology, neurology, etc for further information.

This book intends to cover vascular thromboembolic disorders that are commonly encountered in clinical practice. For example, Section II (Arterial Occlusive Disorders) covers coronary, cerebral, peripheral and mesenteric artery thrombosis; Section IV, peripheral venous thrombosis (deep and superficial venous thrombosis in low extremities) and visceral vein thrombosis (mesenteric, hepatic and portal). In the microvascular thrombosis section, only three major syndromes are included: 1) disseminated intravascular coagulation (DIC), 2) thrombotic thrombocytopenic purpura (TTP) and hemolytic-uremic syndrome (HUS). Obviously, it may be argued that microvascular thrombi may play a role in the pathogenesis of renal disease. However, until the causative role of thrombosis is more clearly defined, it seems unjustified to include it in this section.

Drug therapy of most thromboembolic disorders is empirical and lacks an absolute standard regimen. The dosage and usage schedule of most agents are currently acceptable as of this writing. It must be emphasized, however, that they may be modified in the future in the light of pharmacologic advances.

The author is indebted to Ms Theresa Molynaus, Majorie Jaski and Audrey Papp for their valuable secretarial and editorial assistance.

1 *Historical Perspective*

Kenneth K. Wu

The history of thrombocmoblism perhaps could be dated back to the era of Aristotle when he observed fibers in the blood, which became solidified upon cooling, but frank scientific documentation occurred only some three hundred years ago. Since the history of thrombosis is interwoven with that of basic blood clotting (hemostasis), congenital bleeding problems, platelets, and blood vessels, this discussion will be limited to the events that the author considers to be directly relevant to clinical thrombosis.

In the seventeenth and eighteenth centuries, clot formation and its relation to disease states became recognized. Marcello Malpighi (1628–1694), the noted Italian scientist and physician, of Bologna, Italy, among many of his important contributions noted blood clot formation and distinguished postmortem clots from premortem clots. William Harvey (1578–1657), the great English physiologist, attributed the postmortem clot formation to the blood stasis due to cessation of heart beat. John Hunter (1728–1793), the leading surgeon and medical scientist from Glasgow, Scotland, observed iliac artery clots in a patient with foot gangrene.

Studies with respect to mechanisms of vascular thrombosis flourished in the nineteenth century. In this era we were confronted with the bitter arguments about atherogenesis and the repeated misidentification of platelets as fragments of other cells by great morphologists. Nevertheless, one should be quite enchanted by the remarkable achievements made by people like Virchow, Rokitansky, Bizzozero, Hayem, Zahn, Wharton-Jones, and Eberth. Rudolph Virchow (1821–1902) exerted great influence on the concept of pathology and disease pathogenesis and is considered to be the father of modern pathology. He recognized the importance of blood stasis, vascular injury, and clot formation in the pathogenesis of thrombosis. These three pathogenetic factors are duly termed Virchow's triad. Through his keen observations in performing pathologic examination he put forth a theory for the pathogenesis of atherosclerosis. The imbibing (or infiltration) theory stated that the constituents of the atherosclerotic lesion were derived from blood by way of passing through the endothelium into the intima. His authoritative view was so dominant that it discouraged further investigation into other causes of these lesions for many years, including an important alternative hypothesis advocated

2

by Karl Rokitansky (1804–1878). Rokitansky, born in Königgrätz, Bohemia, studied medicine at Prague and Vienna, where he dedicated his life to the study of pathology. In his famous *Handbuch der pathologischen Anatomie* published in 1842, he postulated that the thickening of arterial walls might be caused by an excessive deposition on the arterial surface, the so-called encrustation (or thrombogenic) hypothesis. This hypothesis was bitterly criticized by Virchow and was suppressed until the early part of the twentieth century when the hypothesis was supported by Duguid's investigations.[1] Both theories are considered to be of equal importance for explaining the pathogenesis of atherosclerosis.

Experimental thrombosis was initiated in England while both atherogenesis theories were being debated in Prussia. Wharton-Jones was credited with making the first direct observations by microscopic examination on thrombus formation in living vessels of frogs.[2] He thought that these cells underwent rapid degeneration to form a mass of amorphous tissues. It is now recognized that the cells attached to the damaged vessel wall are platelets and that they usually remain intact under electronmicroscopic examination. These small blood cells, which are recognized as playing a pivotal role in thrombosis and atherosclerosis, were noted by several great morphologists but were considered artifacts, ie, leukocyte fragments. This viewpoint persisted until 1882 when Bizzozero[3] and Hayem[4] independently observed their role in hemostatic plug formation and identified them clearly as cells distinct from erythrocytes and leukocytes. Bizzozero (1846–1901), born in Varese, Italy, trained with Virchow and spent his academic life at the University of Turin. His vivid description of hemostatic plug formation is a classic example of how astute observations combined with hard work can swiftly correct a hypothesis predominantly based on false impressions. The next revolutionary observation about platelets did not occur until 1960 when Hellem demonstrated the secretion of adenosine diphosphate from platelets.[5] Subsequently, platelet research has moved at a rapid pace and branched into almost every discipline of biomedical research.

The other major constituent of a thrombus is fibrin. Use of the word "fibrin" was credited to Chaptal in 1797[6] and its importance in hemostasis and thrombosis was quickly recognized. However, an understanding of the complex mechanisms which lead to fibrin formation did not begin until the late nineteenth century. Fibrinogen was purified and its clottability by thrombin was identified by Hammerstein around 1880[7–9]; the concept of the presence of an inactive precursor of thrombin had been proposed by Buchanan.[10] The role of calcium in clotting was defined by Arthus and Pagès.[11] These discoveries laid the foundation for Morawitz's classic theory of coagulation, published in 1905.[12] Based on his own observation that tissue juices did not contain prothrombin or thrombin, he postulated that prothrombin was first converted to thrombin by thromboplastin and calcium. Thrombin then converted fibrinogen to fibrin. In the subsequent fifty years, several new coagulation factors were discovered. The history of their discovery and identification illustrates the productivity that can come from studying the experiments of nature. Finding a patient with a bleeding problem whose coagulation defect is different from existing defects set the stage for the discovery of factor V in 1944 by Owren,[13] factor IX in 1952 by Biggs et al[14] and Aggeler et al,[15] factor XI by Rosenthal et al in 1953,[16] factor XII by Ratnoff and Colopy in 1955[17] and factor X by Hougie et al in 1957.[18] The classic theory of Morawitz was no longer considered to be adequate for explaining the coagulation process. Several modern coagulation schemes have been proposed, of which Macfarlane's cascade hypothesis[19] has become the most commonly acceptable.

In the past thirty years we have witnessed the utility of modern sophisticated physical and chemical techniques in the elucidation of biochemical mechanisms of thrombus formation (eg, genetic engineering in the production of powerful fibrinolytic agents and the biological and chemical synthesis of new antithrombotic compounds). The future of thrombus research will be as enlightening as ever!

REFERENCES

1. Duguid JB: Pathogenesis of atherosclerosis. *Lancet* 1949;2:925–927.
2. Wharton-Jones T: Thrombosis in the frog. *Guy's Hosp Rep 2nd Ser* 1851;7:1.
3. Bizzozero G: Über einen neuen Formbestandtheil des Blutes und dessen Rolle bei der Thrombose und der Blutgerinnung. *Virchows Arch Pathol Anat* 1881;90:261.
4. Hayem G: Nouvelle contribution a l'étude des concrétions sanguines intravasculaires. *C R Seances Acad Sci* 1883;97:144.
5. Hellem AJ: The adhesiveness of human blood platelets in vitro. *Scand J Clin Lab Invest* 1960;12(suppl 51):1.
6. Chaptal HA: Des observations sur les de quelques végétaux et sur les moyens dent le carbone circule dans le végétal et s'y dépose pour servir à nutrition. *Ann Chim* 1797;21:284.
7. Hammersten O: Zur Lehre von der Faserstoffgerinnung. *Pflugers Arch* 1877;14:211.
8. Hammersten O: Über das Fibrinogen (Erster Abschnitt). *Pflugers Arch* 1879;19:563.
9. Hammersten O: Über das Fibrinogen (Zweiter Abschnitt). *Pflugers Arch* 1880;22:431.
10. Buchanan A: On the coagulation of the blood and other fibriniferous liquids. *London Med Gas* 1845;1:617.
11. Arthus M, Pagès C: Nouvelle théorie chimique de la coagulation du sang. *Arch Physiol* 1890;2:739.
12. Morawitz P: Die Chemie der Blutgerinnung. *Ergeb Physiol* 1905;4:307.
13. Owren PA: Parahaemophilia: Haemorrhagic diathesis due to absence of a previous unknown clotting factor. *Lancet* 1947;1:446.
14. Biggs R, Douglas AS, Macfarlane RG, et al: Christmas disease: a condition previously mistaken for haemophilia. *Br Med J* 1952;2:1378.

15. Aggeler PM, White SG, Glendening MB, et al: Plasma thromboplastin component (PTC) deficiency: A new disease resembling hemophilia. *Proc Soc Exp Biol Med* 1952;79:692.
16. Rosenthal RL, Dreskin OH, Rosenthal V: New hemophilia-like disease caused by deficiency of a third plasma thromboplastin factor. *Proc Soc Exp Biol Med* 1953;82:171.
17. Ratnoff OD, Colopy JE: A familial hemorrhagic trait associated with deficiency of a clot-promoting fraction of plasma. *J Clin Invest* 1955;34:602.
18. Hougie C, Barrow EM, Graham JB: Stuart clotting defect. I. Segregation of an hereditary hemorrhagic state from the heterogeneous group heretofore called "stable factor" deficiency. *J Clin Invest* 1957;36:485.
19. Macfarlane RG: The basis of the cascade hypothesis of blood clotting. *Thromb Diath Haemorrh* 1966;15:591.

2   *Thrombogenesis, Atherogenesis and Hypercoagulability*

Kenneth K. Wu

Human thrombocmbolic disorders encompass a variety of clinical syndromes with diversified etiologies. Pathogenesis and clinical manifestations, symptoms and signs are influenced greatly by the localization of the thromboembolism. Blocking of large- or medium-sized arteries by thromboemboli results in severe ischemic pain and life-threatening organ infarction. Thromboembolism of the microcirculation leads to subtle symptomatology owing to multiple organ involvement. The clinical presentation of venous thromboembolism, on the other hand, is attributable to inflammation of the involved tissue. Despite the complexity of clinical manifestations, there is a common, basic pathogenetic mechanism by which thromboembolism is developed in these disorders. The general mechanism of thrombogenesis will be depicted in this chapter. Readers are referred to the subsequent chapters for a more detailed description of the key elements and factors involved in this process, ie, platelets and endothelium, chapter 3; coagulation and fibrinolysis, chapter 4; and rheology, chapter 5.

THROMBOGENESIS

Normal endothelial lining of the vascular wall provides an important barrier preventing circulating platelets and coagulation proteins from adhering to the subendothelium, whereby the platelets are activated and a rapid succession of cellular and biochemical events occurs (Figure 2-1).[1] Platelets undergo secretion of their cellular contents, notably adenosine diphosphate (ADP) and serotonin, to induce platelet aggregation.[2] Moreover, the activated platelets provide a catalytic surface for accelerating the coagulation cascade, leading to the generation of thrombin and eventually fibrin formation.[3] Thrombin is a potent platelet aggregating agent which promotes platelet aggregate formation. The platelet mass is further increased by metabolites of the arachidonic acid pathway, ie, thromboxane A_2 and endoperoxides, which are synthesized following platelet activation.[4] The growing platelet mass is interspersed with fibrin strings, which anchor the platelet mass to the damaged vessel wall. The process of thrombotic plug formation appears to be modulated by a number of physiologic factors (Figure 2-2). On the one hand, there are factors that promote platelet and fibrin plug formation. On the other

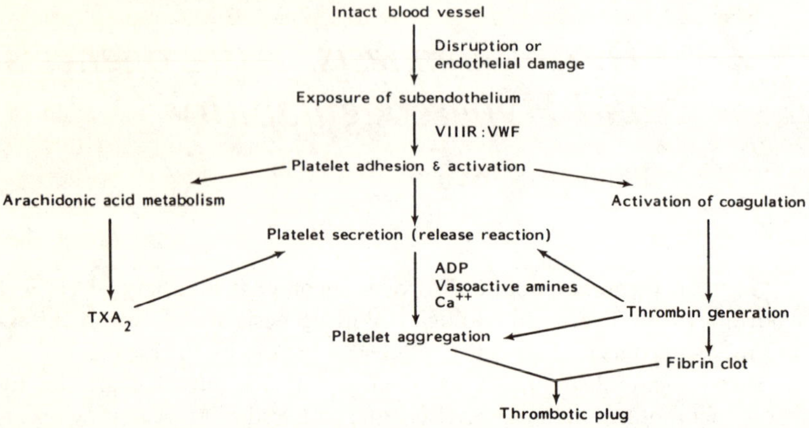

Figure 2-1 Mechanisms of hemostasis and thrombosis.

hand, there exist defense mechanisms that remove platelet aggregates and dissolve fibrin. These factors can be divided into four major categories: (*a*) blood cells, (*b*) plasma proteins, (*c*) rheologic factors, and (*d*) vascular wall function. Most of the factors are intrinsic in nature, but exogenous factors such as immune complexes, viruses, dietary factors, and chemicals may enhance platelet aggregation and therefore contribute to thrombus formation. Balance between the promoting and the defending factors probably plays a pivotal role in the regulation of thrombosis. Thus, an imbalanced state due to perturbation of the defense mechanisms and/or enhancement of the endogenous- or exogenous-promoting factors can lead to a propensity for thrombosis.

Experimental studies have shown that the endothelium can be damaged by dietary factors, chemicals, immune complexes, and viruses. Because of the availability of powerful defense mechanisms, acute vascular damage does not usually cause thrombosis unless there is an underlying vascular disease such as atherosclerosis, repetition of vascular injuries, or a compromised state of defense mechanisms. At least three defense mechanisms are recognized: (1) natural inhibitors of coagulation, ie, antithrombin III (AT-III)[5] and protein C,[6] which can block excessive thrombus formation; (2) prostacyclin and PGD_2, which inhibit platelet aggregation;[6] moreover, PGI_2 disrupts platelet aggregates; and (3) plasminogen activators, which trigger plasmin formation and dissolve fibrin clots.[7] Breakdown of the defense mechanisms is noted to predispose an individual to recurrent thromboembolic disorders. For example, AT-III deficiency[7,8] and protein C deficiency[9] cause recurrent deep vein thrombosis and plumonary embolism. Reduced fibrinolytic capacity may contribute to high risk of thrombosis.[9]

Despite a similar basic mechanism underlying all the human thrombotic disorders, there are substantial differences in the pathogenesis between venous and arterial thrombosis. Venous thrombosis is generally triggered by the stasis of blood flow and the subsequent activation of blood coagulation and vascular damage. A small fibrin-platelet thrombus is deposited at a valvular pocket forming a nidus which grows in size. Because of relatively slow blood flow in the venous system, the thrombi are generally composed of a small white head and prominent red tail, the so-called red clots. Arterial thrombosis is prone to develop on vessels afflicted by atherosclerosis. These diseased vessels possess a reduced capacity for carrying out normal defense functions and their surface is hence thrombogenic. Although the thrombogenic property of the atherosclerotic vessel wall has recently been attributed to reduced PGI_2 production,[10] this hypothesis requires confirmation. Arterial thrombi consist of a large white head composed of platelets and fibrin and a minimal red tail.

Once thrombus formation has begun, it can cause clinical problems by at least three mechanisms. First, the thrombi may grow and propagate in situ and eventually cause significant stenosis and occlusion of the involved vessels. Arterial occlusion leads to symptoms and signs due to organ ischemia and infarction, whereas venous occlusion gives rise to symptomatology related to poor blood return and tissue inflammation. Secondly, the thrombi may become detached and travel to a distant small vessel to cause vascular occlusion. Thirdly, vasoactive substances (eg, thromboxane A_2) may be released into the circulation to promote local platelet aggregation and cause vasoconstriction.

ATHEROGENESIS

Atherosclerosis is a common pathologic process underlying most of the arterial occlusive disorders. This subject has been extensively reviewed

	Promoting Factors	Defense Mechanisms
Endothelium	Subendothelium	Intact endothelial cells
Blood cells	Platelets White blood cells Red blood cells	
Plasma proteins	VIIIR:VWF other coagulation proteins	Protein C Antithrombins Plasminogen activator Plasminogen
Eicosanoids	TXA_2 PGG_2, PGH_2	PGI_2 PGD_2

Figure 2-2 Factors that play a role in modulating vascular thrombosis.

and excellent monographs and review articles are available. The readers are advised to consult them for detailed information.[11-12] A synopsis is given here in the context of the contribution of atherosclerosis to thromboembolic disorders. Observation of atherosclerotic lesions dates back to ancient Egypt. More detailed descriptions appeared in the handbooks of pathology published in the eighteenth and nineteenth centuries. However, the natural history of atherosclerosis was poorly understood until the 1950s when large-scale postmortem examinations were systematically performed.[13] Development of atherosclerosis appears to undergo evolutional changes. The earliest lesions are slightly raised yellowish fatty streaks, which may appear in the aorta in early childhood. These lesions tend to occur in the coronary arteries later in the second decade. Microscopic examinations of the fatty streaks show the characteristic accumulation of foam cells in the intima. These foam cells are derived from macrophages which are filled with cholesterol esters. Fatty streaks are present in isolated spots which may become confluent over time. Moreover, these lesions may evolve into a more raised lesion characterized by fibrous infiltration. These lesions are termed fibrous plaques. They become apparent at the fourth decade in an average American man. The plaques are composed of fibrous tissues in addition to the fatty deposition. The fibrous plaques may become ulcerated with bleeding and thrombotic complications. Eventually the lesions will become calcified. This stage of development is called complicated lesions. Most of the human clinical problems start to appear at this stage.

Atherosclerosis is a chronic disorder. Its pathogenesis is not entirely understood. Neither Rokitansky's encrustation theory nor Virchow's theory of imbibition is sufficient to explain this complex event. The modern theory takes both theories into consideration (Figure 2-3). According to the current view, atherogenesis is initiated by repetitive injury to the vascular endothelium induced by hemodynamic, chemical, immune, viral, and dietary agents.[11] Consequently, platelets adhere to the subendothelium and the activated platelets undergo explosive secretion of a myriad of their endogenous contents to promote atherosclerosis. There substances induce platelet secretion and aggregation and therefore elicit further platelet activation. Moreover, platelets elaborate a mutagenic substance, the so-called platelet-derived growth factor (PDGF), which promotes the vascular smooth muscle cell proliferation.[13,14] Smooth muscle cells, fibroblasts, and macrophages derived from the blood monocytes possess low-density lipoprotein (LDL) receptors on the cell surface.[15] It is believed that once LDL is taken up by the cells, cholesterol is esterified and accumulated in these cells to give a foamy appearance.[16] Esterified cholesterol also appears in the extracellular milieu, which may be bound to the fibrous tissues. There exists a lipid-removing mechanism in the arterial wall mediated probably through the lysosomal

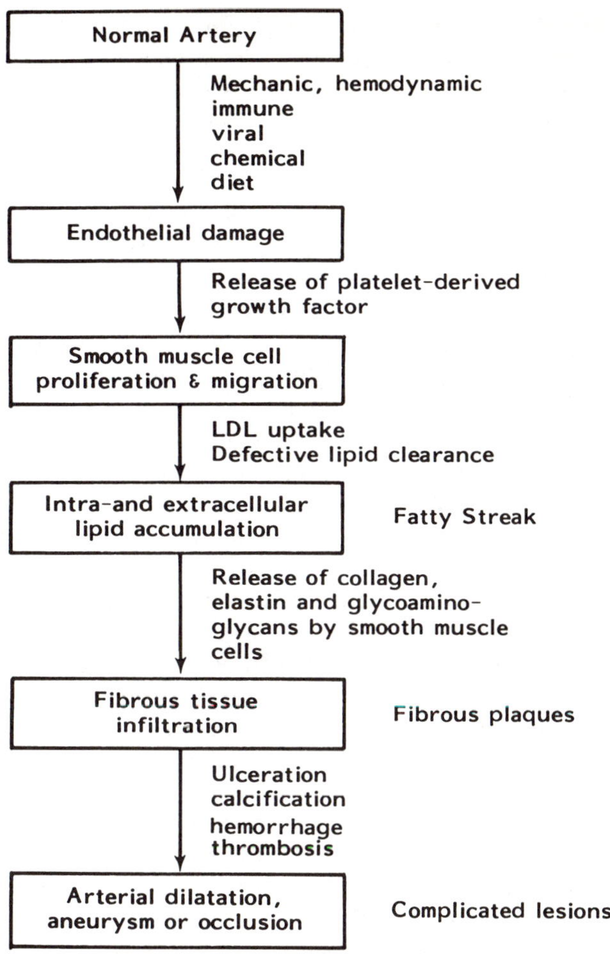

Figure 2-3 Simplistic scheme of atherogenesis.

enzyme, cholesterol ester hydrolase.[17] Lipid accumulation at the vessel wall is therefore determined by the balance between lipid uptake and removal. In human atherosclerosis there is evidence to suggest that the lipid accumulation is mostly due to a combined increased uptake and impaired removal mechanism.[17] Following the appearance of fatty streaks, smooth muscle cells secrete collagen, elastin, glycosaminoglycans, and glycoproteins.[18] These fibrous tissues are accumulated and eventually become the dominant pathologic feature giving rise to the appearance of fibrous plaques. Ulceration of the plaques is thought to be due to the degenerative changes of the elastin fibers in the plaque. The abnormal elastin fibers also play a role in calcification and thrombosis.[18]

10

The rate of atherosclerosis development is determined by multiple factors some of which are beginning to be understood. The recognized factors include genetic factors, diet, habits (cigarette smoking), and disease states (hypertension, diabetes mellitus, and lipoprotein abnormalities).[19] The exact mechanism by which these factors exert their influence over atherogenesis are unclear. Genetic factors represent a multifaceted mechanism which determines the basic capacity of an individual's arteries for resisting insults from food, habits, and disease states. High cholesterol diet appears to accelerate atherosclerosis, particularly in individuals with lipoprotein abnormalities. On the other hand, a diet rich in unsaturated fatty acids seems to have a beneficial effect. For instance, there is the recent observation that inhabitants of certain parts of the world such as the Greenland Eskimos, whose major food is deep-sea fish containing a high concentration of polyunsaturated lipids, have a low incidence of atherosclerosis and a mild bleeding problem.[20] Their platelet function is defective due to the influence of eicosapentaenoic acid (EPA) on the platelet function.[21] EPA is a 20-carbon ("eicosa") fatty acid with five double bonds ("pentaenoic"). Its chemical structure is similar to arachidonic acid, which is also a 20-carbon unsaturated fatty acid containing four double bonds. EPA appears to interfere with platelet arachidonic acid metabolism leading to reduced thromboxane A_2 production and defective release reaction.[22] It is unclear at the present time, however, whether a diet rich in EPA can indeed protect against atherosclerosis.

Although arterial stenosis and/or occlusion, tissue ischemia, and infarction are often attributed to large atheromas on the involved area, the clinical diseases due to atherosclerosis are not strictly related to the size of the atherosclerotic lesions. Acute ischemia may occur when there is only a minimal arterial involvement. Several mechanisms have been identified to account for this. The atheromas may become ulcerated and ulcerated materials may cause occlusion of the distal vessels. Moreover, thrombi are prone to develop on the atheroma which can produce a local detrimental effect by impeding blood flow. Furthermore, the thrombi may become detached and produce distal emboli. Vasoactive substances are produced and further aggravate the ischemia by vasospasm.

HYPERCOAGULABILITY

Thrombogenesis and atherogenesis are controlled by multiple factors. Impairment of these control mechanisms can lead to hypercoagulability and clinically significant thrombotic problems. Despite the recent advances in development of sensitive procedures for the diagnosis of thrombosis, early detection of certain patients who have a preponderance of developing thrombotic problems remains a clinical dilemma. The problem stems from the lack of a clear-cut understanding of the so-called hypercoagulable state on the one hand and lack of sensitive laboratory tests for early detection of the condition on the other. The term "hypercoagulable state" has been used interchangeably with "pre-thrombotic state," "prothrombotic state," and "thrombophilic" to infer certain clinical conditions where patients exhibit a tenacious propensity toward thromboembolism accompanied by evidence of enhanced platelet coagulation activities.[23] Since increased coagulation activities are generally associated with venous thrombosis and pulmonary embolism, whereas platelet hyperaggregability is associated with arterial thromboembolic problems, the thrombophilic states will be divided into "hypercoagulable" and "hyperaggregable" states.

Hypercoagulable State

The hypercoagulable state is probably best defined as any clinical condition exhibiting increased coagulation activities leading to a high preponderance of venous thrombosis and pulmonary embolism. It encompasses a variety of disorders with diversified pathogenetic mechanisms. A tentative classification is listed in Table 2-1. It includes three major categories: (1) hypercoagulable state due to deficiency of natural anticoagulants; (2) hypercoagulable states due to diseases, drugs, or physical conditions; and (3) unclassified. The first category is probably the best defined and most predictable. Both antithrombin III (AT-III) and protein C are physiologically important inhibitors of coagulation. AT-III antagonizes several activated coagulation factors, notably thrombin and factor Xa. Activated protein C inhibits factors Va and VIIIa.[9] Both inhibitors play an important role in the regulation of blood clotting. Their

Table 2-1
Classification of Hypercoagulable State

I. Hypercoagulable states due to deficiency of natural anticoagulants
Antithrombin III deficiency
Protein C deficiency
? Plasminogen abnormality
II. Hypercoagulable states due to certain diseases, drugs, or habitual factors
Malignancy
Myeloproliferative disorders
Paroxysmal nocturnal hemoglobinuria
Surgery
Trauma
Immobilization
Obstetric disorders
Old age
III. Unclassified
Idiopathic recurrent

12

deficiency hence leads to an increased coagulability. A number of families with AT-III deficiency have been reported and the affected members invariably exhibit a high risk for thrombosis.[8] Only a few families with protein-C deficiency have so far been reported[9] and the relationship between its deficiency state and risk for thrombosis has not been entirely clear. Fibrinolysis along with PGI_2 represents the ultimate defense mechanism against excessive clots by dissolving the thrombi. Fibrinolysis is initiated through the conversion of plasminogen to plasmin by plasminogen activators. As abundant plasminogen is present in the blood, the limiting step seems to reside in the quantity of plasminogen activators available for participation in the process. Reduced plasminogen activation has been observed in patients with recurrent thrombosis.[24] The cause-and-effect relationship between reduced plasminogen activation and venous thrombosis has not been clearly documented. Moreover, it remains to be elucidated whether reduced plasminogen activation is due to a congenital deficiency of plasminogen activator synthesis and/or release.

Many diseases and physical conditions are recognized to predispose an individual to venous thrombosis (Table 2-1, category II). The mechanisms by which these conditions trigger venous thrombosis are not entirely clear. As only a small fraction of the population who has these conditions develop thrombosis, it is conceivable that genetic factors may play a part.

Certain young, physically active, and otherwise healthy individuals have a high tendency of developing recurrent venous thrombosis and pulmonary embolism. Despite extensive workup, neither underlying diseases nor predisposing factors can be identified. Several studies have reported reduced plasminogen activation,[25] increased platelet function,[26] and shortened platelet survival time[27] in this group of patients with so-called idiopathic recurrent venous thrombosis. It is unclear whether the blood changes are the consequence or the cause of the increased thrombotic tendency. Further studies are needed to unravel the mechanisms of these disorders.

Strictly speaking, diagnosis of hypercoagulable states must be based on the demonstration of activated coagulation factors such as factor Xa and/or thrombin activities. Assays for these activated coagulation factors are available as experimental procedures but are not yet feasible as routine laboratory procedures. Alternatively, hypercoagulable state may be diagnosed by detecting the thrombin-induced fibrinogen products such as fibrinopeptide A, fibrinopeptide B, and fibrin monomer complex.[28] A hypercoagulable state can also be determined by using the fibrinogen I 125 leg scanning technique for detection of early thrombus formation (see chapter 14). However, under most circumstances, hypercoagulable states are suspected after a patient has had several episodes of overt deep vein thrombosis. Known predisposing factors or underlying diseases are then considered and ruled out while evidence for blood hypercoagulability such as measuring fibrinopeptide A, factor Xa fibrin monomer complexes, AT-III, and protein C is being established. The sensitivity and specificity of these tests remain vague. Activated partial thromboplastin time is often shortened but its reliability has not been established. Elevation of coagulation factors is not considered as evidence for hypercoagulable state. In summary, despite the availability of numerous laboratory tests, hypercoagulable state remains a clinical concept that cannot be precisely diagnosed on the basis of a single or even a battery of laboratory tests. Yet it remains a useful clinical concept for two reasons. First, its detection will alert the physician to perform suitable screening tests to detect the underlying causes including AT-III-and protein C-deficiency. Secondly, establishment of the diagnosis of hypercoagulable state should enable the physician to initiate early the appropriate long-term prophylaxis and treatment. This includes the elimination of the underlying conditions and treatment of the underlying diseases. If the underlying diseases or conditions cannot be completely removed, long-term therapy with mini-dose subcutaneous heparin has been found to be effective (see chapter 14). For AT-III deficiency, subcutaneous heparin is not effective, but warfarin appears to be effective in the prophylaxis of venous thrombosis.

Hyperaggregable State

Numerous diseases have been reported as having enhanced platelet aggregability. A partial list is shown in Table 2-2. The major causes include acute thromboembolic disorders, certain hematologic conditions, and atherogenic and thrombogenic factors. Increased platelet function is measured by a variety of procedures: (1) in vitro platelet aggregability in response to physiologic agonists; (2) proteins secreted by platelets during activation, ie, plasma β-thromboglobulin (βTG), and platelet factor 4 (PF-4); (3) circulating platelet aggregates; and (4) platelet survival time, which does not measure the platelet activity per se but measures the platelet utilization (or surface alteration) due to vascular thrombosis. When the various methods are compared, there is a general agreement between plasma βTG (PF-4) levels and circulating platelet aggregate index, suggesting that these methods measure in vivo platelet activation or extreme sensitivity of platelets to in vitro manipulation during the centrifugation.[29] By contrast, there is poor correlation between the in vitro platelet aggregation and other parameters. Two conclusions may be drawn from the comparative studies. First, the platelet aggregometry measures the platelet reactivity in vitro, while platelet aggregate ratio measures preformed reversible platelet aggregates. Plasma βTG or PF-4 levels represent an in vivo platelet release reaction and aggregation and

14

Table 2-2
List of Conditions Associated with Platelet Hyperaggregability

I. Thromboembolic disorders
    Ischemic cerebrovascular disease (transient ischemic attacks and thrombotic stroke)
    Coronary artery disease (angina pectoris and myocardial infarction)
    Peripheral vascular disease
    Digital ischemia
    Recurrent deep vein thrombosis
II. Hematologic conditions
    Myeloproliferative disorders (essential thrombocythema, polycythemia vera, etc)
    Sickle cell anemia
    Thrombotic thrombocytopenic purpura
III. Atherogenetic and thrombogenic factors
    Type II hyperlipoproteinemia
    Diabetes mellitus
    Homocystinuria
    Cigarette smoking
    Oral contraceptive agents

may also reflect platelet lysis. Second, a battery of tests including at least a test for measuring in vitro aggregability and a test for determining in vivo platelet activity should be utilized in order to detect the wide spectrum of platelet hyperactivity in patients with thromboembolic disorders.

Despite the capability of these procedures for detecting platelet hyperaggregability, pathogenetic mechanisms and clinical implications of platelet hyperaggregability remain unclear. Some recent animal experiments suggest that platelet hyperaggregability may be secondary to vascular damage and represents an early manifestation of vascular thrombosis. On the other hand, there is evidence to suggest that increased platelet aggregation may be induced by exogenous agents such as oral contraceptive agents and hence platelet hyperaggregability may play an important part in contributing to arterial occlusive disorders. Theoretically, increased platelet aggregation may primarily reflect the young age of platelets because of rapid consumption and that young platelets are more reactive. These theories, albeit plausible, remain to be tested and confirmed.

The other key question concerning platelet hyperaggregability is: Can it be reliably used to predict the onset of overt arterial thromboembolism? If so, can the tests be used for selecting patients who are likely to benefit from appropriate antithrombotic therapy? Although anecdotal observations suggest an affirmative answer to these questions, the issues have not been studied in a randomized and controlled fashion. For the practical consideration, however, use of a battery of blood tests to detect both in vitro and in vivo platelet aggregability may have certain clinical usage. In certain patients who have multiple episodes of ischemic attacks such as TIA's, the tests may provide a useful guide for determining whether platelets are involved and whether antiplatelet drug therapy should be initiated. Valuable information may be obtained if sequential clinical and laboratory correlation is carefully documented.

DETECTION OF THROMBUS FORMATION

Diagnosis of arterial and venous thrombotic disorders is based on three basic principles: (1) history and physical examinations, (2) detection of vascular occlusion, and (3) detection of thrombotic activities. Although history and physical examination form the basis for suspicion of these disorders, they should not be relied on as the definitive diagnostic tool. Arteriography and venography are the most accurate tests for localizing the sites of vascular occlusion, but these tests are associated with adverse effects ranging from pain to anaphylactoid reactions. Several noninvasive techniques have consequently been developed over the past decade. These techniques are generally based on two basic principles: electric impedance and ultrasound. These techniques primarily measure the influence of vascular occlusion on blood flow and are therefore more sensitive when major vessels are involved. Their utility in the diagnosis of thromboembolic disorders has been extensively investigated and well established in certain disorders such as deep vein thrombosis. Readers are referred to the respective chapters for the detailed discussions of their clinical use.

The utilization of fibrinogen labeled with iodine 125 or 123 or platelets labeled with chromium 51 or indium 111 adds new dimensions to the diagnosis of vascular thromboembolism. These tests differ from the tests described above in that they are sensitive for detecting active thrombus formation regardless of their size and influence on the blood flow. Hence, these procedures provide a valuable aid for early detection of thrombus formation and follow-up of thrombus progression or regression. Fibrinogen or platelets are injected and the radioactivity incorporated into an active thrombus is detected by a surface counter. Incorporation of platelets labeled with In 111 or fibrinogen I 123 into the thrombus can be detected by an imaging device since these two isotopes possess high energy emission and hence are suitable for imaging.[30-32] The clinical value of fibrinogen I 125 tests has been well established and will be discussed in the chapter on deep vein thrombosis (chapter 14). Preliminary studies on the use of platelets tagged with indium III in testing for detection of arterial thrombi, graft thrombi, and mural thrombi of the heart are promising but their sensitivity and specificity must be established before their consideration as a definite diagnostic test. Platelets labeled

16

with radioactive chromium (^{51}Cr) or indium (^{111}In) can also be used for the measurement of platelet survival time.[33] Ample evidence has indicated that platelet survival time is shortened in thromboembolic disorders. The tests prove to be useful for monitoring the efficacy of antiplatelet agents. However, the diagnostic value of platelet survival time has not been established because its sensitivity and specificity are unclear.

Availability of a myriad of tests for diagnosis of vascular thromboembolic disorders may at times pose a dilemma in decision making. Should the invasive or noninvasive techniques be used as an initial screening test? What tests are suitable for early detection of thrombosis in high-risk patients? How can these tests be used for monitoring the efficacy of antithrombotic drug therapy? Answers to these questions have been provided in certain disorders, notably deep vein thrombosis, by carefully controlled studies (refer to chapter 15) but remain controversial in others such as carotid artery disease. In order to utilize these tests prudently one must be familiar with the sensitivity and specificity of each test. Moreover, the comparative value of each test for the diagnosis of vascular occlusion must be established by prospective studies. Factors giving rise to false-positive and false-negative results must be recognized.

SUMMARY

Despite a tremendous advance in thrombosis research, mechanisms by which various thromboembolic disorders are developed are not entirely clear. Causes for increased thrombotic tendency ("thrombophilia") in certain fractions of the population remain poorly understood. Although the concept of "hypercoagulability" has clinical value, the term has not been well defined and its clinical usage has not been well delineated. Further clinical research must be vigorously pursued in this area in order to accurately identify the hypercoagulable or hyperaggregable states and initiate an effective regimen for prophylaxis or treatment of this group of important diseases.

REFERENCES

1. Michaeli D, Orloff KG: Molecular considerations of platelet adhesion. *Prog Hemost Thromb* 1976;3:29–59.
2. Weiss HJ: Platelet physiology and abnormalities of platelet function. *N Engl J Med* 1975;293:531–540.
3. Walsh PN: Platelets and coagulation proteins. *Fed Proc* 1981;40:2086–2091.
4. Marcus AJ: The role of lipids in platelet function: with particular reference to the arachidonic acid pathway. *J Lipid Res* 1978;19:793–826.
5. Abildgaard U: Antithrombin and related inhibitors of coagulation. *Recent Adv Blood Coag* 1981;3:151–173.

6. Stenflo J: A new vitamin-K dependent protein. Purification from bovine plasma and preliminary characterization. *J Biol Chem* 1976;251:355–363.
7. Egeberg O: Inherited antithrombin deficiency causing thrombophilia. *Thromb Diath Haemorrh* 1965;13:516–530.
8. Johansson L, Hedner U, Hilsson IM: Familial antithrombin III deficiency as pathogenesis of deep vein thrombosis. *Acta Med Scand* 1978;204:491–495.
9. Griffin JH, Evatt B, Zimmerman TS, et al: Deficiency of protein C in congenital thrombotic disease. *J Clin Invest* 1981;68:1370–1373.
10. Szczeklik A, Gryglewski RJ: Low density lipoproteins (LDL) are carriers for lipid peroxides and inhibit PGI_2 biosynthesis in arteries. *Artery* 1980;7:488–495.
11. Ross R, Glomsef JA: The pathogenesis of atherosclerosis. *N Engl J Med* 1976;295:369–376;420–425.
12. Gotto AM: Status Report: plasma lipids, lipoproteins and coronary artery disease. *Atheroscler Rev* 1979;4:17–28.
13. Holman RL, McGill HC Jr, Stron JP, et al: The natural history of atherosclerosis: The early aortic lesions as seen in New Orleans in the middle of the 20th century. *Am J Pathol* 1958;34:209–235.
14. Ross R, Glomset JA: Atherosclerosis and the arterial smooth muscle cell: proliferation of smooth muscle is a key event in the genesis of the lesions of atherosclerosis. *Science* 1973;180:1332–1339.
15. Goldstein JL, Brown MS: The low density lipoprotein pathway and its relation to atherosclerosis. *Annu Rev Biochem* 1977;46:897–930.
16. Smith EB: The relationship between plasma and tissue lipids in human atherosclerosis. *Adv Lipid Res* 1974;12:1–49.
17. Wolinsky H, Fowler S: The participation of lysosomes in atherosclerosis. *N Engl J Med* 1978;299:1173–1178.
18. Morris CJ, Bradby GVH, Walton KW: Fibrous long-spacing collagen in human atherosclerosis. *Atherosclerosis* 1978;31:345–354.
19. Stamler J: Epidemiology of coronary heart disease. *Med Clin North Am* 1973;57:5–46.
20. Dyerberg J, Bang HO: Haemostatic function and platelet polysaturated fatty acids in Eskimos. *Lancet* 1979;2:433–435.
21. Dyerberg J, Bank HO, Stoffersen E: Eicosapentaenoic acid and prevention of thrombosis and atherosclerosis? *Lancet* 1979;2:117–119.
22. Hirai A, Terano T, Hamazaki T, et al: The effects of the oral administration of fish oil concentrate on the release and the metabolism of (^{14}C) arachidonic acid and (^{14}C)-eicosapentaenoic acid by human platelets. *Thromb Res* 1982;28:285–298.
23. Hirsh J, Gallur AS: Hypercoagulability. *Recent Adv Hematol* 1977;2:431–451.
24. Johansson L, Hedner U, Nilsson IM: A family with thromboembolic disease associated with deficient fibrinolytic activity in vessel wall. *Acta Med Scand* 1978;203:477–480.
25. Isacson S, Nilsson IM: Defective fibrinolysis in blood and vein walls in recurrent idiopathic venous thrombosis. *Acta Chir Scand* 1972;138:313–319.
26. Wu KK, Barnes RW, Hoak JC: Platelet hyperaggregability in idiopathic recurrent deep vein thrombosis. *Circulation* 1976;53:687–691.
27. Steele PP, Weily HS, Genton E: Platelet survival and adhesiveness in recurrent venous thrombosis. *N Engl J Med* 1973;288:1148–1152.
28. Nossel HL, Yudelman I, Canfield RE, et al: Measurement of fibrinopeptide A in human blood. *J Clin Invest* 1974;54:43–53.
29. Chen Y-C, Wu KK: A comparison of methods for the study of platelet hyperfunction in thromboembolic disorders. *Br J Haematol* 1980;46:263–268.

30. Thakur ML, Welch MJ, Joist H, et al: Indium-111 labeled platelets: studies on preparation and evaluation of in vitro and in vivo platelet function. *Thromb Res* 1976;9:345–357.
31. Riba AL, Thakur ML, Gottschalk A, et al: Imaging experimental infective endocarditis with indium-III labeled blood cellular components. *Circulation* 1979;59:336–343.
32. Mettinger KL, Larsson S, Ericson K, et al: Detection of atherosclerotic plaques in carotid arteries by the use of ^{125}I fibrinogen. *Lancet* 1978;1:242–244.
33. Heaton WA, Davis HH, Welch MJ, et al: Indium-111 a new radionuclide label for studying human platelet kinetics. *Br J Haematol* 1979;42:613–622.

3 *Platelets and Endothelium*

Elizabeth R. Hall
Max Rafelson

PLATELETS

Platelet Anatomy

Although platelets are but fragments of megakaryocyte cytoplasm, they have evolved a complex machinery to subserve the many functions required of them.

Platelets circulate in the blood as small, biconvex discs (about 2–3 μm in diameter) about one half to one third the diameter of a red cell and only about a thirteenth of its volume. Lacking nuclei, platelets have no DNA and synthesize only minimal protein. Once released from the marrow, platelets have a life span of 7–10 days. Platelets are removed from the circulation either by being engulfed by the reticuloendothelial system when senescent or by incorporation into hemostatic plugs. Platelet size, count, rate of production, and life span can all vary in disease states or be altered by diet and/or drugs. Although platelets may not be considered cells (since they lack nuclei), they have an active metabolism that supplies the energy required for their functions.

The cytoplasm of the unstimulated platelet is surrounded by a plasma membrane that invaginates extensively into the cytoplasm, vastly increasing the surface area of a platelet, to form the surface-connected cannicular system. Intimately associated with the surface-connected cannicular system is a network of dense tubules, believed to be analagous to the calcium sequestering sarcoplasmic reticulum of muscle.[1-4]

Adjacent to the cytoplasmic surface of the plasma membrane and perhaps anchored to it are microfilaments, composed primarily of actin and myosin, and a circumferential band of microtubules. The microtubules apparently serve to help maintain platelet structure and are disrupted when platelets are activated.

The cytoplasm of the platelet contains numerous granules. Their abundance contrasts with the paucity of mitochondria and is consistent with the predominant role of glycolysis in deriving the platelet's metabolic energy. Platelets also contain three types of storage granules, which can be distinguished by density. These are the dense granules (δ), alpha granules (α), and lysosomes (λ granules). Electron-dense granules (δ granules) contain a concentrated mixture of the amines, serotonin, calcium, and the metabolically inactive storage form of adenosine diphosphate (ADP) and adenosine triphosphate (ATP). It should be noted that neither the granule nucleotides nor the granule calcium undergo rapid exchange with the corresponding cytoplasmic pools. Dense granules may also contain large amounts of arachidonic acid-rich phospholipids which may provide a significant source of free arachidonate for the platelet.[5]

α-Granules are a heterogeneous population of granules which are more numerous than the dense ones. They contain a variety of proteins which are probably synthesized in the megakaryocytes. Some of these proteins are specific to platelets such as (1) platelet factor 4 (PF_4), a heparin-neutralizing protein released from platelets bound to a proteoglycan carrier, (2) β-thromboglobulin, and (3) platelet-derived growth factor, a potent mitogen of arterial smooth muscle cells and fibroblasts in culture. Other α-granule proteins can be found in plasma and other cells; these include fibrinogen, factor V, factor VIII-related antigen, and fibronectin. The release of α-granule proteins appears to be a very sensitive measure of platelet activation.[6]

Active Transport in Platelets

Platelets possess the ability to accumulate several compounds by specific active transport processes, notably adenine, adenosine, and vasoactive amines. Adenine and adenosine are transported by separate processes.[7,8] Once transported, adenosine and adenine can be converted to adenosine monophosphate (AMP) and then to ATP. When platelets are incubated with radioactive adenosine or adenine the label is rapidly incorporated into the cytoplasmic pool of adenine nucleotides (chiefly ATP), which is retained intracellularly during secretion. This cytoplasmic pool is sometimes referred to as the metabolic pool to indicate that it provides the energy requirements for the platelet's response to stimuli.[9] A slow exchange between this metabolic pool of adenine nucleotides and those stored in the dense granules and secreted during the release reaction has been shown to occur.[10]

The transport process for serotonin (5-HT) provides a striking example of the cell's ability to concentrate extracellular material. The platelet is capable of taking up and maintaining an intracellular 5-HT concentration that is more than a thousandfold higher than that in the plasma. Once 5-HT has been transported across the plasma membrane into the cytoplasm it is taken up by the dense granules where it is stored in a high-density lattice structure with adenine nucleotides and bivalent cations. Thus, there are two clearly differentiated transport systems for 5-HT in platelets, one across the membrane and the other across the granular membrane.[11]

Platelets accumulate 5-HT by a Na^+-dependent plasma membrane transport system that is inhibited by tricyclic antidepressants such as imipramine.[12] This transport process is thought to be similar or identical to that of serotonergic neurons. Once accumulated by the platelet, the 5-HT is then specifically taken up by the dense granules where an acidic interior (a pH gradient) is the major driving force. This reserpine-sensitive transport system appears to be quite similar to that seen in chromaffin granules in the adrenal medulla.[13]

Other vasoactive amines such as dopamine and norepinephrine can also be transported into platelets and stored in the dense granules. These amines do not have specific transport processes but are transported (although with rather low affinity) by the 5-HT mechanism.[14] Although all of these amines can enter the platelet by simple diffusion, sub-micromolar plasma levels relegate this mechanism to an unimportant position.

Generally there is little metabolism of these amines in the platelets because of the efficiency of their uptake by the dense granules. However, when platelets are deficient in dense storage granules, 5-HT transported into the platelets is metabolized by its cytoplasmic monoamine oxidase and the metabolites diffuse out into the extracelluar medium.

Platelet Adhesion

The term *platelet adhesion* refers to the attachment of platelets to a nonplatelet surface. Platelet adhesion is the initial event in hemostasis following vascular injury. Overlapping endothelial cells form a continuous lining of intact blood vessels, so that during normal blood flow platelets do not come in contact with subendothelial tissue. Platelets do not adhere to the normal endothelial surface of intact blood vessels, vascular segments, or cell cultures. The specific factors that prevent platelet adhesion to the endothelium have not been defined. The discovery that endothelial cells produce an extremely potent platelet-inhibitory substance called prostacyclin (PGI_2) has led to the suggestion that continuous endothelial production of PGI_2 might prevent platelet adhesion to these cells.[15-17] Recent reports indicate that exogenous PGI_2 can inhibit both platelet adhesion and thrombus formation on arterial subendothelium, but that much larger doses of PGI_2 are needed to inhibit the former than the latter process.[18,19] However, PGI_2 synthesis is probably not the entire explanation for endothelial thromboresistance since its inhibition does not lead to increased platelet adhesion.[20,21] Thus, the in vivo mechanism(s) involved in platelet adherence needs to be further investigated.

Since platelets will not adhere to the vascular endothelial lining, it is the disruption of the vascular lining that initiates platelet adhesion. The subendothelial tissue to which platelets adhere consists of four structural components: microfibrils of elastin, basement membrane, collagen fibrils, and elastin.[22,23] Although platelets can adhere to several of these subendothelial components, fibrillar collagen appears to be the major stimulus.[22–24]

Platelet adhesion is a complex process that involves not only subendothelial structures, but also a specific plasma protein and at least one platelet receptor. A significant advance in our understanding of platelet adhesion came with the discovery that a specific plasma factor, shown to be absent in von Willebrand's disease, is required for normal platelet adhesion.[25] Von Willebrand's disease is a hemorrhagic disorder characterized by a deficiency of the von Willebrand factor component of the factor VIII molecule (VIIIR:VWF). VIIIR:VWF is involved in platelet adhesion to subendothelium, while the factor VIII procoagulant (VIIIC) corrects the long clotting time of hemophilic plasma. These two components are separable by gel filtration at high ionic strengths. The importance of VWF activity to hemostasis is readily apparent since patients deficient in this factor have a bleeding problem. VIIIR:VWF protein is produced by endothelial cells, contains carbohydrate, and is a multimer of 230,000 molecular weight (mol wt) subunits joined by disulfide bonds.[26] These subunits associate into a variety of polymers with molecular weights exceeding 5 million.[27,28] Although the mechanism by which VIIIR:VWF mediates platelet adhesion is not known, it has been suggested that it forms a bridge between the platelet and subendothelium. This theory would require that the VIIIR:VWF binds to both the platelet and subendothelium. Quiescent human platelets have a low affinity binding for VWF until they are activated by thrombin or ADP.[29] However, since the amount of VIIIR:VWF binding to the subendothelium correlates with the amount of platelet adhesion,[28,30] two hypotheses are proposed. It has been postulated that VIIIR:VWF binds first to the subendothelium and that the bound VIIIR:VWF is altered and recognizes a specific receptor on the platelet surface. Alternatively, the platelet is first activated and the activated platelet can bind VIIIR:VWF, which will then bind to the subendothelium. Both postulates, however, suggest that VWF acts as a bridge between the platelet and the subendothelium.

The identification of the platelet receptor for VIIIR:VWF was greatly advanced by two observations. The first observation was that the addition of the antibiotic ristocetin to a stirred platelet suspension in the presence of VIIIR:VWF caused platelet agglutination. Ristocetin agglutinates viable or formalin-fixed platelets suspended in normal plasma but not plasma from patients with von Willebrand's disease. In vitro, purified human VIIIR:VWF does not bind to human platelets in the absence of ristocetin; whereas, in the presence of ristocetin, factor VIIIR/VWF binds to the platelet surface.[31] The second observation was that platelets from patients with Bernard-Soulier syndrome did not adhere to the subendothelium, nor did they agglutinate in the presence of ristocetin.[32,33] These patients have normal plasma levels of factor VIIIR:VWF and cannot be corrected by the addition of more factor VIIIR:VWF. It would thus appear that both ristocetin-induced agglutination and adhesion depend on similar (or identical) platelet receptor(s). The concentration of membrane glycoproteins in Bernard-Soulier platelets has been determined by several laboratories. Each has demonstrated that a decreased concentration of glycoprotein Ib is a characteristic defect of Bernard-Soulier platelets.[34,35] Moreover, two preparations of antisera to glycoprotein Ib have been reported to inhibit ristocetin-induced platelet agglutination. One was obtained from a multiply transfused Bernard-Soulier patient and the other was an antiplatelet antiserum adsorbed with chymotrypsin-treated platelets.[36,37] Although these data suggest that glycoprotein Ib is the VIIIR:VWF receptor on the platelet membrane, the exact mechanism of binding awaits further investigation.

Glycoprotein Ib is but one of more than 30 glycoproteins on the surface membrane of human platelets. The current nomenclature is based on early studies of platelet membranes that indicated three major glycoproteins termed I, II, and III.[38,39] Improved methodology has identified many additional glycoproteins. These have been arbitrarily subclassified under groups I and II by using the letters a, b, c, etc. Glycoproteins under the III region are numbered consecutively IV, V etc according to their molecular weight. Glycoprotein Ib has an apparent molecular weight of 170,000 on SDS-polyacrylamide gels under nonreducing conditions. It consists of two disulfide-linked subunits with apparent molecular weights of 143,000 and 22,000.[40] Each subunit contains carbohydrate and is exposed to the outer plasma membrane.

Platelet Aggregation

After the adhesion of platelets to the injured vessel wall, activated platelets then form an aggregate on the adherent layer and initiate the development of the hemostatic plug. The observation that exogenous ADP could initiate platelet aggregation illustrated that platelet function could be stimulated by extrinsic stimuli.[41] Subsequent investigations have shown numerous other platelet agonists such as thrombin, epinephrine, collagen, prostaglandins, immune complexes, and complement components that can induce platelet aggregation by interacting with discrete receptors on the platelet membrane.

Platelet aggregation can be measured in vitro using an aggregometer.[42] The aggregometer is a photometer that measures the transmission of light through platelet-rich plasma during the course of aggregation. When aggregating agents are added to stirred platelets, the platelets become "sticky" such that when they collide they form aggregates. These aggregates leave platelet-poor spaces between them, thereby allowing for increased light transmission. The extent and reversibility of platelet aggregation depends on the nature and concentration of the agonist employed. Primary or "first wave" aggregation is reversible and is not associated with platelet secretion or the generation of platelet prostaglandins. On the other hand, "second wave" aggregation is irreversible and associated with platelet secretion and prostaglandin production. Secreted ADP further stimulates platelet aggregation, while prostaglandin production augments ADP secretion and aggregation.

Physiologically important agonists   The study of collagen-induced aggregation is difficult because of its particulate nature and complex structure. The site(s) of interaction between collagen and the platelet surface have yet to be defined. However, mechanistic studies of collagen-induced aggregation show that collagen exerts its effect by stimulating platelet prostaglandin synthesis and ADP secretion.[43] In addition, collagen can initiate the formation of a prothrombinase complex which can generate thrombin (see section on Platelet Procoagulant Activity). Thrombin causes further platelet activation and aggregation.

Thrombin-induced platelet aggregation is also associated with the release of ADP and prostaglandin formation. However, recent evidence has indicated that another mechanism (or mechanisms) is also involved.[44] Therefore when thrombin is added to the platelets, all three (or more) mechanisms of aggregation contribute synergistically to the platelet response. Inhibition of any one of these mechanisms reduces the extent of induced aggregation and release. Thrombin, at physiologic concentrations (< 10 nm), interacts with approximately 500 high-affinity binding sites with a $K_d \sim 1$ nm and with about 50,000 low-affinity binding sites with a $K_d \sim 100$ nm.[45-48] Whether these two classes of binding sites represent separate molecular entities or a single population showing negative cooperativity remains to be clarified.[49,50] In either case, it is the high-affinity binding that correlates with platelet activation.[45,47] Two of the platelet membrane glycoproteins have been implicated as possible thrombin receptors. Glycoprotein Ib and glycocalicin have been proposed as the thrombin receptor because they will inhibit the binding of thrombin to platelets and the induction of thrombin-induced aggregation.[51,52] While purified glycoprotein Ib will form a reversible complex with thrombin, there are several observations which argue against this glycoprotein being the thrombin receptor that activates platelets. First, anti-glycoprotein Ib has a minimal effect on thrombin-induced aggregation.[37] Secondly, the catalytic activity of thrombin is essential for platelet activation,[45,50] yet glycoprotein Ib and glycocalicin inhibit its proteolytic activity.[51,52] Finally, Bernard-Soulier platelets that are missing glycoprotein Ib and glycocalicin from their platelets show a normal, or only somewhat reduced, response to thrombin.[32,53] Unlike glycoprotein Ib, glycoprotein V (the other membrane glycoprotein implicated as a thrombin receptor) is hydrolyzed by thrombin very rapidly to yield a fragment of an identical molecular weight as that observed in the platelet supernatant after thrombin treatment.[27,54] Clearly, further work will be required to establish the role of glycoprotein V in thrombin-induced aggregation.

Epinephrine can initiate platelet function by binding to α_2-adrenergic receptors.[55,56] Since epinephrine can potentiate platelet response to a variety of stimuli, it has been suggested that this potentiation may enable platelets to respond to stress induced by blood vessel trauma. However, even this potentiation is observed at hormone concentrations that are much higher than those observed during pathologic stress.

Mechanisms of aggregation   There are a number of agents that can trigger platelet aggregation and release. Each of these agents appears to work through one or all of the following mechanisms: ADP release, platelet arachidonate metabolism, and at least one other mechanism, possibly involving the release of platelet activating factor (PAF) and/or lysophosphatidic acid (see section on Platelet Secretion). Probably each of these mechanisms ultimately acts through calcium mobilization from intracellular stores.

The immediate response of platelets when an agonist binds to its receptor is a change in shape. The central body of the platelet becomes spheroidal, extruding long, thin filopodia that facilitate the cell-cell interactions essential for aggregation.[57,58] Platelet aggregation requires platelet-platelet contact and extracellular calcium and fibrinogen to form the intracellular bridges needed to consolidate platelet aggregates.[59,60] Quiescent platelets do not bind fibrinogen; however, upon stimulation by ADP, epinephrine, thrombin or arachidonate, specific fibrinogen binding sites become exposed.[60-62] Fibrinogen binding to these sites is rapid, reversible, and calcium (or magnesium)-dependent.[63] The exact mechanism of fibrinogen binding is unknown, but some evidence suggests that the interplatelet bridge is asymmetrical, ie, different bonds are important on opposite platelets.

One approach toward identifying the fibrinogen binding site has been to characterize glycoprotein abnormalities in platelets from patients with Glanzmann's thrombasthenia. In this disorder, platelets have functional membrane receptors for physiologic stimuli in that they adhere normally to subendothelium, change shape, and undergo secretion; but they fail to aggregate and mediate clot retraction.[64] Thrombasthenic platelets are deficient in glycoprotein IIb and III.[65] Congenital disorders usually involve only one gene and thus one protein, so it is surprising to find apparent deficiencies in two proteins. There are several possibilities: (1) that these two proteins are cleavage products of a single precursor, (2) that there is a defect in a platelet-specific posttranslational process that is common to both proteins, (3) that both glycoproteins are unstable unless inserted together in a stable, membrane complex, and (4) that the two proteins might be specified by different genes having linked expressions.[27] Regardless of the genetic basis for this molecular defect, these observations provided the first evidence that glycoprotein IIb and III are directly involved in platelet aggregation. Therefore, it was of considerable interest when thrombasthenic platelets were shown to bind no fibrinogen in response to ADP, suggesting that one of these two glycoproteins (or both) may be the fibrinogen receptor.[61]

The role of calcium in platelet function and its regulation by cyclic AMP   Calcium is required for each event that occurs during the process of platelet aggregation. Extracellular Ca^{++} is involved in three events. First, it is involved in the interplatelet bridging required for aggregation by participating in fibrinogen binding. Second, it is involved in the interaction of clotting factors with the platelet membrane as described in the section on Platelet Procoagulant Activity. Third, it is required for the in vitro phenomenon of clot retraction, which results from the contraction of platelet actinomyosin. When platelets are stimulated to secrete their granules, the calcium contained in their dense bodies is released to the outside of the cell. The function of this Ca^{++} is unknown as it would contribute little to plasma calcium concentration. However, it may act as a counter-ion for packaging released ADP and/or provide high local concentrations of Ca^{++} to facilitate the membrane events just described.[66]

Cytoplasmic calcium levels are very low in the resting platelet (about 10^{-7} to 10^{-8} M), but may be increased more than a hundredfold upon cell stimulation. The triggering of intracellular calcium mobilization may be the ultimate biochemical mechanism by which platelet aggregation and secretion occurs. Since calcium levels are low in the cytoplasm of quiescent platelets, essentially all of it must be in a bound or stored form. Considerable evidence exists that the dense tubular system represents the primary site of Ca^{++} storage from which the Ca^{++} is released intracellularly upon stimulation of the thromboxane A_2-dependent pathway or the thromboxane-independent pathways used by ADP and thrombin.[66]

Intracellular Ca^{++} mobilization is required for both platelet shape change and secretion. Platelet shape change involves both pseudopod formation and granule centralization. Pseudopod formation probably results from the interaction of actin-binding protein and alpha actinin, while granule centralization is a result of actin-myosin interaction, primarily controlled by a Ca^{++}-calmodulin activation of a protein kinase phosphorylation of myosin light chain. Secretion of platelet granule contents involves granule centralization and the fusion of organelle membranes to the membranes of the surface-connected cannicular system. Although the mechanism is unknown, membrane fusion is facilitated by Ca^{++} and may result from the activation of platelet phospholipases and the generation of lysophosphatidic acid.[66]

If we assume that Ca^{++} represents a common mediator of the various platelet reactions to stimulation, then any compound which regulates Ca^{++} levels could prevent platelet activation. Dibutyryl cAMP or agents that increase cAMP levels will antagonize platelet responses to stimulation. Cyclic AMP not only enhances the sequestration of Ca^{++} by the dense tubular system, but it also inhibits Ca^{++}-dependent reactions. Elevation of cAMP is probably the most important intracellular regulator of platelet responsiveness in general.[67]

Adenylate cyclase stimulants (PGI_2, PGE_1, 6-keto-PGE_1 and PGD_2) exert their inhibitory effects on platelets by elevating cAMP levels. When these compounds are tested for their ability to stimulate platelet adenylate cyclase, PGI_2 is the most potent inhibitor, followed by 6-keto-PGE_1 > PGD_2 > PGE_1.[68] These agents block both primary (thromboxane-independent) and secondary (thromboxane-dependent) aggregation. Prostacyclin is synthesized in the endothelial cells and has been proposed as one factor contributing to the nonthrombogenic properties of vascular endothelium. In fact, it is the most potent endogenous platelet inhibitor known. PGI_2 is unstable in aqueous solutions where it undergoes an acid hydrolysis to the physiologically inactive 6-keto-$PGF_{1\alpha}$. However, its conversion to 6-keto-PGE_1 by several tissues, including platelets, may extend the range and duration of its activities.[69,70] 6-Keto-PGE_1 is more stable than PGI_2 and although not as active as an antiaggregatory agent, it is still quite potent.[68]

Prostaglandin endoperoxides, PGG_2 and PGH_2 and thromboxane A_2 will inhibit the increase in cAMP levels in response to PGI_2, PGD_2, and PGE_1, without affecting basal levels.[71] Regardless of the exact mechanism(s) involved in the inhibition of platelet aggregation by PGI_2 or the stimulation of aggregation by TXA_2, it does appear that these two molecules oppose each other through the regulation of adenylate cyclase.

Platelet Secretion

Secretion of platelet granules involves both a centralization of granules and the fusion of granule membranes with those of the surface-connected cannicular system. Secreted substances can be detected outside the platelet within seconds of stimulation. The different populations of platelet granules do not release their contents with equal facility. Lysosomal enzyme secretion (λ granules) will occur only with a powerful stimulus such as high concentrations of thrombin or collagen. The dense granules (δ) are readily secreted in response to arachidonate, ADP, or epinephrine. However, secretion by epinephrine and ADP will not occur without concomitant aggregation. Some of the contents of the heterogeneous alpha granule (α) population (eg, platelet factor 4, β-thromboglobulin) are secreted even more readily than the dense granule contents.[72,73] Such observations suggest that secretion may be initiated by more than one mechanism. Indeed, thrombin-induced secretion is mediated by both a thromboxane A_2 (TXA_2)-dependent and a TXA_2-independent pathway.[73]

Thromboxane A₂-induced release The synthesis of prostaglandin endoperoxides and TXA₂ by the platelet is required for secretion, in response to ADP, epinephrine, and low concentrations of thrombin and collagen. In resting platelets, the biosynthesis of TXA₂ is insignificant. However, when platelets are activated it is rapidly synthesized and released.[74] The biosynthesis of TXA₂ is a multistep process involving several enzymatic steps (see Figure 3-1). The primary and rate-limiting step in TXA₂ production is the release of arachidonic acid from membrane phospholipids. The platelet contains two enzymatic pathways for

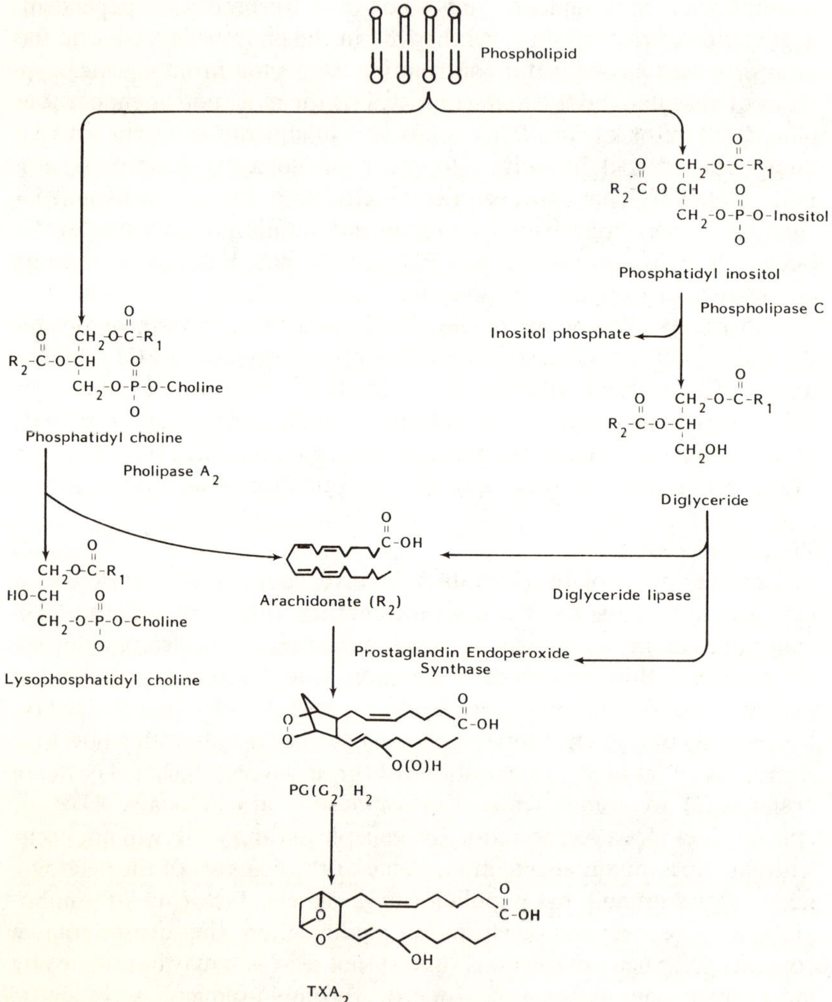

Figure 3-1 A schematic representation of our understanding of the release of arachidonic acid and its metabolism into thromboxane A₂ by stimulated platelets.

the liberation of esterified arachidonate. One is by the activation of phospholipase A_2 (PL-A_2) which will release arachidonate directly.[75,76] Alternatively, phospholipase C (PL-C) first removes inositol-phosphate from phosphatidylinositol, leaving a diglyceride.[77,78] Arachidonic acid is then released from this diglyceride by diglyceride lipase.[79] There is currently a great deal of controversy as to the relative importance of these two enzyme systems. Both systems require Ca^{++}, although the PL-C requires less than does the PL-A_2. Since the hydrolysis of phosphatidylinositol (PL-C-mediated) is more rapid than that of phosphatidylcholine (PL-A_2-mediated), it has been suggested that PL-C is activated first at low Ca^{++} concentrations and that products of its reaction (phosphatidic acid, lysophosphatidic acid, and TXA_2) may exhibit ionophoretic properties such that more Ca^{++} is freed and PL-A_2 is activated. Once released from the membrane phospholipids, arachidonic acid undergoes oxygenation and cyclization to form the prostaglandin endoperoxides, PGG_2 and PGH_2. These reactions are catalyzed by prostaglandin endoperoxide synthase (commonly referred to as cyclooxygenase).[80,81] Then thromboxane synthase catalyzes the rearrangement of the endoperoxides to form TXA_2.[82] TXA_2 is an extremely potent but labile compound ($t\frac{1}{2} = 30$ seconds) that is a key mediator in platelet secretion. The exact mechanism by which TXA_2 induces secretion is not known. However, thromboxane may act both by inhibiting adenyl cyclase and by mobilizing intracellular calcium.

Thromboxane independent release At least one other release mechanism exists in platelets. Both platelet activating factor (PAF) and lysophosphatidic acids have been proposed as possible mediators of this pathway. Human platelets release PAF when stimulated with thrombin, collagen, or A23187. In contrast, arachidonate and ADP were unable to trigger PAF-acether production.[83] PAF is a potent platelet stimulus and its mechanism of action appears to be independent of TXA_2 or ADP.[43,84] However, further studies are needed to establish its physiologic role.

Lysophosphatidic acid can also induce secretion independent of TXA_2 or ADP.[85] Its mechanism of action is unknown, although it can act as a Ca^{++} ionophore. The production of lysophosphatidic acid, like that of PAF, involves the action of platelet phospholipases.

Defects of secretion Bleeding disorders due to platelet-release defects point up the importance of platelet secretion to hemostasis and represent unique experiments in nature which are valuable tools in the investigation of the secretory process. Two distinct subgroups of platelet release disorders have been identified: storage pool deficiency (SPD) and primary release defect (PRD).

Storage pool deficiency (SPD) refers to several diseases that are genetically and phenotypically heterogeneous. SPD is characterized by a decrease in the number and/or content of one or more types of storage granules (especially the dense granules). The overall result of these disorders is a subnormal release of ADP, Ca++, and serotonin and, therefore, a deficiency in "second-wave" aggregation in response to ADP, epinephrine, and low concentrations of collagen and thrombin. The Hermansky-Pudlak syndrome is characterized by a deficiency of dense granules, but a normal content of lysosomes and alpha granules. Other forms of the storage pool disease may have a deficiency of either dense granules or alpha granules or both.[86] These disorders probably result from a defect in granule formation in the megakaryocyte.

The primary release defect (PRD) is related to an abnormal release mechanism per se, despite the presence of adequate dense granules. Investigations of PRD have primarily uncovered defects in platelet arachidonic acid metabolism. Deficiencies of cyclooxygenase and thromboxane synthase have been described, as well as a TXA_2 receptor abnormality.[87]

Platelet Procoagulant Activity

Platelets play a major role in generating various coagulant activities which can promote coagulation in the vicinity of platelet aggregation. Platelets promote coagulation in at least three ways: (1) Platelet membranes contain factor XI, which is activated when platelets come into contact with collagen.[83] (2) Platelet membrane phospholipids become exposed and serve as an active surface for the binding of factor Xa, factor V/Va, and Ca++ to form the "prothrombinase complex," which serves to localize thrombin generation.[89,90] (3) Stimulated platelets secrete the procoagulant proteins fibrinogen and platelet factor 4 from their α-granules.[6] Platelet involvement in coagulation is further discussed in chapter 4.

ENDOTHELIUM AND ENDOTHELIAL CELLS

Anatomy of the Endothelium

The cells of the endothelium form a continuous single cell-layer lining to the plasma face of the entire vascular system and provide a nonthrombogenic surface and a selective barrier between the circulating blood and interstitial spaces. Until rather recently, the endothelium was presumed to be a passive anatomical filter with pores of various sizes, but with little active participation in biochemical and hematologic events. The vascular endothelium is now known as an active and complex entity within the vascular system. It responds to various stimuli, synthesizes a variety of substances including its own basement membrane, transports many substances into and out of the blood, and activates some hormones and inactivates others. It also produces pro- and anticoagulant factors, has important antigenic properties, and is likely to play a pivotal role in hypertension, diabetes angiopathy, tumor angiogenesis, local control of blood flow, tissue nutrition, and host defense, and in other processes yet to be defined.

The evolution and development of our current ideas on the roles of the endothelium have been spurred by the development of techniques for the in vitro culture of endothelial cells from diverse sources. Because endothelial cells in culture retain many of the functional and morphologic properties of the endothelium in vivo, only limited discussion of the properties of the vessel wall will be presented here.

Although the size of blood vessels varies extensively from the capillaries to the veins and arteries, they all have lining the luminal surface a single layer of endothelial cells supported by an underlying extracellular matrix. In general the blood vessel wall is composed of three layers: the *intima, media,* and *adventitia.* The *intima* consists of a single layer of endothelial cells lying on a continuous basement membrane composed of type IV collagen and structural glycoprotein(s). The *media* is composed of smooth muscle surrounded by a connective tissue matrix made up of collagen fibers (types I and III), elastic fibers, glycosaminoglycans, and structural glycoproteins. The *adventitia* is the outer layer containing fibroblasts, adipocytes, mast cells, and an extracellular matrix of collagen fibers (types I and III), glycosaminoglycans, elastic fibers, lipids, and structural glycoproteins.

Morphology of the endothelium[91,92] varies between large and small vessels. In large veins and arteries, the endothelial cells exist as a tightly packed sheet of polygonal cells. In small venules and capillaries, individual endothelial cells form the vessel through which the blood cells pass in single file. Capillaries average some 8 μm in diameter, about the diameter of an erythrocyte. Using junctions and openings as criteria, three main types of endothelia can be distinguished: *continuous endothelium* (brain capillaries, aorta), which is flat and tight and has barely visible cell borders; *fenestrated endothelium* (endocrine glands, renal glomerulus), in which the endothelium is penetrated by fenestrae or pores of some 80–100 nm in diameter; and *discontinuous endothelium* (sinusoids of spleen and bone marrow) with large intercellular and transcellular openings.

Although the morphology of various sized blood vessels varies, the basic functions performed by their endothelial cells are similar in any size vessel. They serve to provide a nonthrombogenic surface, control the passage of solutes and other entities to and from blood and tissues, synthesize vasoactive agents such as prostacyclin (PGI_2), and maintain a patent vessel by growing as a single cell-layer attached to the vessel wall basement membrane. It would, however, be incorrect to assume endothelial cells derived from various sites to be identical. Data are now available which show that certain properties of cultured arterial, venous, and microvascular endothelial cells are indeed different.[93]

32

Properties of Cultured Endothelial Cells

Endothelial cells from human and other species in culture retain many of the morphologic and functional properties of the endothelium in vivo. Methods have been described for the isolation and cultivation of aortic cells,[94-97] venous cells,[97-99] and microvascular cells.[100-102] Whereas the endothelial cell cultures derived from the larger vessels are essentially homogeneous, those derived from the microvasculature are undoubtedly contaminated with pericytes and mast cells. The microvascular cells have been far more difficult to culture than those from larger vessels, suggesting that they may have some fundamentally different properties.

Morphologic characteristics Confluent monolayers of all types of cultured endothelial cells form "cobblestone" monolayers of polygonal-shaped cells which exhibit density-dependent growth inhibition. Figure 3-2 shows the typical growth pattern after 1 hour in culture, after 2 days, and the final confluent appearance after 6 days.[94] The cells are 30–50μm in diameter and closely adjoined to their neighbors. There is a protruding centrally located nucleus containing two or more prominent nucleoli.

Under electron microscopy, cultured endothelial cells have the general characteristics of vascular endothelium. The Weibel-Palade body[103] a rod-shaped organelle 0.1 by 3 μm in size, and containing many tubules 15 nm in diameter, has been observed in endothelial cells. These organelles have not been reported in any other cell type, including fibroblasts and smooth muscle cultured from blood vessel walls.[104,105] Although the function of the Weibel-Palade body is unknown, it is now accepted as a unique ultrastructural marker for endothelium. These organelles have been observed in cultured endothelial cells derived from the aorta,[94,96] arteries and veins,[97,99,106] and the microvessels of the brain, retina,[107] adrenal, skin,[108] lung, kidney, and spleen.[109,110] Pinocytotic vesicles and 60–70 Å filaments are seen in the cytoplasm of both cultured endothelial cells and in vivo. However, these features are seen in other cell types and do not provide definite criteria of identity.

Biochemical and functional characteristics Factor VIII in plasma is a complex of two proteins, the high molecular weight factor VIII–related protein/von Willebrand factor (VIIIR:VWF) and the low molecular weight factor VIII procoagulant (VIIIC). Deficiency of this molecule results in either von Willebrand's disease or hemophilia. VIIIR:VWF is known to be synthesized by the vascular endothelium, whereas VIIIC is not.[111] VIIIR:VWF has been found in cultured endothelial cells derived from the aorta,[94,97] artery and vein,[97,112,113] brain capillaries,[114] and adrenal capillaries.[100] Endothelial cells in vitro synthesize and secrete VIIIR:VWF. The release into the medium is linear for 3 days and endothelial cells are thought to be the major site of synthesis of plasma factor VIIIR:VWF in vivo.[112]

Angiotensin-converting enzyme (ACE) is produced by cultured endothelial cells derived from aorta,[115] umbilical vein,[116] pulmonary

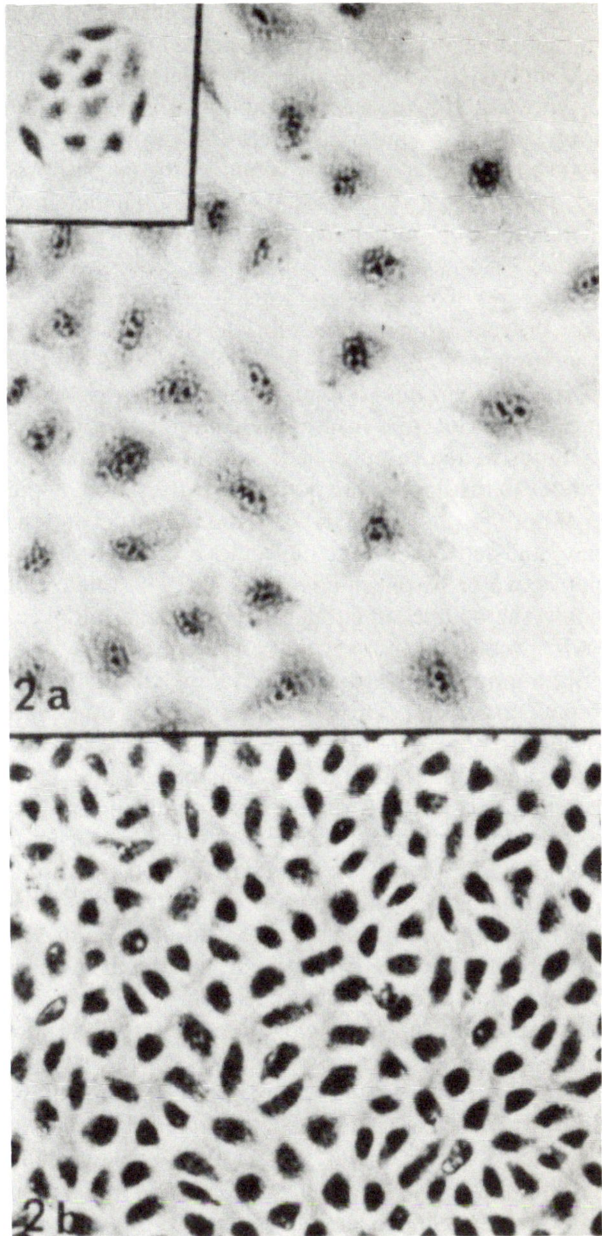

Figure 3-2 **a** Phase contrast micrography of growing edge of primary culture of endothelial cells two days after seeding ($\times$ 345). Endothelial cell patch attached to substratum 1 hour after seeding (inset) ($\times$ 495). **b** Confluent culture seven days after seeding ($\times$ 495).

34

artery and vein,[111] and adrenal[100] and brain capillaries.[101] ACE converts angiotensin I into angiotensin II and also inactivates bradykinin which is the preferred substrate for the enzyme. Angiotensin II is the most potent vasopressor known and is the active component of the renin-angiotensin system. Bradykinin is a powerful arteriolar vasodilator and hence a hypotensive agent. ACE can also be found in the brush border cells of the gut and the proximal tubules of the kidney but not in cultures of smooth muscle cells.[116,117] Other vasoactive substances such as serotonin, norepinephrine, histamine, and adenosine are processed by endothelial cells in vivo and in vitro. Thus, endothelial cells appear to be critically important for the regulation of circulatory levels of vasoactive substances and may play an important role in the regulation of local circulation.

The fibrinolytic enzyme system of plasma is responsible for the dissolution of blood clots and insures the continued circulation of blood through an unobstructed vascular bed. It is now clear that the endothelium contributes to the fibrinolytic potential of the blood by the synthesis and release of both fibrinolytic activators and inhibitors and that the synthesis, release, and activity of these molecules are subject to regulation.[118] The vascular activator of plasminogen produced by the endothelium is most probably the source of circulating blood plasminogen activator responsible for vessel patency by dissolution of fibrin thrombi. The release of plasminogen activator from endothelial cells may be stimulated by anoxia, stress, epinephrine, and possibly by other agents not as yet demonstrated to do so. Endothelial cell cultures produce both plasminogen activators and inhibitors, and it is thought that the interactions between these activities contribute to the overall regulation of this system.[119]

One of the more important products of the endothelial cells is the prostaglandin-like substance prostacyclin (PGI_2). Its importance is related to its action as a potent inhibitor of platelet aggregation and a putative role in preventing platelet–vessel wall interaction.[120] PGI_2 is a metabolite of arachidonic acid which is derived from membrane phospholipids by the action of calcium-dependent phospholipases. Arachidonic acid is converted by the enzyme cyclooxygenase into the endoperoxides PGG_2 and PGH_2 which are converted into PGI_2 by the enzyme prostacyclin synthase. PGI_2 inhibits platelet aggregation by stimulating adenylate cyclase, leading to an increase in cAMP levels in the platelets.[120] PGI_2 production is inhibited by treatment with nonsteroidal antiinflammatory drugs which inhibit the cyclooxygenase enzyme. Aspirin inhibits PGI_2 production by irreversible acetylation of the enzyme. This effect on endothelial cells is short-lived because these cells are capable of enzyme resynthesis. PGI_2 is produced by cultured endothelial cells derived from aorta and umbilical vein.[120,121] It is also produced by cultured capillary cells but in lesser amounts.[122] Production of PGI_2 in endothelial cells is stimulated by a number of agents that include arachidonic acid, trypsin, thrombin, platelet-derived growth factor, and calcium ionophores.[122,123] Some of these effects are species specific. Although PGI_2 could play an important role in platelet-endothelium interaction, it seems unlikely that it plays a major role in maintaining the nonthrombogenic characteristics of the endothelium under normal conditions. It appears to be more important in endothelial injury or in the presence of thrombogenic stimuli.

Endothelial cells in culture synthesize a number of components of their basal lamina. Confluent cultures of endothelial cells show as they do in vivo an asymmetry of cell surfaces. The apical surface is nonthrombogenic, whereas the basal lamina surface is highly thrombogenic and composed mainly of collagen type III and a lesser amount of collagen types IV + V.[124,125] Associated with the basal lamina collagens are proteoglycans and glycoaminoglycans,[126,127] composed mainly of heparin sulfate and dermatin sulfate.[128] Also synthesized in significant quantities are two glycoproteins, fibronectin and laminin. Fibronectin is synthesized and secreted by cultured endothelial cells and accounts for some 15% of the total protein released into the culture medium.[129] In subconfluent cultures, fibronectin is localized on the apical surface, whereas in confluent cultures it is in the matrix beneath the cell monolayer.[130] A second glycoprotein, laminin, in confluent cultures is localized underneath the cells in the basal lamina.[131,132] Fibronectin and laminin are believed to be responsible for cell attachment and the maintenance of contact-inhibited morphology.[128,131] The presence of fibronectin, laminin, and collagens type IV and V in the basal lamina produced by endothelial cells in cultures strongly suggests that this matrix has the in vivo characteristics of a basement membrane.

Platelet–Endothelial Cell Interactions

A critical role of the endothelium is to prevent platelets from adhering to the vessel wall, ie, provide a nonthrombogenic surface. It is widely held that platelets do not interact with intact endothelial cells either in vivo or in vitro. The presence or absence of specific molecules not yet defined are presumed to be responsible for the failure of platelets to adhere.

Endothelial cells in culture derived from aorta,[132] umbilical vein,[133] and brain capillaries[101] all maintain a nonthrombogenic apical surface to which platelets do not attach. This is in contrast to cultured fibroblasts and smooth muscle cells to which platelets readily attach. However, if confluent endothelial cells are treated briefly with agents such as epinephrine, serotonin, or NaCl, there is an extensive alteration in the confluent monolayer structure, resulting in the exposure of a layer or meshwork of microfilaments.[134] Platelets interact extensively with this exposed subendothelial material with very little or no interaction with the endothelial cell per se (Figures 3-3 and 3-4). The nature of these

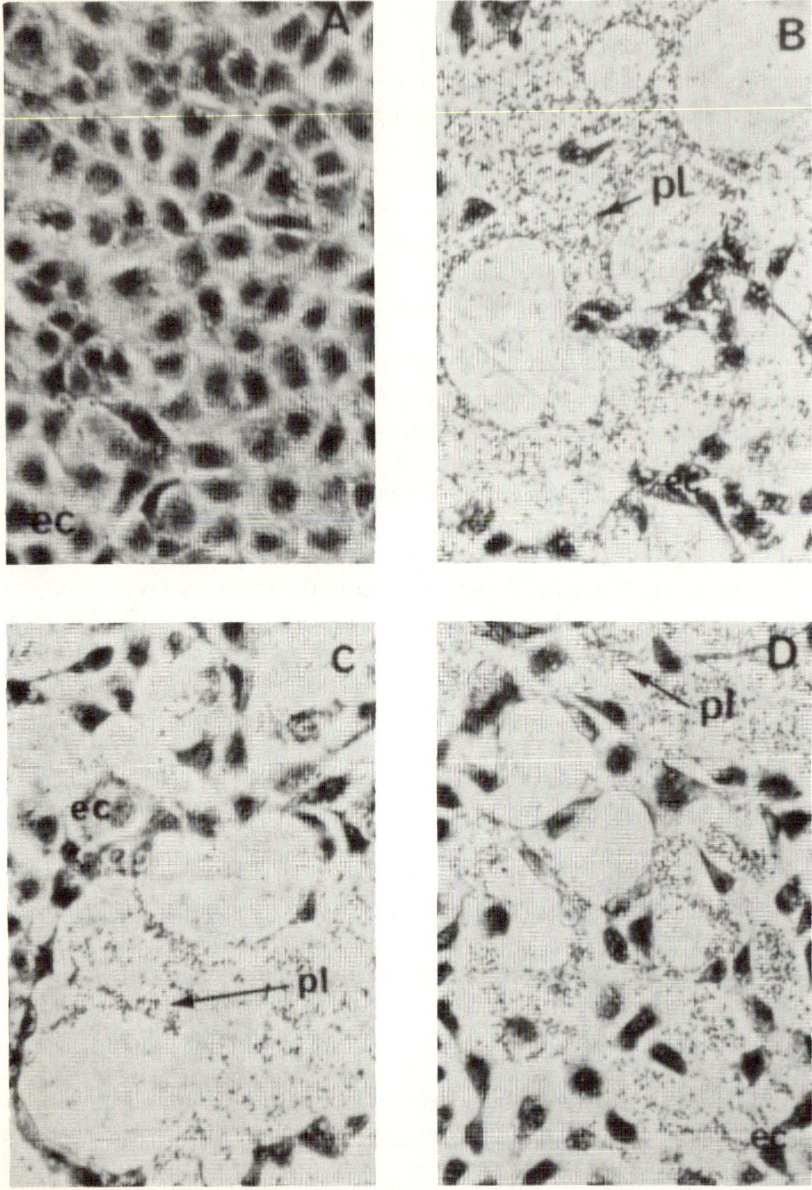

Figure 3-3 Light micrograph of platelets (5×10^5 platelets/μL) interacted with the 4-day postconfluent monolayer of endothelial cells. **A** Unactivated control; **B** activated for 2 minutes with 2×10^{-5} M epinephrine; **C** activated for 2 minutes with 5×10^{-5} M serotonin; **D** 0.15 M NaCl for 15 minutes. Platelets reacted with endothelial cells for 4 minutes, fixed and stained with methylene blue. ec, endothelial cells; pl, platelets. Magnification: $\times$ 233.

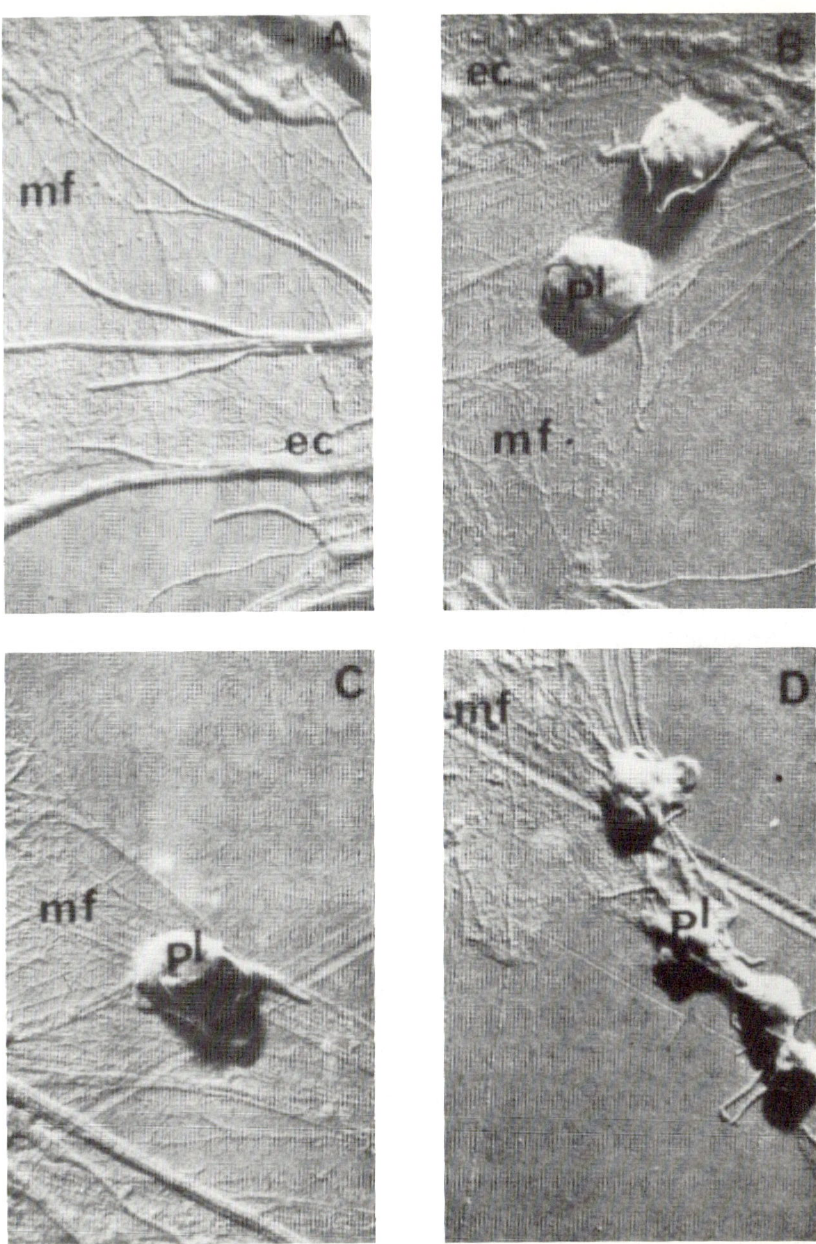

Figure 3-4 Shadow-casted (Pt/C) replicas of extracellular matrix of endothelial microfilaments and interacting platelets. **A** Control, not reacted with platelets ($\times$ 5817); **B** platelets associated with matrix of 100–150 R microfilaments ($\times$ 6380), single platelet associated with matrix ($\times$ 5050). Endothelial cells activated for 2 minutes with 2×10^{-5} M epinephrine and reacted with platelets (5.7×10^{5} platelets/μL) for 4 minutes. mf, microfilaments; ec, endothelial cells; pl, platelets.

microfibrils is not known, but it most probably contains collagens, fibronectin, laminin, proteoglycans, glucosaminoglycans, VIIIR:VWF, and other substances not as yet identified. The interaction of platelets with the exposed subendothelial microfilaments is abolished by trypsin treatment, aspirin, and prostaglandin E_1.[134]

Interaction of platelets with the vascular subendothelium in vivo has been studied by removing the endothelial cells of the aorta with a balloon catheter.[135-138] Platelets adhere initially to the denuded subendothelium as a monolayer, followed by spreading to cover the extent of the injury. Small thrombi formed in the first few minutes are swept away by the bloodstream within one hour, leaving a single monolayer of platelets. Fibrin formation is usually not present in the aorta, but is seen in veins which have a lower shear rate.[139]

It seems clear that platelets do not adhere to an intact, undamaged endothelial cell layer, either in vitro or in vivo. Endothelial cells can limit the formation of a thrombus (1) by forming PGI_2 (a potent inhibitor of platelet aggregation) in response to a number of stimuli, (2) by contributing to the activation of the fibrinolytic system through the secretion of plasminogen activator, (3) by binding thrombin and accelerating its inactivation by antithrombin III, and (4) by providing a cofactor for the activation of protein C, a potent anticoagulant.[140] On the other hand, damage to the endothelium can initiate thrombus formation as a result of the altered endothelium stimulating coagulation or the exposure of the subendothelial structures to which platelets can adhere. Blood flow will also determine the extent of thrombus formation. The balance between thrombus-promoting and -inhibiting factors will determine the extent of the final event.

REFERENCES

1. Weiss H: Platelet physiology and abnormalities of platelet function (Part 1). *N Engl J Med* 1975;293:531–541.
2. White JG, Gerrard JM: Ultrastructural features of abnormal blood platelets: a review. *Am J Pathol* 1976;83:590–614.
3. Shattil SJ, Bennett JS: Platelets and their membranes in hemostasis: physiology and pathophysiology. *Ann Intern Med* 1980;94:108–118.
4. Gordon JL: Platelets in perspective, in Gordon JL (ed): *Platelets in Biology and Pathology*, ed 2. New York, Elsevier/North Holland Biomedical Press, 1981, pp 1–17.
5. Skaer RJ: Platelet degranulation, in Gordon JL (ed): *Platelets in Biology and Pathology*, ed 2. New York, Elsevier/North Holland Biomedical Press, 1981, pp 321–348.
6. Kaplan KL: Platelet granule proteins: localization and secretion, in Gordon JL: (ed): *Platelets in Biology and Pathology*, ed 2. New York, Elsevier/North Holland Biomedical Press, 1981, pp 77–90.
7. Sixma JJ, Holmsen H, Trieschnigg CM: Adenine nucleotide metabolism of

blood platelets. VIII. Transport of adenine into human platelets. *Biochim Biophys Acta* 1973;298:460–468.

8. Sixma JJ, Lips JPM, Trieschnigg MC, et al: Transport and metabolism of adenosine in human blood platelets. *Biochim Biophys Acta* 1976;443:33–48.

9. Holmsen H, Day HJ, Storm E: Adenine nucleotide metabolism of blood platelets. VI. Subcellular localization of nucleotide pools with different functions in the platelet release reaction. *Biochim Biophys Acta* 1969;186:254–266.

10. Reimers HJ, Mustard JF, Packham MA: Transfer of adenine nucleotides between the releasable and nonreleasable compartments of rabbit blood platelets. *J Cell Biol* 1975;67:61–71.

11. Rudnick G, Fishkes H, Nelson PJ, et al: Evidence for two distinct serotonin transport systems in platelets. *J Biol Chem* 1980;255:3638–3641.

12. Talvenheimo J, Nelson PJ, Rudnick G: Mechanism of imipramine inhibition of platelet 5-hydroxytryptamine transport. *J Biol Chem* 1979;254:4631–4635.

13. Wilkins JA, Greenawalt JW, Huan L: Transport of 5-hydroxytryptamine by dense granules from porcine platelets. *J Biol Chem* 1978;253:6260–6265.

14. Gordon JL, Olverman HJ: 5-Hydroxytryptamine and dopamine transport by rat and human blood platelets. *Br J Pharmacol* 1978;62:219–226.

15. Moncada S, Gryglewski R, Bunting S, et al: An enzyme isolated from arteries transforms prostaglandin endoperoxides to an unstable substance that inhibits platelet aggregation. *Nature* 1976;263:663–665.

16. Weksler BB, Marcus AJ, Jaffe EA: Synthesis of prostaglandin I_2 (prostacyclin) by cultured human and bovine endothelial cells. *Proc Natl Acad Sci USA* 1977;74:3922–3928.

17. Baenziger NL, Dillender MJ, Majerus PW: Cultured human skin fibroblasts and arterial cells produce a labile platelet-inhibitory prostaglandin. *Biochem Biophys Res Commun* 1977;78:294–301.

18. Higgs EA, Moncada S, Vane JR, et al: Effect of prostacyclin (PGI_2) on platelet adhesion to rabbit arterial subendothelium. *Prostaglandins* 1978;16:17–22.

19. Weiss HJ, Turitto VT: Prostacyclin (prostaglandin I_2, PGI_2) inhibits platelet adhesion and thrombus formation on subendothelium. *Blood* 1979;53:91–105.

20. Dejana E, Cazenave J-P, Groves HM, et al: The effect of aspirin inhibition of PGI_2 production on platelet adherence to normal and damaged rabbit aortas. *Thromb Res* 1980;17:453–464.

21. Curwen KD, Gimbrone MA, Handin RI: In vitro studies of thromboresistance. The role of prostacyclin (PGI_2) in platelet adhesion to cultured normal and virally transformed human vascular endothelial cells. *Lab Invest* 1980;42:366–374.

22. Stemmerman MB: Vascular intimal components: precursors of thrombosis. *Prog Hemost Thromb* 1974;2:1–47.

23. Baumgartner HR, Muggli R: Adhesion and aggregation: morphological demonstration and quantitation in vivo and in vitro, in Gordon JL (ed): *Platelets in Biology and Pathology*. New York, North Holland Publishing Company, 1976, pp 23–60.

24. Jaffe RM: Interaction of platelets with connective tissue, in Gordon JL (ed); *Platelets in Biology and Pathology*. New York, North Holland Publishing Company, 1976, pp 261–292.

25. Tschopp TB, Weiss HJ, Baumgartner HR: Decreased adhesion of platelets

to subendothelium in von Willebrand's disease. *J Lab Clin Med* 1974;83: 296–300.

26. Jaffe EA, Hoyer LW, Nachman RL: Synthesis of von Willebrand factor by cultured human endothelial cells. *Proc Natl Acad Sci USA* 1974;71:1906–1909.

27. Berndt MC, Phillips DR: Platelet membrane proteins: composition and receptor function, in Gordon JL (ed): *Platelets in Biology and Pathology*, ed 2. New York, Elsevier/North Holland Biomedical Press, 1981, pp 43–75.

28. Counts RB, Paskell SL, Elgee SK: Disulfide bonds and the quaternary structure of factor VIII/von Willebrand factor. *J Clin Invest* 1978;62:702–709.

29. Fujimoto T, Hawiger J: Adenosine diphosphate induces binding of von Willebrand factor to human platelets. *Nature* 1982;297:154–156.

30. Kao KJ, Pizzo SV, McKee PA: Demonstration and characterization of specific binding sites for factor VIII/von Willebrand factor in human platelets. *J Clin Invest* 1979;63:656–664.

31. Kao KJ, Pizzo SV, McKee PA: Platelet receptors for human factor VIII/von Willebrand protein: functional correlation of receptor occupancy and ristocetin-induced platelet aggregation. *Proc Natl Acad Sci USA* 1979; 76:5317–5320.

32. Howard MA, Hutton RA, Hardisty RM: Hereditary giant platelet syndrome: a disorder of a new aspect of platelet function. *Br Med J* 1973;2: 586–588.

33. Weiss HJ, Tschopp TB, Baumgartner HR, et al: Decreased adhesion of giant (Bernard-Soulier) platelets to subendothelium: further implications on the role of the von Willebrand factor in hemostasis. *Am J Med* 1974;57:920–925.

34. Jankins CSP, Phillips DR, Clemetson KJ, et al: Platelet membrane glycoproteins implicated in ristocetin-induced aggregation. *J Clin Invest* 1976;57:112–124.

35. Jamieson GA, Okumura T, Fishback B, et al: Platelet membrane glycoproteins in thrombasthenia, Bernard-Soulier syndrome and storage pool disease. *J Lab Clin Med* 1979;93:652–660.

36. Tobelem G, Levy-Toledano S, Nurden AT, et al: Further studies on a specific platelet antibody found in Bernard-Soulier syndrome and its effects on normal platelet function. *Br J Haematol* 1979;41:427–436.

37. Nachman RL, Jaffe EA, Weksler BB: Immuninhibition of ristocetin-induced platelet aggregation. *J Clin Invest* 1977;59:143–148.

38. Phillips DR: Effect of trypsin on the exposed polypeptides and glycoproteins in the human platelet membrane. *Biochemistry* 1972;11:4582–4588.

39. Nachman RL, Ferris B: Studies on the proteins of human platelet membranes. *J Biol Chem* 1972;4468–4475.

40. Phillips DR, Agin PP: Platelet plasma membrane glycoproteins: evidence for the presence of nonequivalent disulfide bonds using nonreduced-reduced two-dimensional gel electrophoresis. *J Biol Chem* 1977;252:2121–2126.

41. Haslam RJ: Role of adenosine diphosphate in the aggregation of human blood platelets by thrombin and fatty acids. *Nature* 1964;202:765–768.

42. Born GVR: Aggregation of platelets by adenosine diphosphate and its reversal. *Nature* 1962;194:927–929.

43. Packham MA, Kinlough-Rathbone RL, Reimers H-J, et al: Mechanisms of platelet aggregation independent of adenosine diphosphate, in Silver MJ, Smith JB, Kocsis JJ (eds): *Prostaglandins in Hematology*. Cocheton, NY, Spectrum Publications, 1977, pp 247–276.

44. Macfarlane DE, Mills DCB: The effects of ATP on platelets: Evidence

against the central role of released ADP in primary aggregation. *Blood* 1975;46:309–320.

45. Tollefsen DM, Feager JR, Majerus PW: The binding of thrombin to the surface of human platelets. *J Biol Chem* 1974;249:2646–2651.

46. Shuman MA, Majerus PW: The measurement of thrombin in clotting blood by radioimmunoassay. *J Clin Invest* 1976;58:1249–1258.

47. Martin BM, Wasiewski WW, Fenton JW II, et al: Equilibrium binding of thrombin to platelets. *Biochemistry* 1976;15:4886–4892.

48. Tam SW, Detwiler TC: Binding of thrombin to human platelet plasma membranes. *Biochim Biophys Acta* 1978;543:194–201.

49. Tollefsen DM, Majerus PW: Evidence for a single class of thrombin-binding sites on human platelets. *Biochemistry* 1976;15:2144–2148.

50. Workman EF Jr, White GC II, Lundblad RL: Structure-function relationships in the interaction of α-thrombin with blood platelets. *J Biol Chem* 1977;252:7118–7123.

51. Okumura T, Hasitz M, Jamieson GA; Platelet glycocalicin: interaction with thrombin and role as thrombin receptor of the platelet surface. *J Biol Chem* 1978;253:3435–3443.

52. Ganguly P, Gould NL: Thrombin receptors of human platelets: thrombin binding and anti-thrombin properties of glycoprotein I. *Br J Haematol* 1979;42:137–146.

53. Jamieson GA, Okumura T: Reduced thrombin binding and aggregation in Bernard-Soulier platelets. *J Clin Invest* 1978;61:861–864.

54. Phillips DR, Agin PP: Platelet plasma membrane glycoproteins; identification of a proteolytic substrate for thrombin. *Biochim Biophys Res Commun* 1977;75:940–947.

55. Newman KD, Williams LT, Bishopric NH, et al: Identification of α-adrenergic receptors on human platelets by [^{3}H]-dihydroergocryptine binding. *J Clin Invest* 1978;61:395–402.

56. Grant JA, Scrutton MC: Positive interaction between agonist in the aggregation response between ADP, adrenaline and vasopressin. *Brit J Haematol* 1980;44:109–125.

57. Feinberg H, Michel H, Born GVR: Determination of the fluid volume of platelets by their separation through silicone oil. *J Lab Clin Med* 1974;84;926–934.

58. Nachmias V, Sullender J, Asch A: Shape and cytoplasmic filaments in control and lidocaine-treated human platelets. *Blood* 1977;50:39–53.

59. Mustard JF, Packham MA, Kinlough-Rathbone RL, et al: Fibrinogen and ADP-induced platelet aggregation. *Blood* 1978;52:453–466.

60. Harfenist EJ, Guccione MA, Packham MA, et al: Arachidonate-induced fibrinogen binding to thrombin-degranulated rabbit platelets is independent of release ADP. *Blood* 1982;59:956–962.

61. Bennett JS, Vilaire G: Exposure of platelet fibrinogen receptors by ADP and epinephrine. *J Clin Invest* 1979;64:1393–1401.

62. Hawiger J, Parkinson S, Timmons S: Prostacyclin inhibits mobilization of fibrinogen-binding sites on human ADP and thrombin-treated platelets. *Nature* 1980;283:195–197.

63. Harfenist EJ, Packham MA, Mustard JF: Reversibility of the association of fibrinogen with rabbit platelets exposed to ADP. *Blood* 1980;56:189–198.

64. Caen J: Glanzmann's thrombasthenia. *Clin Haematol* 1972;1:383–392.

65. Phillip DR, Agin PP: Platelet membrane defects in Glanzmann's thrombasthenia. *J Clin Invest* 1977;60:535–545.

66. Gerrard JM, Peterson DA, White JG: Calcium mobilization, in Gordon JL (ed): *Platelets in Biology and Pathology*, ed 2. New York, Elsevier/North Holland Biomedical Press, 1981, pp 407–436.

67. Feinstein MB, Rodan GA, Cutler LS: Cyclic AMP and calcium in platelet function, in Gordon JL (ed): *Platelets in Biology and Pathology*, ed 2. New York, Elsevier/North Holland Biomedical Press, 1981, pp 437–472.

68. Miller OV, Aiken JW, Shebuski RJ, et al: 6-Keto-Prostaglandin E_1 is not equipotent to prostacyclin (PGI_2) as an antiaggregatory agent. *Prostaglandins* 1980;20:391–400.

69. Wong PY-K, Malin KU, Desiderio DM, et al: Hepatic metobolism of prostacyclin (PGI_2) in the rabbit: formation of a potent novel inhibitor of platelet aggregation. *Biochem Biophys Res Commun* 1980;93:486–494.

70. Wong PY-K, Lee WH, Chao PH-W, et al: Metabolism of prostacyclin by 9-hydroxyprostaglandin dehydrogenase in human platelets. *J Biol Chem* 1980;255:9021–9024.

71 Gorman RR, Fitzpatrick FA, Miller OV: Reciprocal regulation of human platelet cAMP levels by thromboxane A_2 and prostacyclin, in George WJ, Ignarro LJ (eds): *Advances in Cyclic Nucleotide Research*. New York, Raven Press, 1978, vol 9, pp 597–609.

72. Witte LD, Kaplan KL, Nossel HL, et al: Studies on the release from human platelets of the growth factor for cultured human arterial smooth muscle cells. *Circ Res* 1978;42:402–409.

73. Kinlough-Rathbone RL, Packham MA, Reimers H-J, et al: Mechanisms of platelet shape change, aggregation and release induced by collagen, thrombin, or A23,187. *J Lab Clin Med* 1977;90:707–719.

74. Marcus AJ: The role of lipids in platelet function with particular reference to the arachidonic acid pathway. *J Lipid Chem* 1978;19:793–826.

75. Bills TK, Smith JB, Silver MJ: Selective release of arachidonic acid from the phospholipids of human platelets in response to thrombin. *J Clin Invest* 1977;60:1–6.

76. Rittenhouse-Simmons S, Russell FA, Deykin D: Mobilization of arachiodonic acid in human platelets: Kinetics and Ca^{2+} dependency. *Biochim Biophys Acta* 1977;488:370–380.

77. Mauco G, Chap H, Douste-Blazy L: Characterization and properties of a phosphatidylinositol phosphodiesterase (phospholipase C) from platelet cytosol. *FEBS Lett* 1979;100:367–370.

78. Rittenhouse-Simmons S, Russell FA, Deykin D: Production of diglyceride from phosphatidylinositol in activated platelets. *J Clin Invest* 1979;63:580–587.

79. Bell RL, Kennerly DA, Stanford N, et al: Diglyceride lipase: a pathway for arachidonate release from human platelets. *Proc Natl Acad Sci USA* 1979;76:3238–3241.

80. Miyamoto T, Ogino N, Yamamoto S, et al: Purification of prostaglandin endoperoxide synthetase from bovine vesicular gland microsomes. *J Biol Chem* 1976;251:2629–2636.

81. Hembler M, Lands WEM, Smith WL: Purification of the cyclooxygenase that forms prostaglandins. Demonstration of two forms of iron in the holozyme. *J Biol Chem* 1976;251:5575–5579.

82. Hamberg M, Svensson J, Samuelsson B: Thromboxanes: a new group of biologically active compounds derived from prostaglandin endoperoxides. *Proc Natl Acad Sci USA* 1975;72:2994–2998.

83. Chignard M, LeCouedic JP, Vargaftig BB, et al: Platelet-activating Factor

(PAF-Acether) secretion from platelets: effect of aggregating agents. *Br J Haematol* 1980;46:455–464.

84. Cazenave JP, Benveniste J, Mustard JF: Aggregation of rabbit platelets by platelet activating factor is independent of the release reaction and the arachidonate pathway and inhibited by membrane-active drugs. *Lab Invest* 1979;41:275–285.

85. Benton AM, Gerrard JM, Michiel T, et al: Are lysophosphatidic acids or phosphatidic acids involved in stimulus activation coupling in platelets. *Blood* 1982;60:642–649.

86. Weiss HJ, Witle LD, Kaplan KL, et al: Heterogeneity in storage pool deficiency: studies on granule-bound substances in 18 patients including varients deficient in α-granules, platelet factor 4, β-thromboglobulin, and platelet-derived growth factor. *Blood* 1979;54:1296–1319.

87. Wu KK: Bleeding disorders due to abnormalities in platelet prostaglandins, in Wu KK, Rossi EC (eds); *Prostaglandins in Clinical Medicine: Cardiovascular and Thrombotic Disorders.* Chicago, Year Book Medical Publishers, 1982, pp 81–92.

88. Walsh PN, Tuszynski GP: Factor XI, platelets and hemostatic control, in Mann KG, Taylor FB (eds): *The Regulation of Coagulation.* New York, Elsevier/North Holland Biochemical Press, 1980, pp 251–257.

89. Tracey PB, Peterson JM, Nesheim ME, et al: Interaction of coagulation factor V and factor Va with platelets. *J Biol Chem* 1979;254:10354–10361.

90. Kane WH, Lindhout MJ, Jackson CM, et al: Factor Va-dependent binding of factor Xa to human platelets. *J Biol Chem* 1980;255:1170–1174.

91. Rodin JAG: *Histology, Text and Atlas.* New York, London, Toronto, Oxford University Press, 1974, pp 340–370.

92. Thorgursson G, Robertson AL: The vascular endothelium-pathologic significance—a review. *Am J Pathol* 1978;93:803–847.

93. Zetter BR: The endothelial cells of large and small blood vessels. *Diabetes* 1981;30(suppl):24–28.

94. Booyse FM, Sedlack B, Rafelson ME: Culture of arterial endothelial cells. *Thromb Diath Haemorrhagica* 1975;34:825–839.

95. Slater DN, Sloan JM: The porcine endothelial cell in tissue culture. *Atherosclerosis* 1975;21:259–272.

96. Schwartz AM: Selection and characterization of bovine aortic endothelial cells. *In Vitro* 1978;14:966–980.

97. Eskin SG, Sybers HD, Trevino L, et al: Comparison of tissue culture bovine endothelial cells from aorta and saphenous vein. *In Vitro* 1978;14:903–910.

98. Jaffe EA, Nachman RL, Becker AG, Minick CR: Culture of human endothelial cells derived from umbilical veins. *J Clin Invest* 1973;52:2745–2756.

99. Gimbrone MA: Culture of vascular endothelium, in Spaet TH (ed): *Progress in Hemostasis and Thrombosis.* New York, Grune & Stratton, 1976, pp 1–28.

100. Folkman J, Haudenschild CC, Zetter BR: Long-term culture of capillary endothelial cells. *Proc Natl Acad Sci USA* 1971;76:5217–5221.

101. Bowman PD, Betz AL, Ar D, et al: Primary culture of capillary endothelium from rat brain. *In Vitro* 1981;17:353–362.

102. Bowman PD, Betz AL, Goldstein GW: Primary culture of microvascular endothelial cells from bovine retina. *In Vitro* 1982;18:626–632.

103. Weibel ER, Palade GE: New cytoplasmin components in arterial endothelia. *J Cell Biol* 1964;23:101–112.

44

104. Gimbrone MA, Cotran RS: Human vascular smooth muscle in culture. *Lab Invest* 1975;33:16–27.
105. Haudenschild CC, Cotran RS, Gimbrone MA: Fine structure of vascular endothelium in culture. *J Ultrastruct Res* 1975;50:22–32.
106. Santolaya RC, Bertini F: Fine structure of endothelial cells of vertebrates. *Z Anat Entwicklunsgesch* 1970;131:148–155.
107. Buzney SM, Massicotle SJ: Retinal vessels: proliferation of endothelium in vitro. *Ophthalmol Vis Sci* 1979;18:1191–1195.
108. Davison PM, Bensch K, Karasek MA: Isolation and growth of endothelial cells from the microvessels of the newborn human foreskin in cell culture. *J Invest Dermatol* 1980;75:316–321.
109. De Bault LE, Lahn LE, Frommes SP, et al: Cerebral microvessels and derived cells in tissue culture. *In Vitro* 1979;15:473–487.
110. Sherer BK, Fitzharris TP, Faulk WP, et al: Cultivation of microvascular endothelial cells from human preputial skin. *In Vitro* 1980;16:675–684.
111. Chan V, Chan TK: Characterization of factor VIII related protein synthesized by human endothelial cell. *Thromb Haemost* 1982;48:177–181.
112. Jaffe EA: Endothelial cells and the biology of factor VIII. *N Engl J Med* 1977;296:372–383.
113. Johnson AR: Human pulmonary endothelial cells in culture: activities of cells from arteries and cells from veins. *J Clin Invest* 1980;65:841–850.
114. Philips P, Kumar P, Kumar S, et al: Isolation and characterization of endothelial cells from rat and cow brain white matter. *J Anat* 1979;129:261–272.
115. Hayes LW, Goguen CH, Ching SF, et al: Angiotensin converting enzyme: Accumulation in medium from cultured endothelial cells. *Biochem Biophys Res Commun* 1978;82:1147–1153.
116. Heal V: Angiotensin metabolism by cultured human vascular endothelial and smooth muscle cells. *Microvasc Res* 1979;17:314–321.
117. Johnson AR, Erdos EG: Metabolism of vasoactive peptides by human endothelial cells in culture. *J Clin Invest* 1977;59:684–695.
118. Loskutoff DJ, Levin EG: Fluctuation in the fibrinolytic activity of cultural endothelial cells caused by routine culture manipulations, in Mann K, Taylor FB (eds): *The Regulation of Coagulation*. New York, Elsevier/North Holland, 1980, pp 589–595.
119. Loskutoff DJ, Levin E, Mussoni L: Fibrinolytic components of cultured endothelial cells, in Mosel H, Vogel H (eds): *Pathology of the Endothelial Cells*. New York, Academic Press, 1982, pp 167–182.
120. Moncada S, Vane JR: Arachidonic acid metabolites and the interaction between blood vessel walls. *N Engl J Med* 1979;300:1142–1147.
121. Weksler BB, Marcus AJ, Jaffe EA: Synthesis of prostaglandin I_2 (prostacyclin) by cultured human and bovine endothelial cells. *Proc Natl Acad Sci USA* 1977;74:3922–3926.
122. Coughlin SR, Moskowitz MA, Zetter BR, et al: Platelet dependent stimulation of prostacyclin synthesis by platelet-derived growth factor. *Nature* 1980;288:600–602.
123. Weksler BB, Ley CW, Jaffe EA: Stimulation of endothelial cell prostacyclin production by thrombin, trypsin and the ionophore A23187. *J Clin Invest* 1978;62:923–930.
124. Howard BV, Macarak EJ, Gunson D, et al: Characterization of the collagen synthesized by endothelial cells in culture. *Proc Natl Acad Sci USA* 1976;73:2361–2364.
125. Jaffe E, Adelman B, Minuk CR, et al: Synthesis of basement membrane collagen by cultured human endothelial cells. *J Exp Med* 1976;144:209–225.

126. Buonassesi V, Root M: Enzymatic degradation of heparin related muco-polysaccharides from the surface of endothelial cell cultures. *Biochim Biophys Acta* 1975;385:1–100.

127. Burch C, Lyjcingman C, Helden CM, et al: Surface properties of cultured endothelial cells. *Haemostasis* 1979;8:142–148.

128. Gospodarowicz, D, Fujii D: *Miami Winter Symposium* 1981;18:113–135.

129. Jaffe E, Mosher DF: Synthesis of fibronectin by cultured human endothelial cells. *Ann NY Acad Sci* 1978;312:122–130.

130. Waxler B, Schumacher B, Eisenstein R: Cell stroma interactions in aortic endothelial cell cultures. *Lab Invest* 1979;41:128–134.

131. Templ R, Rhode H, Robey PG, et al: Laminin — A glycoprotein from basement membranes. *J Biol Chem* 1979;254:9933–9937.

132. Gospodarowicz D, Greenburg H, Froidart JM, et al: Laminin and fibronectin production by cultured vascular and corneal endothelial cells. *J Cell Physiol* 1981;107:173–183.

133. Curwen CA, Gimbrone MA, Handin RJ: In vitro studies of thromboresistance. *Lab Invest* 1980;42:366–374.

134. Booyse FM, Bell S, Sedlak B, Rafelson ME: Development of an in vitro vessel wall model for studying certain aspects of platelet-vessel wall (endothelial) interactions. *Artery* 1975;1:517–527.

135. Stemmerman MB: Vascular intima components: precursor in thrombosis, in Spaet TH (ed): *Progress in Haemostasis and Thrombosis*. New York, Grune & Stratton, 1974, vol 2, pp 1–47.

136. Baumgartner HR, Haudenschild C: Adhesion of platelets to subendothelium. *Ann NY Acad Sci* 1972;201:22–36.

137. Baumgartner HR, Muggli R: Adhesion and aggregation: morphological demonstration and quantitation *in vivo* and *in vitro*, in Gordon JL (ed): *Platelets in Biology and Pathology*. New York, North Holland Publishing Company, 1976, pp 23–60.

138. Baumgartner HR, Studer A: Folgen des Gefässkatheterismus am normo- und hypercholinesterinämischen Kaninchen. *Pathologie et Microbiologie* 1966;29:393–412.

139. Baumgartner HR: The role of blood flow in platelet adhesion, fibrin deposition and formation of mural thrombi. *Microvasc Res* 1973;5:167–179.

140. Esmon ET, Esmon NL, Saugstad J, et al: Activation of protein C by a complex between thrombin and endothelial cell surface protein, in Nossel H, Vogel H (eds): *Pathobiology of the Endothelial Cell*. New York, Academic Press, 1982, pp 122–136.

4 *Coagulation and Fibrinolysis*

Edmond R. Cole

PHYLOGENETIC ASPECTS OF HEMOSTASIS

The coagulation mechanism of man and other mammals has its origin far back in the evolutionary process. Conservation of vital fluids is a prime requisite for maintenance of life processes, and even unicellular organisms are capable of preserving their intracellular fluids after injury to their cell wall. These organisms employ a surface precipitation reaction (SPR) which has a remarkable similarity to some reactions in mammalian blood coagulation. SPR is calcium ion–dependent; injuries to cells grown in calcium ion–free media result in loss of intracellular fluid. A thrombin-like enzyme is generated in the SPR process, and in some organisms, such as the giant amoeba, the SPR reaction is inhibited by dilute heparin solutions. Therefore, SPR is a common defense mechanism for the preservation of cellular protoplasm and can be considered as hemostasis at the cellular level or a rudimentary coagulation system. This subject has been reviewed by Heilbrunn.[1]

Primitive prototype hemostatic systems are to be found in organisms further advanced in evolution than the unicellular organisms. In the horseshoe crab, nucleoted thrombocytes (hemocytes) contain a clotting protein similar to fibrinogen. These cells undergo aggregation following injury to the vascular system of these organisms.[2,3] In another divergent path of hemostasis, the hemolymph of the lobster contains a fibrinogen-like protein which, after the proper stimulus, is crosslinked by a muscle enzyme similar in action to factor XIII (fibrin stabilizing factor), producing a hemostatic gel.[4]

As organisms became more complex, more extensive vascular systems developed requiring higher blood pump output and increased intravascular pressures to provide oxygen and nutrients to specialized tissues for locomotion, grasping of prey, and for the more complex brain required for higher intelligence. However, higher intravascular pressures also increased the risk of rapid loss of intravascular fluids if any injury to the vascular system occurred. At the same time, the need arose to protect the vascular system of complex organisms from occlusion in the absence of a proper stimulus. A balanced hemostatic mechanism obviously is crucial to the survival of any species and nowhere is this better exemplified than in man and in other mammalian species. The term *hemostasis* as used here refers not only to all the reactions that maintain blood in a freely circulating state in the vascular system in the absence of injury, but also, in the event of vascular injury, to those reactions that lead to the formation of a hemostatic plug to prevent life-threatening hemorrhage as well as to the removal of these products from the vascular system after repair of the hemorrhage site. Therefore, hemostasis involves platelets, the vessel wall, the coagulation and fibrinolytic components of blood plasma, and several inhibitors that modulate procoagulant and profibrinolytic processes.

The series of reactions involved in the arrest of bleeding from an injured vessel is commonly divided into primary and secondary hemostasis. The properties of platelets, their activation, adhesion, and aggregation, and their interaction with the endothelium and subendothelium have been presented in a previous chapter of this book, and need not be further discussed here, aside from the statement that primary hemostasis involves the reaction leading to formation of the platelet plug and involves those interactions between the vessel wall, platelets, and a specific blood plasma factor (von Willebrand factor).

The second major mechanism of hemostasis is the coagulation system. This system is expressed by the activation of a number of coagulation factors and the formation of an insoluble protein, fibrin, which reinforces the hemostatic properties of the platelet plug. The third major mechanism is the fibrinolytic system which has to do with the dissolution of fibrin deposited in the vascular system as a consequence of activation of the coagulation system. In all three systems (platelet plug formation, coagulation, and fibrinolysis) the components necessary for each system to be activated are compartmentalized, which has the advantage of minimizing the activation of that system, except after a proper and sustaining stimulus. In a major injury to the vascular system, all three mechanisms participate. However, under certain circumstances, each may become the major mechanism with minimal involvement of the other two. This is especially true in the case of primary hemostasis. It is probably that most episodes of hemostasis arising from minor day-to-day trauma are of this type, especially if such trauma occurs in the smaller vessels and capillaries. As an example, a penetration injury of a capillary resulting in escape of blood into the subendothelium leads to the axon reflex, causing an initial vasoconstriction of the vessel. For a period of a few seconds only a small amount of blood flows from the injured vessel. This vasoconstriction may result in closing of the injured vessel and this may be sufficient for hemostasis. However, more often the intravascular pressure is sufficient to overcome the vasoconstriction and cause blood to flow out of the vessels and into contact with the basement membrane and the collagenous fibers in the perivascular tissues, where platelet adhesion and aggregation result in the formation of a platelet plug. This stage, known as primary hemostasis, is often followed by activation of the coagulation system and consolidation of the platelet plug, but hemostasis in the small vessels may occur even in the absence of fibrin formation, as evidenced by the fact that individuals with severely impaired coagulation systems (hemophiliacs) have normal bleeding times, a measure of primary hemostasis.

THE COAGULATION SYSTEM

Our basic understanding of the sequence of reactions which constitute the coagulation mechanisms was considerably improved in 1964 when MacFarlane,[5] as well as Davie and Ratnoff[6] independently proposed that coagulation involved a series of proenzyme-to-enzyme transformations, each catalyzed by the action of the active enzyme preceding it in a scheme. This biological amplification system hypothesis has been modified with the discovery of additional factors and newer knowledge of the properties of coagulation factors participating in this mechanism.

Table 4-1 lists the factors currently known to be involved in the coagulation mechanism. With the exception of Ca^{++} and tissue factor, all

Table 4-1
Factors Participating in Coagulation

Factor	Synthesis Site	Approximate Plasma Concentration $\mu g/ml$	Half-life (h)
Factor I (fibrinogen)	Liver	3000	90
Factor II (prothrombin)	Liver	100	65
Factor III (thromboplastin, tissue factor)	Endothelium, other cells	—	—
Factor IV (Ca^{++})		—	—
Factor V (labile factor, accelerator globulin)	Liver	15	15
Factor VII (stable factor, SPCA)	Liver	1	5
Factor VIII:C (antihemophilic factor)	Unknown	—	10
Factor IX (Christmas factor)	Liver	5	25
Factor X (Stuart factor)	Liver	5	40
Factor XI (plasma thromboplastin antecedent)	Liver	7	45
Factor XII (Hageman factor)	Liver	29	50
Factor XIII (fibrin stabilizing factor, fibrinoligase)	Liver	6	120
Fletcher Factor (prekallikrein)	Liver	50	—
Fitzgerald Factor (high mol wt kininogen)	Liver	70	—

are known to be present in blood plasma in the unactivated forms. Conversion to the active forms with resulting formation of thrombin may proceed through either of two pathways, the intrinsic or the extrinsic coagulation cascade. Both pathways are initiated by a common event — damage to the endothelium and contact of blood with subendothelium components.

The Intrinsic Pathway

Initiation of coagulation by the intrinsic pathway is through activation of factor XII when this factor comes into contact with a foreign surface.[7,8] Physiologically, this foreign surface may be collagen, basement membrane, or microfibrillar material underlying the endothelium. On contact with these surfaces, factor XII undergoes a conformation change with appearance of enzymatic activity but not change in its molecular weight (80,000).[9] With the discovery that Fletcher factor (prekallikrein) and Fitzgerald factor (HMW kininogen) actively participate in a feedback loop to enhance the conversion of factor XII to factor XIIa, by proteolytic cleavage, to a smaller fragment,[10,11] the participation of factor XII in the initiation of coagulation, fibrinolysis, and kinin formation appears to have been elucidated. Prekallikrein and HMW-kininogen are known to circulate in plasma as a complex and it is this complex that acts as a cofactor for activation of factor XI.[12,13] It can be readily demonstrated that contact of plasma with negatively charged surfaces also results in a pronounced fibrinolytic activity.[14] Although both XIIa and kallikrein have been implicated in this plasminogen activation reaction, the exact mechanism has not been elucidated. The contact activation scheme is illustrated in Figure 4-1.

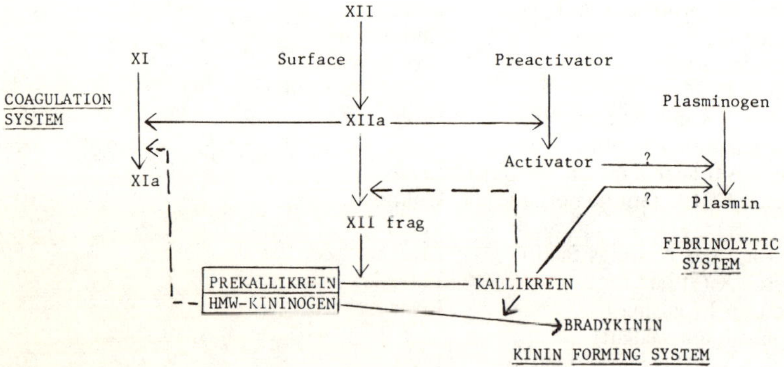

Figure 4-1 The contact phase of blood coagulation which also initiates the fibrinolytic- and kinin-forming systems. Solid arrows indicate major pathways; Dashed arrows indicate positive feedback loops where kallikrein and HMW-kininogen accelerate the conversion of factor XIIIa to factor XII frag and the activation of factor XI to factor XIa, respectively.

The remainder of the intrinsic pathway of coagulation is shown in Figure 4-2. The activation of factor XI completes the contact phase of coagulation, which does not require calcium ion. However, in subsequent steps leading to thrombin generation, calcium is an obligatory ion which participates in formation of procoagulant complexes of vitamin K–dependent factors (IX, X, and prothrombin), phospholipids, and cofactor proteins. These complexes function to greatly amplify thrombin generation in this pathway by concentration of reactants at the vascular

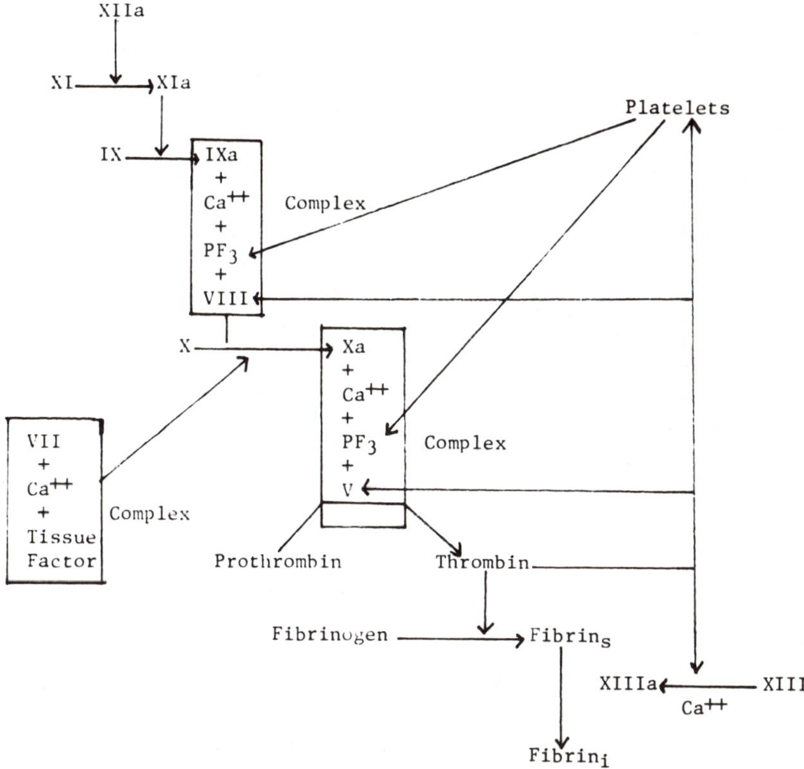

Figure 4-2 Coagulation pathways. The formation of complexes of activated coagulation factors, calcium, and cofactors are represented by boxes. Plasma coagulation factors listed by Roman numerals are as follows: XII, Hageman factor; XI, plasma thromboplastin antecedent; IX, Christmas factor; VIII, antihemophilic factor; X, Stuart factor; VII, stabile factor or proconvertin; V, labile factor; XIII, fibrin stabilizing factor. Prothrombin is factor II and fibrinogen is factor I. Fibrin$_s$ and Fibrin$_i$ represent non-crosslinked and crosslinked fibrin, respectively. Also illustrated is the control rate of thrombin in platelet activation to make phospholipid (platelet factor 3, PF$_3$) available for complex formation, in the conversion of factors VIII and V to more active forms, in the activation of factor XIII, and in the fibrinogen-fibrin transition. Activation of enzymatic factors is indicated by the letter a.

injury site. Activation of factor IX is initiated when factor XIa catalyzes the hydrolysis of a specific peptide bond in factor IX to form an inactive two-chain disulfide-linked intermediate and further proteolytic cleavage by factor XIa removes a 9000-dalton polypeptide from the heavy chain of the intermediate to produce the active serine protease, factor IXa.[15]

The catalytic efficiency of factor IXa and of the other vitamin K–dependent factors is greatly increased through formation of enzyme-phospholipid-calcium-cofactor complexes. The recent elucidation of the vitamin K-dependent, postribosomal incorporation of carboxyl groups into the N-terminal regions of the vitamin K–dependent factors[16,17] has provided the understanding of how these complexes form. The γ-carboxy glutamic acid residues in the functional forms of the vitamin K–dependent factors are required for calcium ion binding and for complexing of these factors to phospholipid micelles through calcium ion bridges. This phospholipid-calcium-enzyme complex also provides a hydrophobic surface for adsorption of a cofactor and subsequent binding of the substrate. In the activation of factor X by factor IXa, factor VIII is the cofactor for this step in the intrinsic coagulation pathway. The cofactor activity of factor VIII is greatly increased by the proteolytic action of thrombin. Thus thrombin participates in a positive feedback loop to enhance the effect of factor VIII on factor IXa–catalyzed activation of factor X.[18] However, further action of thrombin on factor VIII results in a destruction of the cofactor activity of factor VIII, resulting in an important control mechanism of the coagulation system.

The Extrinsic Pathway

Factor X can be activated through another pathway, the extrinsic coagulation system. A ubiquitous component of cells, tissue factor, is released when the endothelium surface is disturbed and the subendothelium exposed.[19] Tissue factor is a complex of phospholipids and a specific protein with the ability to activate another of the γ-carboxy glutamic acid residue–containing vitamin K–dependent factors, factor VII. Binding of factor VIIa to tissue factor through calcium bridges generates an activity which is capable of rapidly converting factor X to factor Xa.

The Common Pathway

The remainder of the coagulation system is termed the common pathway where factor Xa, derived from either the intrinsic or extrinsic system, forms a calcium bridge-mediated complex with phospholipids and a cofactor, factor V. Factor VIII and factor V are similar in properties and function in that their activities are initially stimulated by thrombin and are eventually destroyed by this enzyme.[18,20] Evidence of the latter phenomenon is observed in the plasma of patients with acute, decompensated intravascular coagulation where the levels of these two factors may be markedly reduced.

In the last step of sequential activation of the serine proteases that comprise the coagulation system, the factor Xa–calcium-phospholipid-factor V complex then acts as the catalytic surface upon which the substrate prothrombin binds and is converted to thrombin. In contrast to the activated vitamin K–dependent factors IX, VII, and X, which remain localized to the phospholipid complex, prothrombin is proteolytically activated in such a way that thrombin is split from the γ-carboxy glutamic acid–containing portion of the prothrombin molecule, allowing thrombin to diffuse away from the thrombus and participate in reactions which further stimulate the formation of a stabilized hemostatic plug. Thrombin is a very active stimulant of platelet aggregation and release reactions resulting in the release of platelet factor 3, the source of phospholipids participating in the intrinsic system; of platelet factor 4, the heparin-neutralizing factor; of several vasoactive amines which cause vasoconstriction of the injured vessel; and for viscous metamorphosis in which there is a breakdown of individual platelet membranes and formation of a nonreversible platelet plug. Platelet-contractile protein, thrombasthenin, also is exposed and contributes to clot retraction. In addition, thrombin is responsible for the formation of fibrin and the activation of factor XIII, the fibrin stabilizing factor,[21] to further consolidate the thrombus.

The interaction of thrombin with fibrinogen to form fibrin and the stabilization of the fibrin network is the final phase of blood coagulation. Fibrinogen is present in blood plasma in the highest concentration (200–400 mg/ml) of any coagulation factor. It is a 340,000-dalton rod-shaped molecule consisting of two monomeric units each containing an α-, β-, and γ-chain.[2] At the amino terminal ends of the α- and β-chains are sequences of amino acid residues which are proteolytically removed by thrombin.[23] These are called fibrinopeptide A and fibrinopeptide B, arising from the α- and β-chains, respectively.[24] The specific point of hydrolysis by thrombin is the same in both chains; an arginyl-glycine peptide bond. Fibrinopeptide A is removed first, causing a conformational change in the fibrinogen molecule, allowing an end-to-end association of the dimeric units and exposure of the B peptide to thrombin action.[24] Upon removal of fibrinopeptide B,[25] there is then a side-to-side association of the dimeric units, called fibrin monomers. Thus, end-to-end and side-to-side aggregation of the fibrin monomeric units allows the formation of an extended highly branched fibrin network. At this point the attactive forces holding the monomers together are of relatively weak hydrogen bonds and ionic, hydrophobic, and von der Waals types,[26] and the polymer is susceptible to disruption by fibrinolytic enzymes and flow shear forces. That further stabilization of this polymer is necessary is exemplified by the serious bleeding syndrome in individuals who have normal fibrin-forming systems but are deficient in factor XIII (fibrin-stabilizing factor).

54

Fibrin stabilization is initiated by thrombin activation of factor XIII,[21] a plasma zymogen with a molecular weight of 320,000 daltons and composed of two A-chains (mol wt 75,000) and two B-chains (mol wt 88,000).[27,28] Interestingly, platelet factor XIII consists of only two A-chains.[28] Thrombin in the presence of calcium ion removes a 4000-dalton polypeptide from the N-terminal region of each of the A-chains by hydrolysis of an arginyl-glycine bond, inducing a conformational change in the altered A subunits, in the presence of calcium ion, with a subsequent dissociation from the catalytically inactive B-subunits.[21] The B-chain dimer thus is not important for the catalytic action of factor XIIIa, but is necessary for secretion of the 320,000-dalton form at the synthesis site, and may prolong the survival of the zymogen within the circulation.

Factor XIIIa is a transamidase enzyme with a single sulfhydryl group at its active site, exposed during the conformational transition stage of activation. The active enzyme catalyzes the formation of peptide bonds between specific lysine residues and specific glutamyl residues of adjacent fibrin polypeptide chains. The peptide bonds most rapidly formed are between pairs of γ-chains, with peptide linkages between pairs of α-chains forming less rapidly.[29] The net effect is to bring the α- and γ-chains of fibrin monomers together in close proximity and linked by peptide bonds which are not easily dissociable, producing a fibrin network with greater mechanical strength and with greater resistance to dissolution by fibrinolytic enzymes.

Modulation of Coagulation Pathways

It should be obvious that inappropriate production of procoagulant substances, either too little or in excess, is life-threatening to the organism. While the hemorrhagic disorders are most often a consequence of deficiency of one of the hemostatic elements of plasma, platelets, or vessel wall, the circumstances leading to thrombosis are often less understood. From the description of the coagulation system in this chapter, one may surmise that once a proper stimulus for activation of coagulation is generated, an uncontrolled generation of procoagulant activities ensues. This is not the case for there are present in plasma inhibitors which modulate the procoagulant response and limit its effect. The major inhibitor of plasma is antithrombin III, also known as heparin cofactor.[30] Antithrombin III, a 56,000-dalton protein,[31] can, in the absence of heparin, slowly neutralize the enzymatic activity of thrombin and some other serine proteases of the coagulation mechanism as well (factors XIIa, XIa, IXa, Xa, and VIIa).[32-36] It is also capable of inactivating the fibrinolytic enzyme, plasmin.[37] It is known to form a 1:1 stoichemetic complex with thrombin.[38] Although it is a slow, progressive type of inhibition, the modulating effect on thrombus formation and action can be appreciated. Therefore, the feedback loop stimulation of the activity of factors VIII and V by thrombin, the thrombin-stimulated aggregation of platelets, and release of procoagulant platelet elements, as well as the fibrin-forming and factor XIII–activation properties of thrombin are kept under control, especially in the early stage of coagulation system activation. Antithrombin III inhibition of other serine proteases provides additional control of thrombin generation. The role of antithrombin III in modulation of coagulation is exemplified by the observation that a deficiency is associated with a tendency of humans to develop a recurrent thrombotic syndrome.[39–40]

Antithrombin III also has been identified as the heparin cofactor.[31] Heparin is a sulfated mucopolysaccharide with a very high negative charge density and is a component of mast cells and basophils.[41] It has been isolated from a number of organs, and the heparin isolated from beef lung and porcine intestine are important clinical agents for the treatment of intravascular thrombosis. Interaction of the negatively charged group of heparin and positively charged lysyl residues in antithrombin III results in a complex which is two thousand- to ten thousandfold more rapid in neutralizing the enzymatic activity of thrombin than is antithrombin III alone.[38] Similar enhancement of inhibitor activity against other serine proteases of the coagulation and fibrinolytic systems has been observed.

α_2-Macroglobulin, although present in blood plasma in much larger quantities (2.5 mg/ml) than antithrombin III,[42] plays a lesser role in maintaining hemostatic balance. It does, however, inhibit many proteolytic enzymes such as thrombin, trypsin, kallikrein, elastase, plasmin, and cathepsin,[43] but the substrates for these enzymes appear to have partial access to the active site of the enzyme in the enzyme-α_2-macroglobulin complex since limited proteolysis can be observed.[44] Therefore, the enzyme-α_2-macroglobulin complex may play a role in the initial stages of coagulation by converting factors VIII and V to their more active forms, thereby accelerating the production of thrombin through the intrinsic coagulation pathway. In a similar manner, plasmin-α_2-macroglobulin complex may be able to exert a small plasmin effect on plasminogen, releasing the activation peptide and accelerating the fibrinolytic system.

THE FIBRINOLYTIC SYSTEM

Fibrinolysis is the major defense mechanism against permanent occlusion of the blood vessels, and therefore has an important role in hemostatic balance. Historically, our understanding of fibrinolytic mechanisms has developed more slowly than that of the coagulation system, but recent investigations have demonstrated that the fibrinolytic systems may be as complex as those leading to the formation of stabilized fibrin in the vascular system, and, analogous to coagulation pathways, there exists both an intrinsic and extrinsic pathway of fibrinolysis.

Physiologic Activators of Plasminogen

Intrinsic activation of fibrinolysis implies that the elements required for the initiation of fibrinolysis are present in blood. Contact activation of factor XII appears to be the initial event (discussed in the section on coagulation). Evidence to support the concept of a plasminogen activator existing normally as the inactive precursor form was reported by Iatridis and Ferguson[14] who demonstrated that glass activation of plasma resulted in activation of factor XII and generation of a pronounced fibrinolytic activity. Whether the plasminogen activator is factor XIIa, or kallikrein or an activator generated from a proactivator by factor XIIa proteolysis is as yet undetermined. The physiologic importance of this fibrinolytic pathway has to be questioned, however, since an overt fibrinolytic deficit in individuals with deficiencies of the contact factors has not been demonstrated.

The physiologic activators of the extrinsic fibrinolytic system are of two types: the urokinase-type and the tissue-type plasminogen activators, both serine proteases which are direct activators of plasminogen. Urokinase, an enzyme of 54,000-dalton mol wt is synthesized by epithelial cells of the renal tubules and excreted into the urine from which it has been purified on a commercial basis.[45] Urokinase also has been isolated and purified from human fetal kidney cell culture medium.[46-48] Both products are used for the treatment of thrombotic disorders (see chapter 6). Until recently, kidney cells were believed to be the only site of synthesis of urokinase-type plasminogen activator, but more recent investigations indicate that the urokinase type is found in some malignant cells[49-52] and in the circulation itself, as evidenced by its recent detection[53] and isolation in a latent form from human plasma fraction.[54]

Tissue-type plasminogen activator is a ubiquitous activator found in many tissues and organs.[55] The development of the fibrin autograph technique by Todd[56] has shown that the endothelium is a particularly rich source of tissue-type plasminogen activator, and this site of synthesis is probably the most important in terms of hemostatic balance. Numerous reports in the literature have indicated that the activator is released by a number of stimuli such as vasodilators, exercise, epinephrine, and vascular stasis.[57] Brandykinin-induced release of activator[58] from endothelial cells may be of particular importance since this vasodilator is generated from HMW-kininogen via the coagulation contact system. Tissue-type activator is a 70,000-dalton serine protease, although higher and lower molecular weight forms released in human cell cultures have been reported.[59] The affinity for binding of the activator to fibrin is much greater for tissue-type than urokinase-type activator.[60]

Plasminogen Activation

Plasminogen is the principal fibrinolytic pathway zymogen in plasma with a molecular weight of 81,000 daltons and present at about 200 μg/ml.[61] In its native form, it is a single chain polypeptide with an N-terminal glutamic acid residue.[62,63] In the N-terminal portion of the molecule are five looped structures called kringles which are essential for binding to lysine residues in fibrin.[64] These lysine-binding sites have the function of localizing the plasminogen (plasmin) molecule to specific areas of fibrin, insuring efficient localized lysis of fibrin and minimizing diffusion of plasmin away from the fibrin deposition site and the occurrence of generalized systemic fibrinolysis.[65]

Plasmin itself may initiate plasminogen activation by proteolytic cleavage of a lysine-lysine bond in the N-terminal portion of plasminogen, producing a 9000-dalton polypeptide fragment termed the preactivation peptide and a degraded form of plasminogen with a N-terminal lysine residue.[66] This is not the only cleavage site since plasminogen molecules with N-terminal methionine and N-terminal valine are known.[66] In any case, the removal of the preactivation peptide renders plasminogen more susceptible to cleavage of an arginine-valine bond by a plasminogen activator, resulting in the formation of a plasmin molecule with a heavy and light chain connected through disulfide bonds with the active site on the light chain. The plasmin found can then participate in a feedback loop to cleave activation peptide from additional plasminogen molecules and render them susceptible to activation (see Figure 4-3).

Modulation of Fibrinolysis

The principal inhibitor of fibrinolysis is α_2-antiplasmin. This is a rapidly acting inhibitor of the serine esterase plasmin and is present in normal plasma at a concentration of approximately 70 μg/ml and has a molecular weight of about 67,000 daltons.[67,68] A genetically transmitted deficiency of α_2-antiplasmin results in a hemorrhagic syndrome due to excessive fibrinolysis.[69] The mechanism of action of α_2-antiplasmin is a two-stage process: in the first reaction, a $1:1$ stoichimetric complex[68] of plasmin and inhibitor forms which involves interactions of the inhibitor with one of the kringle structures of plasmin and with the serine active site plasmin.[70] At this point, the interaction is reversible. However, the second stage involves the proteolytic cleavage of a peptide from α_2-antiplasmin by the active site of plasmin resulting in a nondissociable complex. The level of α_2-antiplasmin in plasma is sufficient to neutralize approximately one half of all the plasmin that can potentially be generated. Although the full potential of plasmin probably is never achieved in the physiologic situation, the kringle structures of plasmin, with their lysine-binding properties, insure adequate interaction of plasmin at specific lysine residues of fibrin, localizing it for lysis of the

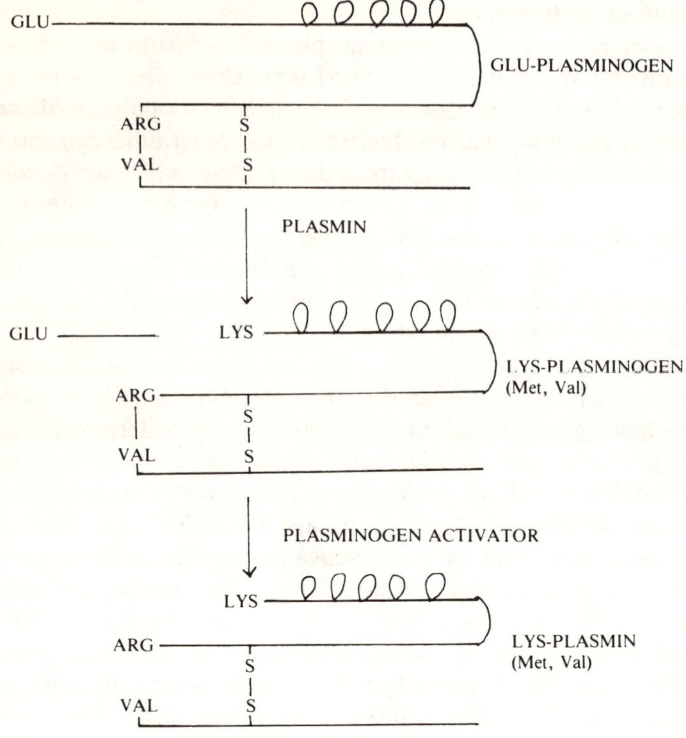

Figure 4-3 Conversion of the native plasminogen form (GLU-PLASMINOGEN) to enzymatically active plasmin. Removal of an N-terminal peptide (activation peptide) by plasmin action induces a conformational change in LYS-PLASMINOGEN which makes the ARG-VAL peptide bond more accessible to plasminogen activator. N-terminal lysine or methionine plasminogens and plasmins also may be formed, depending on the location of plasmin attack. The loops indicated in this diagram represent the kringle structures which are important in interactions with fibrin and α_2-antiplasmin.

fibrin network and protecting it from the inhibitory effect of α_2-antiplasmin. The secondary role of α_2-macroglobulin in the maintenance of fibrinolytic balance has been discussed previously.

Fibrin Degradation

The final step in hemostasis is the lysis of the fibrin network. While the specificity of peptide bond hydrolysis in fibrinogen by thrombin is quite limited, resulting in the cleavage of four arginyl-glycine bonds to release fibrinopeptides A and B, the specificity of peptide-bond hydrolysis of plasmin is, theoretically, less limited. However, the lysis of fibrin monomer to its degradation products is quite predictable. Figure 4-4 depicts the sequence of proteolytic cleavage that occurs when fibrinogen is subjected to plasmin action.[71-73] Conversion to fragment X involves the removal of three 15,000-dalton polypeptides (fragments A,B,C) from the carboxy-terminal ends of the two α-chains and cleavage of smaller peptides from the C-terminal ends of the β-chains. The β-chains also undergo some proteolytic degradation at the N-terminal end, with

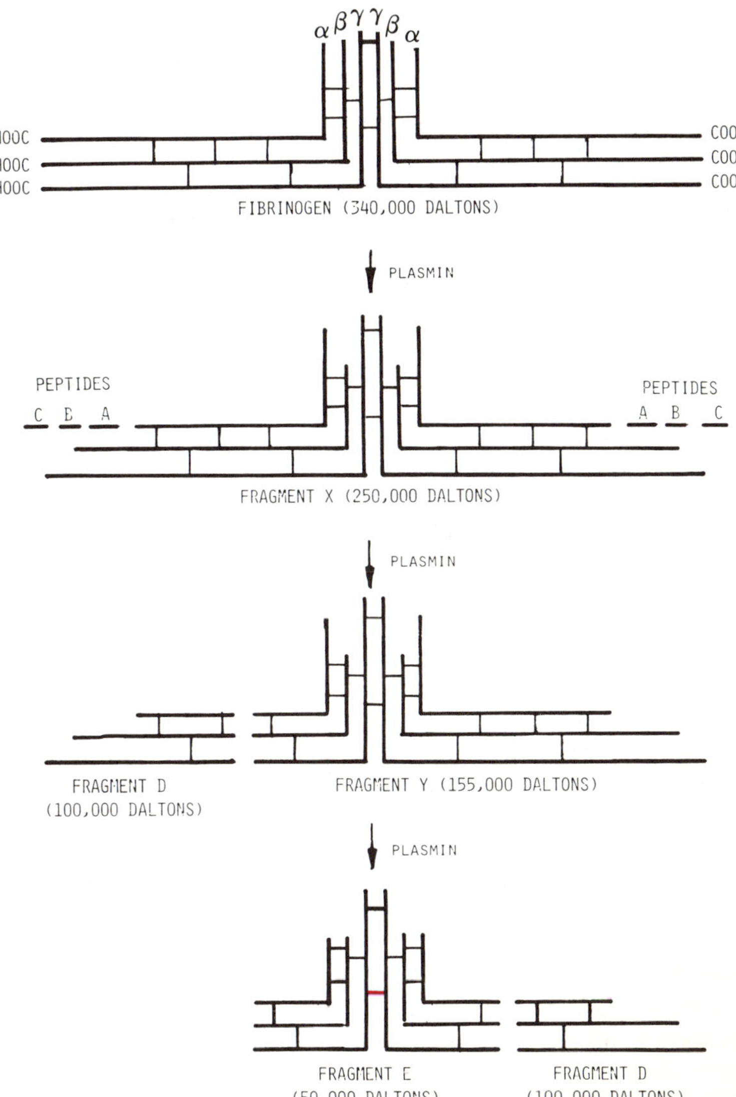

Figure 4-4 A representation of plasmin-catalyzed degradation of fibrinogen to fibrinogen degradation products. The pathway for fibrinolysis is similar except for crosslinked fibrin (see text).

cleavage of a peptide containing fibrinopeptide B. Fragment X, 250,000-dalton mol wt, remains slowly clottable by thrombin when fibrinopeptide A is removed, and can act as an inhibitor of thrombin action on fibrinogen. Further plasmin action results in the removal of one Fragment D which contains parts of the α-, β-, and γ-chains of fibrinogen and the resultant formation of fragment Y. From fragment Y, another fragment D molecule and fragment E are generated. Fragment E is composed of the "disulfide knot" region of fibrinogen. If a fibrinopeptide A has not already been liberated by thrombin action, it is liberated from fragment E by plasmin at this stage. The process thus described is for fibrinogenolysis. Plasmin action on fibrin may generate degradation products which are somewhat different, especially if factor XIIIa–induced crosslinking has occurred. In this event, fragment D dimers are obtained. Nevertheless, plasmin degradation results in fibrin clot lysis, followed by clearance of degradation products from the circulation. However, fragments Y, D, and E may modulate the hemostatic process by forming soluble complexes with fibrin monomer,[74] interfering with fibrin monomer polymerization, or with platelet adhesion, aggregation, and release reactions.[75]

CONCLUSION

In the introduction to this chapter, an attempt was made to emphasize the evolutionary development of hemostatic processes according to the requirements of the organism for an efficient, yet controlled means of preserving the vital circulating fluids of that organism. The diversity of the serine proteases which participate in coagulation and fibrinolysis is evident, yet the common glycine-asparagine-serine-glycine active site peptide sequence for proteolytic enzymes such as trypsin, chymotrypsin, elastase, and the serine proteases of the coagulation and fibrinolytic pathways, as well as considerable amino acid sequence homology in other parts of these enzymes, makes one believe that all of these may have evolved from a common ancestral gene. Further evidence that hemostatic mechanisms have evolved according to the physiologic requirements of an organism can be found in the extremely low levels of factors IX and XII as well as Fletcher factor in the deep-diving Sei whales.[76] Retarded blood flow and acidosis are known to contribute to thrombogenesis, and a deficiency of these contact coagulation factors may serve to protect this mammal from the development of thrombosis.

REFERENCES

1. Heilbrunn LV: The evolution of the haemostatic mechanism, in Macfarlane RG, Robb-Smith ATH (eds): *Functions of the Blood*. New York, Academic Press, 1961, pp 283–301.

2. Levin J, Bang FB: Clottable protein in *Limulus* blood: Its localization and kinetics of its coagulation by endotoxin. *Fed Proc* 1966;25:497.

3. Levin J, Bang FB: A comparison between human blood platelets and *Limulus* amebocytes. *Blood* 1966;28:984–985.

4. Morand L, Doolittle RF, Konishi K, et al: A new class of blood coagulation inhibitors. *Arch Biochem Biophys* 1963;102:171–179.

5. MacFarlane RG: An enzyme cascade in the blood clotting mechanism and the function as a biochemical amplifier. *Nature* 1964;202:498–499.

6. Davie EW, Ratnoff OD: Waterfall sequence for intrinsic blood clotting. *Science* 1964;145:1310–1312.

7. Niewiarowski S, Bankowski E, Rogowicki J: Studies on the adsorption and activation of Hageman factor (factor XII) by collagen and elastin. *Thromb Diath Haemorrh* 1965;14:387–400.

8. Griffin JH, Harper E, Cochrane CG: Studies on the activation of human blood coagulation factor XII by soluble collagen. *Fed Proc* 1975;34:860.

9. MacMillan CR, Saito H, Ratnoff OD, et al: The secondary structure of human Hageman factor (factor XII) and its alteration by activating agents. *J Clin Invest* 1974;54:1312–1322.

10. Kaplan AP, Austen KF: A pre-albumin activator of prekallikrein form active Hageman factor by digestion with plasmin. *J Exp Med* 1971;133:672–712.

11. Weupper KD, Cochrane CG: Isolation and mechanism of activation of components of the plasma kinin forming system, in Austen KF, Becker EL (eds): *Biochemistry of the Acute Allergic Reactions. Second International Symposium*. Oxford, Blackwell Scientific Publishers, 1971, pp 299–320.

12. Mandle R Jr, Colman RW: Identification of prekallikrein and high molecular weight kininogen as a circulating complex in human plasma. *Proc Nat Acad Sci USA* 1976;73:4179–4183.

13. Thompson R, Mandle R Jr: Interaction of factor XI and kallikrein with high molecular weight kininogen. *Thromb Haemost* 1977;38:13.

14. Iatrides SG, Ferguson JH: Active Hageman factor: a plasma lyokinase of the human fibrinolytic system. *J Clin Invest* 1962;41:1277–1287.

15. Fukikawa K, Coan MH, Legaz ME, et al: The mechanism of activation of bovine factor IX by bovine factor XI_a. *Biochemistry* 1974;13:5290–5299.

16. Stenflo J, Fernlund P, Egan W, et al: Vitamin K dependent modifications of glutamic acid residues in prothrombin. *Proc Nat Acad Sci USA* 1974;71:2730–2733.

17. Nelsestuen GL, Zytkovicz TH, Howard JB: The mode of action of vitamin K: identification of γ-carboxy glutamic acid as a component of prothrombin. *J Biol Chem* 1974;249:6347–6350.

18. Hultin MB, Nemerson Y: Activation of factor X by factor IX_a and factor VIII. *Blood* 1978;52:928–940.

19. Nemerson Y, Pitlick FA: The tissue factor pathway of blood coagulation, in Spaet TH (ed): *Progress in Hemostasis and Thrombosis*. New York, Grune & Stratton, 1972, vol 1, pp 1–37.

20. Colman RW: The effects of proteolytic enzymes on bovine factor V. *Biochemistry* 1969;8:1438–1445.

21. Takagi T, Doolittle RF: Amino acid sequence studies on factor XIII and the peptide released during its activation by thrombin. *Biochemistry* 1974;13:750–756.

22. Blomback B, Blomback M: The molecular structure of fibrinogen. *Ann NY Acad Sci* 1972;202:77–97.

23. Lorand L: "Fibrinopeptide." New aspects of the fibrinogen-fibrin transformation. *Nature* 1951;167:992–993.

24. Doolittle RF: Structural aspects of the fibrinogen to fibrin conversion. *Adv Protein Chem* 1973;27:1–109.
25. Blomback B: Selectional trends in the structure of fibrinogen of different species, in MacFarlane RG (ed): *The Hemostatic Mechanism in Man and Animals*, New York, Academic Press, 1970, pp 167–187.
26. York LL, Blomback B: Interaction of fragments of fibrinogen with in-solubilized fibrin monomer. *Thromb Res* 1976;8:607–618.
27. Schwartz ML, Pizzo SV, Hill RL, et al: The subunit structures of human plasma and platelet factor XIII. *J Biol Chem* 1971;246:5851–5854.
28. Schwartz ML, Pizzo SV, Hill RL, et al: Human factor XIII from plasma and platelets. Molecular weights, subunit structure, proteolytic activation and crosslinking of fibrinogen and fibrin. *J Biol Chem* 1973;248:1395–1407.
29. McKee PA, Mattlock P, Hill RL: Subunit structure of human fibrinogen soluble fibrin and cross-linked insoluble fibrin. *Proc Nat Acac Sci USA* 1970; 66:738–744.
30. Harpel PC, Rosenberg RD: α_2-Macroglobulin and antithrombin-heparin cofactor: modulators of hemostatic and inflammatory reactions, in Spaet TH (ed): *Progress in Hemostasis and Thrombosis*. New York, Grune & Stratton, 1976, vol 3, pp 145–189.
31. Abildgaard U: Highly purified antithrombin III with heparin cofactor activity prepared by disc electrophoresis. *Scand J Clin Lab Invest* 1968;21:89–91.
32. Seegers WH, Cole ER, Harmison CR, Monkhouse FG: Neutralization of autoprothrombin C activity with antithrombin. *Can J Biochem* 1964;42: 359–364.
33. Damus PS, Hicks M, Rosenberg RD: Anticoagulant action of heparin. *Nature* 1973;246:355–357.
34. Rosenberg JS, McKenna PW, Rosenberg RD: The inhibition of human factor IX_a by human antithrombin. *J Biol Chem* 1975;250:8883–8888.
35. Godal HC, Rygh M, Laake K: Progressive inactivation of purified factor VII by heparin and antithrombin III. *Thromb Res* 1974;5:773–775.
36. Stead N, Kaplan AP, Rosenberg RD: The inhibition of activated factor XII by antithrombin-heparin cofactor. *J Biol Chem* 1976;251:6481–6488.
37. Rosenberg RD: The effect of heparin on factor XI_a and plasmin. *Thromb Diath Haemorrh* 1974;33:51–62.
38. Rosenberg RD, Damus PS: The purification and mechanism of action of human antithrombin-heparin cofactor. *J Biol Chem* 1973;248:6490–6505.
39. Egeberg O: Inherited antithrombin deficiency causing thrombophilia. *Thromb Diath Haemorrh* 1965;13:516–530.
40. Odegard OR, Abildgaard U: Antifactor X_a activity in thrombophilia. Studies in a family with AT-III deficiency. *Scand J Haematol* 1977;18:86–90.
41. Cifonelli JA, King J: Structural studies on heparins with unusually high N-acetylglucosamine contents. *Biochim Biophys Acta* 1973;320:331–340.
42. Harpel PC: Human α_2-macroglobulin, in Lorand L (ed): *Methods in Enzymology: Proteolytic Enzymes*. New York, Academic Press, 1976, vol 45, part B, pp 639–652.
43. Starkey PM, Barrett AJ: α_2-Macroglobulin: a physiological regulator of protease activity, in Barrett AJ (ed): *Proteases in Mammalian Cells and Tissues*, Amsterdam and New York, North Holland Publishing Co, 1977, pp 663–696.
44. Barrett AJ, Starkey PM: The interaction of α_2-macroglobulin with proteases. *Biochem J* 1973;133:709–724.
45. White WF, Barlow GH, Mozen MM: The isolation and characterization of plasminogen activators from human urine. *Biochemistry* 1966;5:2160–2169.

46. Schleicher JB, Weiss RE: Application of a multiple surface tissue culture propagator for the production of cell monolayers, virus and biochemicals. *Biotechnol Bioeng* 1968;10:617–624.
47. Barlow GH, Lazer L: Characterization of the plasminogen activator isolated from human embryo kidney cells. *Thromb Res* 1972;1:201–208.
48. Bernik MB, White WF, Oller EP, et al: Immunologic identity of plasminogen activator in human urine, heart, blood vessels and tissue culture. *J Lab Clin Med* 1974;84:546–558.
49. Naito S, Sueishi K, Hattori F, et al: Immunological analysis of plasminogen activators from cultured human cancer cells. *Virchows Arch Pathol Anat* 1980;387:251–257.
50. Svanberg L, Astedt B: Release of plasminogen activator from normal and neoplastic endometrium. *Experimentia* 1979;35:818–819.
51. Tucker WS, Kirsch WM, Martinez-Hernandez A, et al: In vitro plasminogen activator activity in human brain tumors. *Cancer Res* 1978;38:297–302.
52. Astedt B, Holmberg L: Immunologic identity of urokinase and ovarian carcinoma plasminogen activator released in tissue culture. *Nature* 1976;261:595–597.
53. Shakespeare M, Wolf P: The demonstration of urokinase antigen in whole blood. *Thromb Res* 1979;14:825–835.
54. Wun T-C, Schleuning W-D, Reich E: Isolation and characterization of urokinase from human plasma. *J Biol Chem* 1982;257:3276–3283.
55. Astrup T, Sterndorff I: The plasminogen activator in animal tissues. *Acta Physiol Scand* 1956;36:250–255.
56. Todd AS: Fibrinolysis autographs. *Nature* 1958;181:495–496.
57. Brozovic M: Physiological mechanisms in coagulation and fibrinolysis. *Br Med Bull* 1977;33:231–238.
58. Markwardt F, Klocking HP: Studies on the release of plasminogen activator. *Thromb Res* 1976;8:217–223.
59. Rijken DC, Hoylaerts M, Collen D: Fibrinolytic properties of one-chain and two-chain extrinsic (tissue type) plasminogen activator. *J Biol Chem* 1982;257:2920–2925.
60. Thorsen S, Glas-Greenwalt P, Astrup T: Differences in the binding to fibrin of urokinase and tissue plasminogen activator. *Thromb Diath Haemorrh* 1972;28:65–74.
61. Barlow GH, Summaria L, Robbins KC: Molecular weight studies on human plasminogen and plasmin at the microgram level. *J Biol Chem* 1969;244:1138–1141.
62. Wallen P, Wiman B: Characterization of human plasminogen. I. On the relationship between different molecular forms of plasminogen demonstrated in plasma and found in purified preparations. *Biochim Biophys Acta* 1970;221:20–30.
63. Wallen P, Wiman B: Characterization of human plasminogen. II. Separation and partial characterization of different molecular forms of human plasminogen. *Biochim Biophys Acta* 1972;257:122–134.
64. Scottrup-Jensen L, Claeys H, Zajdel M, et al: The primary structure of human plasminogen: Isolation of two lysine binding fragments and one "mini"-plasminogen (M.W. 38,000) by elastase-catalyzed-specific limited proteolysis, in Davison JF, Rowan RM, Samama MM, Desnoyers PC (eds): *Progress in Chemical Fibrinolysis and Thrombolysis*. New York, Raven Press, 1970, vol 3, pp 191–209.
65. Wiman B: Biochemistry of the plasminogen to plasmin conversion, in

Gaffney PJ, Balkuv-Ukitin S (eds): *Fibrinolysis: Current Fundamental and Clinical Concepts*, New York, Academic Press, 1970, pp 47–60.
66. Robbins KC, Summaria L, Hsieh B, et al: The peptide chains of human plasmin. Mechanisms of activation of human plasminogen to plasmin. *J Biol Chem* 1967;242:2333–2342.
67. Aoki N, Norsi M: Distinction of serum inhibitor of activator-induced clot lysis from α_1-antitrypsin. *Proc Soc Exp Biol Med* 1974;146:567–570.
68. Moroi M, Aoki N: Isolation and characterization of α_2-antiplasmin from human plasma. *J Biol Chem* 1976;251:5956–5965.
69. Koie K, Kamiya T, Ogata K, et al: α_2-plasmin inhibitor deficiency (Miyasato disease). *Lancet* 1978;2:1334–1336.
70. Moroi M, Aoki N: On the interaction of α_2-plasmin inhibitor and proteases. Evidence for the formation of a covalent crosslinkage and non-covalent weak bondings between the inhibitor and proteases. *Biochim Biophys Acta* 1977;482:412–420.
71. Marder VJ, Budzynski AZ: Data for defining fibrinogen and its plasmic degradation products. *Thromb Diath Haemorrh* 1975;33:199–207.
72. Furlan M, Kemp G, Beck EA: Plasmic degradation of fibrinogen. III. Molecular model of the plasmin-resistant disulfide knot in monomeric fragment D. *Biochim Biophys Acta* 1975;400:95–111.
73. Gaffney PJ, Dobos P: A structural aspect of human fibrinogen suggested by its plasmic degradation. *FEBS Lett* 1971;15:13–16.
74. Arensen H: The effect of purified products D and E on the conversion of fibrinogen to fibrin as studied by N-terminal amino acid analysis. *IVth International Congress on Thrombosis and Haemostasis*, Abstract 253, Vienna, 1973.
75. Kopec M, Budzynski A, Stachurska J, et al: Studies on the mechanism of interference of fibrinogen degradation products (FDP) with the platelet function role of fibrinogen in the platelet atmosphere. *Thromb Diath Haemorrh* 1966;15:476–490.
76. Saito, H Poon M-C, Goldsmith GH, et al: Studies on the blood clotting and fibrinolytic system in the plasma from a Sei (baleen) whale. *Proc Soc Exp Biol Med* 1976;152:503–507.

5 *Blood Rheology and Thromboembolic Disorders*

Richard J. Sassetti

The preceding chapters have dealt with the interaction between the cells and proteins of the coagulation system and the endothelial lining of the blood vessels. All this is with the recognition that in vivo this interaction occurs as the blood flows past the altered endothelial surface of the vessel. Since Virchow's studies of white and red thrombi there has been the recognition that thrombosis is a hemodynamic event but until recently very little has been investigated or understood about the role of the dynamics of blood flow in the initiation and propagation of coagulation either in normal or pathologic states.

The purpose of this chapter is to inquire into the dynamic properties of blood and attempt to illuminate the characteristics of flowing blood and relate them to the initiation and/or the propagation of coagulation.

Blood flow or hemorheology, like any other biomechanical process, is susceptible to rigorous mathematical analysis and the precise definition of phenomena in crisp mathematical notation. It is not the purpose of this chapter to analyze hemorheologic phenomena in that fashion; however, in order to provide the reader with a foundation for reading a literature filled with a terminology often loosely used, expressing subtle but profound differences in superficially similar terms, it is necessary to describe some basic principles, definitions, and methodologies. Readers interested in a more vigorous mathematical approach are referred to Merrill,[1] Goldsmith and Mason,[2] and Meiselman.[3]

Rheology in its broadest definition is the study of flow. In a more narrow sense it is the study of flow of non-ideal (non-Newtonian) fluids.

Viscosity is the resistance of a fluid to changes in the dimension relations of its volume elements, or more simply it is the resistance to flow. Since rheology deals with non-ideal fluids it follows that the viscosity with which we will be mainly concerned is also non-ideal, or non-Newtonian. As will be shown later, Newtonian liquids are those whose viscosity is constant for a given set of conditions whereas non-Newtonian refers to liquids whose viscosity is not constant over the same given set of conditions.

The resistance to flow manifest by a liquid is determined by five independent parameters: pressure, temperature, physicochemical nature of the substance, shear rate, and time. Pressure is not of significance in biologic systems because all events occur at or near ambient pressure and whatever pressure differences exist are not of a magnitude to effect viscosity. A second, temperature, is also of relatively little consequence for our discussion since all events take place at or near body temperature. However in certain conditions, the cryopathies, temperature is important.

Three other parameters — the physicochemical nature of the substance, shear rate, and time — are very important and will be the major consideration in this section.

The physicochemical nature of the liquid is of paramount importance. Whether it is a pure chemical which happens to be liquid at ambient temperature, a solution either dilute or concentrated, or a suspension either stable or unstable, the resistance to flow will depend upon the interaction between the components of the liquid. Pure liquids tend to be ideal or Newtonian. Solutions can be either ideal or non-ideal (non-Newtonian). Suspensions generally are non-Newtonian.

The degree of non-ideality depends on several factors: the volume fraction of the disperse phase, the interactions between the units of the disperse phase (molecules or particles), the interactions between the disperse phase and the continuous phase, and finally the interactions between the liquid and the vessels containing it.

The shear rate, which also will be defined below, is a very important parameter since it is the common property by which most rheologic phenomena are described.

Liquids whose viscosity is independent of the shear rate are called Newtonian; those in which viscosity is dependent on shear rate are non-Newtonian. Virtually all liquids in biologic systems are basically non-Newtonian. Normal plasma demonstrates Newtonian behavior. Plasma with markedly increased proteins, especially paraproteins, may show non-Newtonian behavior.

Time is the third important parameter in hemorheology. As will become apparent in the subsequent discussion, the flow characteristics of blood at a given time and circumstance will often depend on the circumstances of flow just preceding.

The definition of the basic elements of flow can be developed by deriving the Newtonian equation for viscosity. Consider a liquid layer of thickness y (Figure 5-1). This layer can be viewed as being composed of a large number of very thin layers or lamellae. If one applies a force (F) to the uppermost layer (A) in a direction perpendicular to the thickness of the layer, shearing will take place. The force (F) applied to the lamella of surface area (A) will impart a velocity (V) to the lamella so that it will move relative to the stationary lamella below it. The force (F) in newtons per unit area in square meters (A) is the shear stress (T), which is expressed in pascals (Pa). The rate of change of V (m/s) relative to y (m) is the shear rate (D), which is expressed in units of reciprocal seconds (s^{-1}).

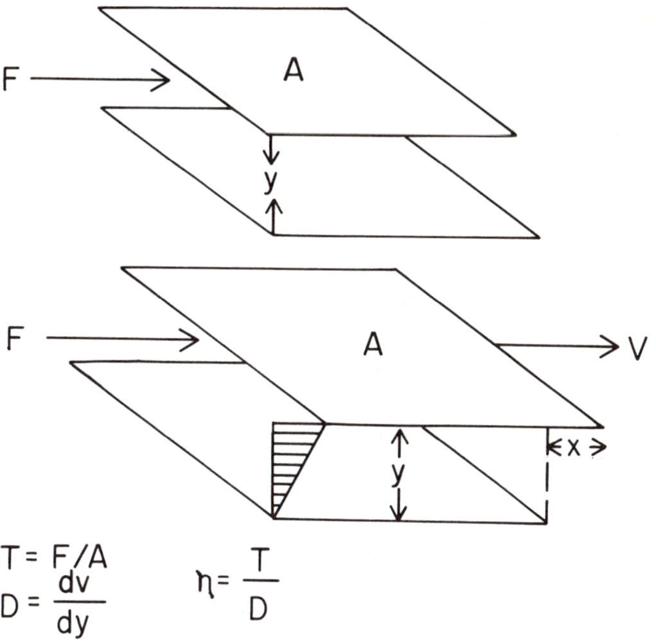

$$T = F/A$$
$$D = \frac{dv}{dy}$$
$$\eta = \frac{T}{D}$$

Figure 5-1   The derivation of the equation for the viscosity of laminar flow.

The ratio of T to D (shear stress to shear rate) is the viscosity, which is expressed in units of pascal seconds (this replaces the poise, the old unit of viscosity). The ratio T/D = Newton's law of viscosity. A liquid whose viscosity is constant over the entire range of shear rates, ie, independent of shear rate, is a Newtonian liquid. If the viscosity is dependent on the shear rate, the liquid is non-Newtonian.

At this point it might be of value to alert the reader to the need for wariness and skepticism when comparing or extrapolating from data in the literature on viscosity. The reason for this caveat is twofold. The first is that there are a large number of devices, generally capillary flow viscometers, for the measurement of viscosity of Newtonian liquids that are relatively cheap and simple to operate and all too often are used by the uninitiated to study non-Newtonian liquids with totally invalid results. Secondly, even if studies are validly done, unless sufficient data are supplied to fully define the non-Newtonian nature of the liquid, viscosities of non-Newtonian fluids are not comparable. This will be made clearer in the discussion immediately following.

There are four overlapping categories of non-Newtonian liquids: pseudoplastic, plastic, dilitant, and thixotropic. The viscosity–shear rate relationships of the first three are compared to a Newtonian liquid in Figure 5-2. The rarest of these types is dilitant. The characteristic of dilitancy is an increase in viscosity as shear rate increases. A dilitant

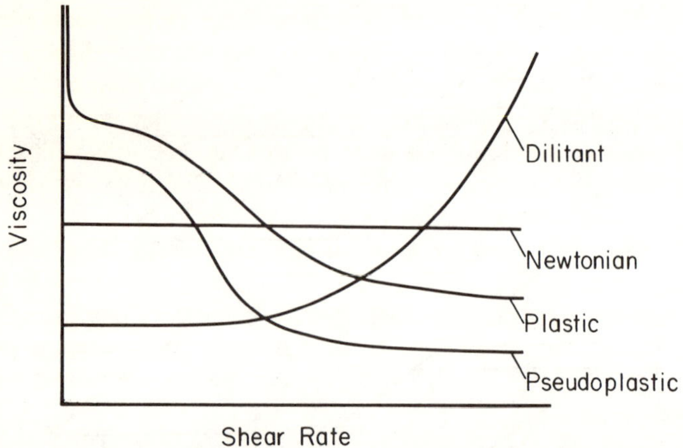

Figure 5-2 Flow characteristics of the four most common types of liquids.

liquid usually is a suspension of semirigid particles at high volume fractions; it is rare in biologic systems and will not be discussed further. Liquids which have a viscosity which decreases as the shear rate increases are common in biologic systems and are called pseudoplastic. Meaningful data about both dilitant and pseudoplastic liquids require pairs of data points (viscosity and shear rate). Plastic liquids are essentially pseudoplastic liquids; the viscosity decreases as the shear rate increases. However, in a plastic liquid there is a minimum shearing stress necessary to initiate flow. These liquids are characterized by a viscosity which aproaches infinity as the shear rate decreases toward zero. In addition to the viscosity–shear rate pairs, meaningful data on plastic, pseudoplastic, and dilitant liquids require extrapolation of low shear rates to zero to determine the presence or absence of a yield stress. Except for the initial yield stress, plastic and pseudoplastic liquids are the same. Blood is a plastic liquid.

The characteristic of decreasing viscosity with increasing shear rate is called shear thinning and is due to an instantaneous, shear rate–dependent change in orientation of the units of the disperse phase (red cells, platelets, fibrinogen molecules, etc) from random orientation at zero or low flow to axial orientation to the direction of flow at high flow rates with an immediate return toward the random orientation when flow is decreased. Shear thinning must be differentiated from thixotropy which will be discussed more fully below. Shear thinning is an instantaneous, immediately reversible process limited to the individually suspended elements of the disperse phase whereas thixotropy refers to the organization and subsequent disorganization of a network of elements of the disperse phase; it is not instantaneous in either direction.

For a pseudoplastic liquid, the fine structure of the curve in Figure 5-2 showing the relationship of shear stress to shear rate contains three phases. The earliest phase at the lowest shear rates reveals Newtonian behavior where the liquid has begun to flow while the disperse phase is randomly oriented. The second phase is non-Newtonian and depicts the phase during which the viscosity decreases as the elements of the disperse phase undergo orientation along the axis of flow. The third phase is Newtonian and represents the minimum attainable viscosity as the elements have undergone maximum axial orientation.

In a graphic representation of viscosity versus shear rate (Figure 5-2), the trace of increasing viscosity as the shear rate decreases from the high values at the right will exactly follow the trace of decreasing viscosity as the shear rate increases from zero. This is an important difference from the next form to be discussed, thixotropic liquids. Blood is a plastic thixotropic liquid.

Thixotropic liquids are either plastic or pseudoplastic liquids which undergo a change more profound than shear thinning during flow. In a thixotropic liquid at rest, the elements of the disperse phase undergo organization over a period of time to form a network structure. This structure forms as the elements of the disperse phase, either molecules or particles, come in contact with each other and form a variety of linkages. The linkage may take the form of simple interdigitation of complementary topologic structures or the stronger linkage of molecular bonding such as hydrogen bonding or other non-covalent interactions. The extent of organization will depend on the degree and nature of the interaction between the dispersed units, their concentration, and the length of time at rest. When a shearing stress is applied this organization of the disperse phase imparts a high viscosity. As the stress is applied over time the organization is disrupted and the viscosity drops as the shear rate is either held constant or increases until the viscosity reaches a minimum value. While it is not separable from thixotropy, as the elements of the disperse phase become disengaged from the meshwork they undergo axial orientation. Thus shear thinning is also a property of thixotropic liquids. When the shear rate is then decreased the viscosity increases but not at the same rate. The path taken by the plot of the viscosity against decreasing shear rate falls below that of the viscosity versus increasing shear rate. In a plot of shear stress and shear rate, the bidirectional trace produces a hysteresis or thixotropic loop (Figure 5-3). (This is in sharp contrast to the results mentioned above with nonthixotropic pseudoplastic liquids.) Since the product of the coordinates of the plot (shear stress versus shear rate) can be expressed in units of work per volume, the area inside the loop can be considered to represent the energy necessary to disrupt the bonding between the elements of the disperse phase.

When the shear rate returns to zero as flow ceases, the liquid undergoes reorganization over a period of time so that the viscosity slowly returns to its original value. The rate at which the viscosity attains its original value is specific to the liquid in question. This phenomenon is

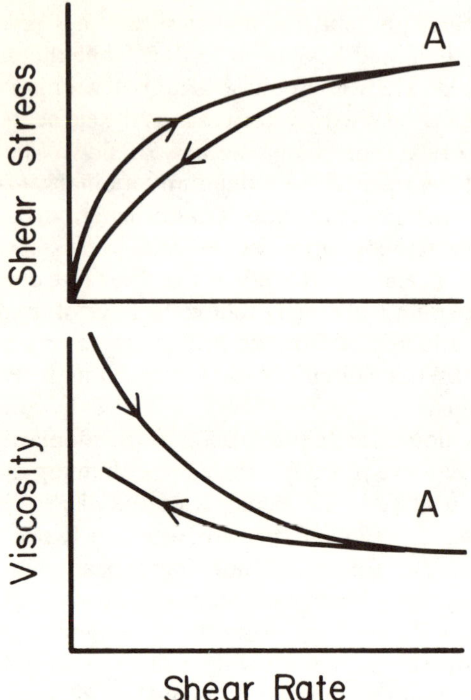

Figure 5-3 Flow characteristics of a thixotropic liquid.

called "sol-gel transformation." As opposed to the transition from random to axial orientation of shear thinning, this represents a disruption of a more highly organized structure with strong interparticle or intermolecular interactions to create a more random orientation of the disperse phase. Because the particles undergo axial orientation as they are individually disengaged from the meshwork, there is no separately detectable shear thinning.

Meaningful data about the thixotropic liquids must include the viscosities and shear rates for both the outbound and inbound limbs of the loop as well as whether or not shear rates had been achieved at the upper limit of the loop where the outbound and inbound plots overlay each other indicating that the disperse phase has undergone maximum disorganization (point A in Figure 5-3). For two comparable liquids at a given shear rate the times of flow necessary to reach this point can be compared and from this an estimate of their relative degree of thixotropy can be compared.

From the foregoing it can be seen that the flow characteristics of different liquids can be markedly dissimilar and that flow characteristics of the same fluid can be markedly different at different shear rates.

As can be seen in Figure 5-2 the viscosity at a single shear rate does not characterize non-Newtonian liquids. There are shear rates at which two types of liquids would have the same viscosity but at another shear rate each would have a different viscosity. For this reason it is customary to use the term apparent viscosity for non-Newtonian liquids.

These facts are important for at least two reasons: they make comparisons between studies difficult because reported shear rates often vary from study to study; and as we shall see later, since the shear rates and flow rates vary widely from site to site in the vascular space, it is extremely difficult to make any generalizations about the role of viscosity in the pathogenesis of various disease states.

Since the various components of a solution or suspension contribute to the viscosity of the whole in a complex fashion, it is often desirable to attempt to treat the contribution of the components separately. For this reason it is necessary to introduce the concept of relative viscosity. (η_r).

If η is the viscosity of the solution or suspension and η_o is the viscosity of the solute or continuous phase:

$$\eta_r = \frac{\eta}{\eta_o}$$

If η_o is subtracted from both numerator and denominator:

$$\frac{\eta}{\eta_o} + \frac{\eta_o}{\eta_o} = \frac{\eta}{\eta_o} + 1 \qquad \frac{\eta}{\eta_o} - 1 = \eta_r - 1$$

$\eta_r - 1 = \eta_{sp}$, the specific viscosity of the disperse phase. If η is the viscosity of whole blood and η_o is the viscosity of plasma, then $\eta_r - 1$ expresses the contribution to the viscosity of whole blood made by the red cells alone. This expression captures the effect of red cell–plasma interaction as part of the red cell viscosity and therefore cannot be considered as identical to the viscosity of red cells. This restriction is true of any relative viscosity determination.

The specific viscosity can be used to derive the intrinsic viscosity $[\eta]$ of the dispersed phase.

The intrinsic viscosity divided by the concentration yields the reduced specific viscosity. Extrapolation to zero concentration yields the intrinsic viscosity $[\eta]$.

$$[\eta] = \lim_{\mathrm{conc} \to 0} \frac{\eta_{sp}}{\mathrm{conc}}$$

This derivation is of value in the determination of the viscosity of solutions and represents the contribution of solute-solvent interactions to the viscosity of solutions. It is important to note that in this simple form this expression for intrinsic viscosity cannot be used for suspensions, so that while it is useful for plasma protein studies it cannot be applied to whole blood or red cell suspensions without modification to a more complex form.

The wide variety of instruments available for the determination of viscosity merit some discussion and will lead to the definition of some additional terms.

The first instruments were gravity-driven capillary flow devices based on the principles elucidated by Poiseuille. Jean Poiseuille was a French physiologist interested in the study of blood flow. After many attempts to study blood by capillary flow viscometry he abandoned blood out of frustration and switched to salt solutions. From this work he divised his function for viscosity.

$$\eta = \frac{H \cdot g \cdot \varrho \cdot R^4 \cdot t}{-8 \times 1}$$

where $H \cdot g$ = pressure head
ϱ = density of liquid
R = capillary radius
t = flow time
L = capillary length

H, g, R, t, and L can be combined as the instrument constant (k), then:

$$\eta = \varrho t k$$

or

$$\eta/\varrho = tk$$

the kinematic viscosity.

For Newtonian liquids whose density approaches 1.0, the kinematic viscosity is an easy, valid measure. That is also true of any solutions whose density approaches that of the solvent and allows the rapid determination of relative viscosity.

$$\eta_r = \frac{\eta}{\eta_o} = \frac{\varrho t k}{\varrho_o t_o k_o}$$

For a given instrument, k is constant and can be dropped from the expression:

$$\eta_r = \frac{\varrho t}{\varrho_o t_o}$$

Since ϱ approaches ϱ_o, their ratio approaches 1 and can be dropped from the expression:

$$\eta_r = \frac{t}{t_o}.$$

Unfortunately, non-Newtonian liquids cannot be studied in such a simple instrument because the shear rate is not constant across the lumen of the tube but is parabolic with zero shear at the center and very high shear rates at the wall. This limitation can be overcome by more complex instrumentation which either measures flow under constant pressure or the pressure necessary to achieve constant flow.

The more common instruments for the measurement of viscosity of non-Newtonian liquids are adaptations of the moving parallel plates concept used in the derivation of the Newtonian equation. The most common types of instruments are the concentric cylinder and the cone and plate viscometers. The basic principle involves the movement of one surface relative to the other. A liquid in the gap between the surfaces retards their relative motion. The retardation can be measured and is a function of the viscosity of the liquid in the gap. These instruments have the important characteristic that the shear rate is constant at any point across the gap between the two surfaces.

The variety of capillary-flow and moving-plate instruments is large and for a detailed discussion of their structure, applicability, and limitations, the reader is referred to the works of Whorlow[4] and Schramm.[5]

A few other terms merit definition and discussion. Hemorheology, a term introduced by Alfred Copley in 1958, implies the study of the flow of blood and the relationship of its flow properties to the interaction of its various components, their function, and the immensely varied, complicated, non-ideal structure of the vascular tree in both normal and pathologic states. Since the rheologic properties of blood are also very much a function of the size and character of the vessels in which it flows, it is necessary, for conceptual reasons at least, to consider blood as having two sets of rheologic characteristics. Macrorheology deals with the flow properties of blood as a bulk liquid with no significant compositional differences across the diameter of the vessel, flowing in vessels of large bore with a high ratio of vessel diameter to cell diameter and with relatively low shear rates and velocities sufficiently high to minimize interaction between components of the disperse phase. Microrheology deals with the flow properties of blood in vessels in which the cell diameter approaches the vessel diameter and shear rates are high. In this circumstance blood becomes a more heterogeneous liquid in which there are significant compositional differences along the diameter of the vessel, and the internal viscosity of the cells begins to influence the flow characteristics of blood. There is probably a third, intermediate set of flow properties which make the boundaries between macro- and microrheology vague and suggests that blood, more correctly, has a continuum of flow properties that vary with the vessel involved.

While these definitions may serve only to confuse, they should also remind the reader that in the field of hemorheology extrapolation of data from one set of circumstances to another, from in vitro to in vivo, and from the laboratory to the bedside, is especially dangerous. The introduction of these concepts and definitions allows a consideration of the viscosity of whole blood, the factors that account for it, and its role in normal physiology, which will in turn serve as a point of departure for the discussion of the role of hemorheology in the pathogenesis of thromboembolic diseases.

HEMORHEOLOGY

Blood makes up about 7.5% of a human's body weight and serves a variety of physiologic functions which are in turn best served by its great heterogeneity in composition both in size and concentration of its components. Whole blood is an unstable suspension of cells in plasma, a protein-rich electrolyte solution. The cellular elements make up approximately 45% of its volume and have a tenfold variation is size and a thousandfold variation in concentration. Red cells with an average diameter of 8 μm account for 95% of the cellular elements, leukocytes with an average diameter of 15 μm account for 0.1% and platelets with an average diameter of 2 μm make up approximately 5%.

The formed elements are unstably suspended in plasma made up of water, electrolytes, and proteins, which are rheologically its most important components (purists might argue that since the rheologic behavior of pure water is so anomolous the electrolytes in plasma which "normalize" it are the major contribution to the rheologic character of blood). The plasma proteins number about 150 of which approximately 70 are well characterized.[6] These vary in molecular weight from approximately 1000 to 6,000,000 daltons and in concentration from a few nanograms (ng) to 5 grams (g) per deciliter. The proteins of greatest direct rheologic importance are fibrinogen, IgM, and IgG. Of the three, fibrinogen, which makes the greatest contribution, has a molecular weight of 340,000 daltons, an intrinsic viscosity of 0.25 dl/g, a frictional ratio of 2.34, and occurs in the highest concentration, 2.5 g/dl. IgG has a molecular weight of 150,000 daltons, an intrinsic viscosity of 0.06 dl/g and a frictional ratio of 1.38, while IgM has a molecular weight of 900,000 daltons, an intrinsic viscosity of 0.16 dl/g, and a frictional ratio of 1.5. Their plasma concentrations are 1.5 and 0.1 g/dl, respectively.

The variation in the concentration of fibrinogen, an acute phase reactant, accounts for the most common variation in blood viscosity in a wide variety of pathologic states. The fibrinogen molecule is rod-shaped; this accounts for its high frictional ratio and its high intrinsic viscosity. Its intrinsic viscosity contributes only to a small degree to increasing whole blood viscosity. Its interaction with red cells enhances their aggregability. This in turn increases the viscosity of whole blood. This interaction will be discussed below.

IgM and IgG are very important contributors to viscosity only when they are present in extremely large quantities as occurs in neoplastic conditions of the lymphocytes and plasma cells, but not in the frequent hypergammaglobulinemia seen in infections or collagen vascular diseases.

The contribution of other plasma proteins to whole blood viscosity is not well known. While it is very likely that they do not contribute in any major way it is possible that they may alter the protein-cell or protein-protein interactions of those proteins which do contribute to whole blood viscosity and thus serve in some indirect modulating capacity. For example, lipoproteins interacting with red cells may alter their membrane in such a way as to either enhance or reduce the red cell contribution to viscosity.

The interaction of the various components of blood is, to say the least, complex. In any given condition, the contribution to viscosity of changes in one component may very well neutralize the contribution of changes in another component. It is necessary then to discuss the contribution of each component separately before undertaking an analysis of their interaction as it may be seen in pathologic states. For example, in sickle cell disease, the hyperviscosity of the cells is compensated for to a large extent by their low concentration.

Table 5-1 lists five factors that affect the viscosity of whole blood. These factors will be discussed in some detail below. It must be remembered that these factors act separately and conjointly and their effects may be additive, synergistic, or antagonistic.

Red Cell Aggregability

All cellular elements of blood interact with each other and undergo aggregation or adhesion. The adhesion of platelets to other platelets

Table 5-1
Factors Affecting Whole Blood Viscosity

Aggregability of red cells
Internal viscosity of red cells
Volume fraction of cellular components
Plasma viscosity
Temperature

(aggregation) or to the endothelial surface of blood vessels is essential to their function, both in the normal state of hemostasis and in the abnormal state of thrombosis. Granulocytes adhere to vessel walls as part of their initial response to inflammation. These two cases of adhesion are part of the normal function of the cells. Circulating tumor cells also are capable of adhering to the endothelial surface of vessels and such adherence is probably an integral part of the metastatic process.

While the formation of close contacts between cells is a widespread and fundamental phenomenon in biology, the meaning of red cell aggregation is not at all clear. Red cells tend to aggregate but do so spontaneously and not, in any way that is apparent, as part of their normal function. This tendency to aggregate is enhanced in a wide variety of disease states and its clinical correlates are fairly well defined. However, its mechanism, explainable in biophysical terms, is not well understood in biochemical terms.[7,8] It is clear that it makes a significant contribution to the non-Newtonian behavior of blood and for that reason will be considered here.

When a suspension of red cells is at rest the cells undergo sedimentation. This occurs whether the cells are suspended in unmodified native plasma, as in freshly drawn unanticoagulated blood, or in saline solution. The rate of sedimentation is much slower in saline solution than in plasma.

The explanation for the nature of sedimentation and aggregation of red cells, and generally all living cells is still lacking. The colloidal theory explaining the suspension of rigid nonliving particles falls far short of explaining red cell aggregation. Estimates based on the known parameters of red cell shape, surface size, and content also fall wide of the mark. These variances suggest that not all the relevant forces are understood.[3] The most reasonable additional force that can be implicated in aggregation is that of macromolecular bridging.

Red cells by virtue of their surface composition carry a negative charge at or near physiologic pH. This charge generates a cloud of counterions and provides a mutually repulsive force acting over a distance of several tenths of a nanometer creating a minimum approach distance. The macromolecules in plasma are sufficiently large to bridge this minimum allowable approach distance. This bridging mechanism has been demonstrated with inert colloidal particles both with the addition of proteins derived from plasma and nonphysiologic biopolymers such as dextran and is the basis of agglutination with anti–red cell antibodies.

The plasma protein that figures most prominently as the natural macromolecular bridge is fibrinogen. Fibrinogen has long been considered in the phenomena of erythrocyte sedimentation and rouleaux formation, and appears to be the single most important contributor to the accleration of sedimentation.[9] In those circumstances where there is elevation of α_2- and γ-globulins as either acute phase reactants or as paraproteins, these can augment the contribution of fibrinogen and in many cases overshadow it.[7] The rate of erythrocyte sedimentation is affected by the size of the aggregates, the density of both the cells and plasma, the viscosity of plasma, and the concentration of the cells (the hematocrit). The sedimentation is proportional to the degree of aggregation and to lower values of the viscosity of the plasma and inversely proportional to the concentration of the cells and the very high value of plasma viscosity produced by large amounts of paraproteins.

The degree of sedimentation is influenced by red cell deformability for as the red cells sediment their concentration is increased by virtue of plasma exclusion in the sedimented or packed portion. As plasma exclusion progresses, cell-to-cell contact increases. Continued sedimentation will ultimately depend on cell deformability, which will be the limiting factor in further red cell packing. The size of the aggregate formed as red cells sediment determines the final sedimented volume of the cells. This fully sedimented volume is greated than the hematocrit by the volume of trapped plasma. From the volume of sedimented erythrocytes and the hematocrit, the size of the red cell aggregated can be derived.[10] Hematocrit has the largest effect on the rate at which red cells sediment and hence aggregate. It is clear, then, as the concentration of particles increases, the frequency of collision and adherence should increase. This should lead to increased sedimentation through aggregate formation. However, hematocrit has the opposite effect. The rate of sedimentation decreases rapidly with the square of the hematocrit. This is important to note because the deterrent effect of hematocrit on aggregation tends to decrease its contribution to viscosity while hematocrit increases viscosity by its direct contribution.

Plasma viscosity has a retarding effect on red cell aggregation by inhibiting the movement of red cells toward one another through the thicker medium. Fibrinogen, which increases plasma viscosity, provides another example of a bidirectional effect since the increase in aggregation secondary to fibrinogen due to the macromolecular bridging has an effect of greater magnitude than the direct effect of elevation of plasma viscosity per se. The maximum increase in plasma viscosity due to increases in fibrinogen is relatively small compared to the increases in plasma viscosity due to paraproteins, but in either case the enhancement of aggregation by macromolecular bridging outweighs the deterrence of aggregation due to increased plasma viscosity. The exception is in the very high ranges of viscosity due to paraproteins, in which case it is possible to have decreased erythrocyte sedimentation because the viscous plasma retards sedimentation so much that it overshadows the enhancing effect of red cell aggregation.

It may become clearer to the reader if the increased plasma viscosity is viewed as a secondary, retarding effect on aggregation caused by the presence of large amounts of protein which enhance aggregation primarily through intercellular bridging.

The non-Newtonian viscosity of blood appears to be due in large part to the aggregation of red cells. This effect, while generally most pronounced at lowest shear rates, can be seen at shear rates as high as 100 s^{-1}. This is especially so when there is marked red cell aggregation. Each sample of whole blood, then, can have a unique critical shear rate at which complete red cell aggregate dispersion is achieved depending on the summation of those factors responsible for red cell aggregation. Because of the distribution of shear rates in tubular flow, the distribution of aggregates will vary along the radius of the vessel. In the center where the shear rate is zero and red cell concentration is highest, aggregation will be at its relative maximum. Near the vessel wall where shear rates are very high, the red cells will be completely disaggregated. Further, the profile of aggregation across the tube will vary according to the velocity of flow. At low flow, the locus of points of shear rates critical to the full dispersion of aggregates (100 s^{-1}) will be closer to the wall than at high flow. This reaches its maximum when flow goes to zero. The aggregates then are equally distributed throughout the lumen from the center to the wall. This is the phenomenon observed as "sludging" in vascular collapse. The aggregation will impart a yield stress to the stagnant blood in the vessel. This implies that sludged blood will not flow when reestablishment of flow is attempted until the shear stress applied exceeds some minimum value. Furthermore, aggregation makes the blood thixotropic which means that the shearing force necessary to initiate flow will be greater than the force necessary to maintain flow.

If flow is reestablished immediately, the blood will behave as a simple plastic liquid. If flow disruption allows the aggregation to progress or become more organized, thixotropy will manifest itself, ie, a greater shearing force will be necessary to disrupt the organized aggregates and establish flow at a given velocity. The extra energy needed to reestablish flow will be determined by the degree of organization of the red cell aggregates, which will in turn, be dependent on the time during which the aggregation took place.

At shear rates below 100 s^{-1} aggregation is incompletely disrupted so that even with steady-state measurements of viscosity the values obtained will contain a component due to aggregation. In this circumstance an increase in shear rate to greater than 100 s^{-1} will demonstrate the residual thixotropy.

The pathophysiologic effect of non-Newtonian flow at low shear rates will be discussed below. Suffice it to say at this point that it may be important in thromboembolism and vascular ischemic conditions.

A discussion of the role of aggregation is not complete without mention of the variation in size of the vessels and its impact on aggregation, and the effect of aggregation on blood flow. The role of the vasculature will be discussed more fully below.

Where the diameter of the vessel is much greater than the diameter of the red cell, there is a large portion of the vessel cross section in which shear rates are below the critical value for aggregation to take place. In these vessels there is the phenomenon of axial streaming where the red cells, singly or in aggregates, tend to flow in the center of the vessel lumen and cell-poor plasma flows along the wall. If the plasma proteins (fibrinogen, etc) are in such concentration as to enhance aggregation, most of the cells will be in the aggregated state. When these aggregates enter a vessel of lesser diameter, the flow rate must increase. Disaggregation will occur because of the higher shear rate. However, since shear rates are a resultant of velocity and vessel radius, if the degree of aggregation is such that velocity does not increase, the increase in shear rate will be due only to the decrease in vessel diameter. The shear rates necessary for optimal disaggregation may not be achieved and flow will continue more slowly than expected with the cells only partially disaggregated. This can lead to further slowing of flow downstream as the vessel bore decreases further.

Hematocrit

The effect of red cell concentration on the viscosity of blood has been known since the beginning of this century and the effect of increasing concentrations of leukocytes has been known since the 1950s. Other than the hyperviscosity associated with Waldenström's macroglobulinemia, the most widely recognized hyperviscous state is that associated with elevations in the hematocrit in patients with either primary or secondary erythrocytosis.

At a given shear rate the viscosity is a function of the hematocrit raised to approximately the power of 3:2 so that the rise in viscosity is rapid with an increase in hematocrit.[10] The clinically critical value of hematocrit appears to be approximately 60%. Because of the variety of factors affecting the viscosity at low rates of shear, the range of values for the viscosity at high hematocrits and low shear rates is very wide, thus making it difficult to assess whole blood viscosity at a given shear rate in the low range (less than 1 s⁻¹) and at low hematocrit.

Using multivariate regression analysis, equations have been developed which relate the logarithm of the viscosity to the hematocrit at various shear rates with high degrees of correlation.[11] At lower shear rates there was significant correlation between log viscosity and both hematocrit and fibrinogen content. This additional parameter probably reflects the role of red cell aggregation secondary to fibrinogen content, as discussed earlier.

The increase in viscosity at elevated hematocrits is not proportionate at all shear rates.[12] At low shear rates the increase is less than would be extrapolated from higher shear rates. This is felt to be due to the inhibitory effect of hematocrit on red cell aggregation, the largest contributor to the non-Newtonian behavior at low shear rates.

The role of increased concentrations of leukocytes on the viscosity of whole blood has not been studied systematically. That such studies should be undertaken is clear from the recognition of leukostasis syndromes in leukemia patients with very high leukocytes counts. From the little data available it appears that both the viscosity and shear rate dependence of the viscosity increase as the volume fraction of white blood cells (leukocrit) increases. The increase in shear rate dependence is accompanied by a marked increase in thixotropy. This observation suggests that the internal viscosity of white cells is greater than the internal viscosity of red cells.

The nature of the structure and function of platelets make it impossible with current technology to study the viscosity of platelet suspensions at any approximation of their natural resting states.

Internal Viscosity of the Red Cell

Blood is a remarkably fluid liquid. Fluidity is a term occasionally encountered in the rheology literature and is the expression of the ease with which a liquid flows. A physical property that is the opposite of viscosity, fluidity (ϕ) is expressed mathmatically as the reciprocal of the viscosity ($1/\eta$). The fluidity of blood is such that for a suspension of particles of 8 μm diameter with a concentration normally close to 50%, it flows remarkably well even when the concentration of cells reaches 98%. The viscosity of packed red cells stays well below 100 millipascalseconds (mPas) even when the hematocrit reaches 99%. It can even be as low as 2–3 mPas.

A suspension of rigid particles of dimensions similar to red cells develops an infinite viscosity, ie, it effectively becomes solid, if the volume fraction approaches 65%. Recognition of this led to the discarding of the rigid particle as a model of the red cell and the adoption of the view that the red cell behaves as a highly deformable, nearly perfectly resiliant fluid drop. This model permits a fuller understanding of the rheologic characteristics of capillary flow and the physiologic consequences of conditions which result in decreasing red cell deformability. This remarkable fluidity is due to the low internal viscosity of the red cell. The term internal viscosity is taken to include the viscosity of the red cell membrane as well as the viscosity of the intracellular content.

Low internal viscosity makes red cell deformability as important for the production of low blood viscosities at high shear rates as is red cell aggregation for the production of high viscosity at low shear rates. It is also the most important factor in determining the microrheologic characteristics of blood.

Red cell deformability depends on the flexing and stretching of the red cell membrane, the ratio of membrane surface to cell volume, and the flow characteristics of its internal fluids, mainly hemoglobin. Numerous investigations of red cell deformability have been reported using a variety of techniques including aspiration into micropipettes, filtration through paper, or polycarbonate sieves.

Each of these three components of internal viscosity has been analyzed to some extent. Alterations in each have been shown to produce a decrease in red cell deformability and an increase in blood viscosity.

Before discussing these factors in more detail, it would serve well to examine some details of microrheology in vitro in tubes of a diameter similar to the capillary component of the vascular system. Capillary diameters vary by about 3 μm. Obviously, deformability is a necessary property for a red cell if it is to accomplish its capillary transit. It appears that red cell deformability contributes to a decrease in blood viscosity in capillaries through the Fahraeus-Lindqvist effect. The Fahraeus-Lindqvist effect is the reduction of viscosity of blood flowing through capillaries of decreasing diameter. The effect is seen in capillaries of less than 1000 μm. The viscosity continues to decrease as the capillary diameter decreases until the lower limit of 2 μm is reached. At that point there is a sharp increase in viscosity known as the inversion effect. This effect is illustrated in Figure 5-4.

The decrease in viscosity is due to the reduction of the hematocrit due to wall effects. Since red cells are discoid, near the point in the radius of the vessel equal to the radius of a red cell, their concentration decreases by the exclusion of red cells along the wall. As the vessel radius decreases the fraction of volume from which red cells are excluded increases until the vessel diameter is that of the red cell. At this point blood flow is characterized by single cells separated by boluses of plasma. Below this diameter the same phenomenon continues with the red cell undergoing progressively greater deformation until it reaches a maximum at the inversion point. Below that diameter greater force is

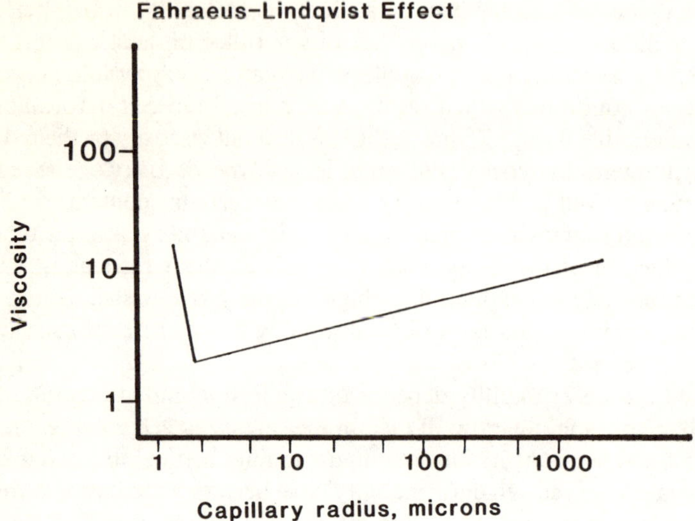

Figure 5-4 The Fahraeus-Lindqvist effect.

required to move the red cell through the capillary. Hence the increase in viscosity.

A number of factors decrease red cell deformability. The most common physiologic factor is red cell senescence. Depletion of adenosine triphosphate (ATP) results in increased membrane rigidity. In stored blood, membrane deformability progresses with age and can be restored to normal by restoration of red cell ATP.

High hematocrits shift the inversion point toward higher capillary diameters and raise the viscosity throughout the range of capillaries studied. It follows that red cell aggregation will also shift the inversion point and raise the viscosity throughout. The shift of the Fahraeus-Lindqvist effect due to all factors is probably the most important microrheologic effect that will account for increased viscosity of blood in a variety of conditions. Spherocytosis, whether congenital or acquired, will alter the Fahraeus-Lindqvist effect in the same manner. Simple reduction in blood pH will decrease deformability and result in increased viscosity. Sickle cell disease is a most remarkable example of red cell deformation. As the cell undergoes the shape change of sickling its deformability in response to external forces decreases until the cell reaches its maximum intrinsic deformation. At this point it becomes totally rigid and undeformable.

Plasma Viscosity

Increases in plasma viscosity result in increases in whole blood viscosity. However, the increase in viscosity is not as great as would be expected from a simple summation of plasma and red cell viscosities. This is due to the interaction of the macromolecules with red cells in a way which reduces the viscosity of the mixture while the macromolecules raise the viscosity of the plasma. This is accounted for by a number of factors. The most relevant are the effects on red cell deformation, axial alignment of flowing cells, and contact between red cells.

Red cells flowing in solutions of macroglobulins or dextran show greater deformation at a given shear rate than those flowing in saline. This accounts for the lower viscosity of red cells in plasma than red cells in saline. In addition, as deformed, ellipsoidal red cells flow, they orient themselves with their longest diameter parallel to the axis of flow. The fraction of cells aligned with the axis of flow is proportional to the shear rate and viscosity. The higher the viscosity the greater proportion that are aligned. Under the conditions of high viscosity and high shear rate the red cell membrane undergoes "tank treading," ie, the rotation of the membrane around the red cell contents, which transmits the velocity gradient to the inside of the cell affecting the internal viscosity of the cells.

Further, an increase in plasma viscosity would result in a decrease in the shear rate; this would reduce the likelihood of cellular interaction. At a given shear rate the shear stress would increase. These two events serve to hinder aggregation and to enhance disaggregation. However, this effect is modulated in the opposite direction by the macromolecular enhancement of aggregation. Therefore, at low shear rates the intercellular bridging would dominate and increase viscosity. At high shear rates, interaction inhibition, flow orientation, and tank treading would dominate and serve to decrease the viscosity.

Temperature

As indicated earlier, viscosity of liquids varies inversely with temperature. However in the physiologic temperature range, the magnitude of viscosity change is relatively small. A decrease in temperature from 37 °C to room temperature results in a viscosity increase of approximately 75%, from 4 mPas at 37 °C to 7 mPas at 22 °C at a shear rate of 200 s^{-1} and from approximately 6 mPas to 11 mPas at 20 s^{-1}. The viscosity of normal plasma increases from 1.5 mPas to 2.5 mPas with the same temperature changes.

Important changes in plasma viscosity in response to temperature variation occur in patients whose plasma contains cryoglobulins. In these cases the plasma shows thixotropic behavior at a temperature below 37 °C. As the temperature decreases to near the precipitation point of these proteins, they undergo aggregation with a concommitant increase in viscosity, which may abruptly increase to infinity in vitro. This marked increase in viscosity is due to sol-gel transformation which occurs while the plasma is at rest. Under conditions of continuous flow the temperature can be lowered well below the critical point with only a moderate increase in viscosity. The failure of the viscosity to undergo a dramatic increase is due to the fact that under conditions of continuous flow the constant motion prevents the formation of the intermolecular bridging necessary for the sol-gel transformation.

The effect of cooling of blood in vivo as blood flows from the central vessels into the distal extremities, the fingers, toes, ears, and nose, leads to increases in viscosity and slow blood flow. However, continuous flow modulates this effect and while it may lead to microrheologic alterations it is not likely to produce macrorheologic changes of significance.

In summary, a number of factors influence the viscosity of blood. These factors may work independently or in concert and may be synergistic or antagonistic in their effect on blood viscosity. These factors may be of prime significance in macrorheology and of minor significance in microrheology or vice versa. These may increase viscosity on the one hand and decrease it on the other, and finally it is very difficult to assess how closely the phenomena observed in vitro parallel or mimic the in vivo function.

Vascular Components in Hemorheology

The extrapolation of rheologic data obtained in either moving-plate or capillary viscometers to in vivo conditions cannot be attempted in any way without consideration of the unique characteristics of the vascular system and their effect on blood flow. Blood vessel radii vary from approximately 2 cm for the aorta to 3 μm for capillaries. The velocity of flow varies from 100 cm/s in the aorta to 0.4 mm/s for capillaries, and the wall shear rates vary from 200 s^{-1} for the aorta to 1000 s^{-1} for capillaries.

The vascular apertures vary from relatively rigid circles for arteries to partially collapsible circles for capillaries and partially collapsible rectangular capillaries in the lungs. The spleen is a special case with the central arteries having right-angled branches which promote plasma skimming. This will be discussed later. Further, there is a difference of flow rate through the red pulp and the cords. The slowest flow is through the red pulp while there is both fast and slow flow through the cords. The slow flow is probably related to the filtering process and the fast flow to a shunting process.

It is in the spleen that decreases in erythrocyte deformability have their most immediate effect, for in order to traverse the splenic sinus the red cell must pass through orifices that require maximum red cell deformability.

Increased hematocrit due to plasma skimming, retarded flow in the sinuses, both of which reduce axial streaming and bring red cells closer to the sinus wall, and slow progression of the red cell through the sinus interstices, all promote the filtering function of the spleen by increasing red cell contact with macrophages and the removal of intracellular debris, or the less deformable senescent cells.

Axial flow, which is responsible in part for the Fahraeus-Lindqvist effect, also produces plasma skimming, which creates the converse effect in larger vessels, ie, it results in increases in the hematocrit of blood flowing downstream of perpendicular branches into which plasma has been skimmed.

A further contribution to the nonhomogeneity of flow in small blood vessels which is becoming well recognized as an important facet of coagulation and thrombosis is that while red cells tend to flow in the center of the vessel lumen, platelets and leukocytes in the presence of red cells tend to be displaced toward the margin of the stream and are likely to undergo skimming.

The already complex relationship of vessel diameter, flow rate, and shear rate are further complicated in vivo by such factors as vessel tortuosity, variation of branching angles, variation in diameter of branching vessels, localized narrowings, and dilitations or other disruptions of luminal architecture. These all result in flow patterns that deviate widely from the ideal and can lead to flow separation with eddies and turbulence at various sites creating local areas of flow with shear stresses, shear rates, and widely varying flow rates. Vessels which are characterized generally by high flow and low viscosity may have circumscribed areas in which low flow and high viscosity are present.

Venous flow, characterized by low pressure, low shear stress, and variability of flow tends toward conditions of high viscosity under which disturbances of flow may be important to the initiation of coagulation and thrombosis, especially in areas where there is an alteration in the geometry of the vessel that promotes stasis.

Thrombosis

The effect of blood flow on the activation of platelets and the intiation of coagulation is beginning to be understood as the biochemical changes of platelets and coagulation proteins are correlated with morphologic and rheologic concommitants in the process of thrombus formation. Whether these changes are the result or the cause of alterations in the viscosity of blood remains to be elucidated.

It appears that the two aspects of coagulation, platelet aggregation and fibrin formation, have different relationships to viscosity. High shear rates tend to enhance platelet thrombus formation while low shear rates tend to favor fibrin formation.[13] The rate of platelet adhesion and the magnitude of platelet thrombus formation are directly proportional to the wall shear rate while the rate of fibrin formation is inversely proportional.

Perfusion chamber experiments on platelet thrombus formation with denuded vascular endothelium suggest two phases.[13] The first phase is the increase in platelet adhesion as the shear rate increases from 50 to 150 s⁻¹ and a leveling at shear rates above 150 s⁻¹. This increase in platelet adhesiveness is paralleled to some extent by the platelet release reaction. At low shear stress (below 1000 Pa) there is a clear increase in platelet aggregation but no loss of platelet granules; at higher shear stress platelet granules are released.[14] The second phase is platelet thrombus formation which progresses slowly at shear rates below 150 s⁻¹ but accelerates rapidly and levels off at shear rates above 1000 s⁻¹.

This suggests that in arteries and arterioles where shear rates are high, platelet aggregation and thrombus formation are prominent features, whereas in veins with low flow, low shear rates, and high viscosity, fibrin formation will predominate. Factors that raise viscosity and lower blood flow, such as high hematocrit, rapid erythrocyte sedimentation rate, red cell aggregation, or marked leukocytosis, will obviously have their greatest pathophysiologic effects in those parts of the circulation characterized by low flow rates. Since these factors are interrelated, vascular conditions promoting low flow or stasis with enhanced red cell aggregation lead to increased viscosity and thereby initiate a circular, self-propagating set of pathophysiologic conditions all conducive to thrombus formation.

The formation of platelet aggregates during flow have an effect on the Farhaeus-Lindqvist effect similar to that of increased hematocrit, ie, the curve of Figure 5-4 shifts in the direction of larger capillary radius and the whole curve is raised, the critical radius is larger, and the viscosity is higher throughout the range studies.[15] The shift in the curve due to platelet aggregation is superadded to the shift due to increased hematocrit with the result that when these occur together the critical radius for the inversion phenomenon shifts even further to the vascular dimensions of small arterioles. Moreover, the decreasing pH also causes the curve to shift up and to the right as a result of decreasing red cell deformability and its effect is also in additon to the above. In clinical situations associated with increased platelet adhesiveness, increases in hematocrit or red cell aggregation cause a similar deleterious shift in the Farhaeus-Lindqvist curve and will lead to retarded flow through larger vessels, thus creating conditions favorable to fibrin formation, which, along with increased platelet aggregability, may precipitate thrombus formation. If tissue acidosis is an added factor, the conditions are even more favorable for low flow, low shear rate, high viscosity, and enhanced fibrin formation.

A variety of investigators have reported the observation of increased platelet adhesiveness and elevated whole blood viscosity in patients who have clinical states associated with thrombosis. Not all reports have been consistent. One study, for example, reported that patients with myocardial infarction, major artery occlusion, acute thrombophlebitis, or valvular heart disease have elevations of blood viscosity.[16] Patients with myocardial infarction have a tendency toward elevated platelet adhesiveness, but those with valvular heart disease have platelet adhesiveness values that are the same as those in the normal control group. Patients with acute thrombophlebitis have platelet adhesiveness increased to values greater than normal but less than those in patients with myocardial infarction or major artery occlusion. There is a wide range of values of platelet adhesiveness in each of the three groups with abnormal results; however, many patients with thrombophlebitis cluster into the normal or high normal range. The patients with myocardial infarction fall into two evenly divided groups. One has values above and the other below the mean. Patients with acute thrombophlebitis have values that cluster in the moderately abnormal range, but some have values in the high abnormal range suggesting two subsets of patients. The viscosity data are expressed only as a mean value and a similar assessment regarding heterogeneity cannot be made. In spite of these shortcomings these data are consistent with the earlier statement that circumstances of high flow and high shear rate enhance platelet adhesiveness whereas low flow and low shear rate enhance fibrin formation and are associated with measurable increases in viscosity. The effect of low flow or stasis on the soluble coagulation factors is not known, but it is tempting to speculate that coagulation inhibitors which normally are in a dynamic state of activation and degradation are not replenished and are consequently reduced to levels below those necessary to prevent the initiation of the intrinsic coagulation system.

The role of red cells in the enhancement of thrombus formation is not fully understood. The effect of increasing hematocrit and viscosity in the transport of platelets from the midstream to the wall is clear; however, the enhancement of platelet adhesiveness and thrombus formation may be due to red cell membrane effects such as a release of adenosine diphosphate (ADP) or some other red cell membrane component which might result if red cell aggregation were a significant factor.

In this context it is worth exploring the possible role of the red cell at the very low flows necessary to produce the low shear rates at which blood demonstrates the property of thixotropy. This occurs at shear rates below 10 s^{-1}. Under these conditions the tendency of red cells to sediment is not overshadowed by laminar flow and they tend to aggregate. The aggregation will be proportional to the duration of the low flow. The reduction in axial streaming will allow the aggregates to migrate toward the vessel wall, and with time the vessel will be entirely filled with a highly organized network of red cell aggregates in intimate contact with platelets, soluble coagulation factors, and the vessel wall. It is possible that the degree of aggregation will be such that the reinstitution of flow may be precluded because the yield stress for dispersion may not be normally achievable in that particular blood vessel. Under these circumstances of uninterrupted stasis, eventual deterioration of red cell membrane components might provide the ADP necessary to initiate platelet adhesion.

While it is clear that whole blood viscosity, especially the special condition of thixotropy, is involved in the activation of coagulation and that shear stress has a role in the activation of platelets, these aspects of rheology are still a long way from being assigned a specific place in the scheme of blood coagulation.

Other Pathologic States

A number of diseases have an increased incidence of thrombotic events and elevation of blood viscosity in which the primary disorder does not reside either in abnormality of platelets or in coagulation proteins. Although it is tempting to impute a cause-and-effect relationship, in some cases the hyperviscosity is well explained while in others it is not. Those diseases in which the hyperviscosity is considered to be well explained are those with a marked increase in plasma protein concentration (either normal or abnormal forms), marked increase in cellular elements, or marked decreases in red cell deformability.

Sickle cell disease is the most severe example of hyperviscosity due to decreased red cell deformability and increased tendency to thrombosis. There are two components to this process. The first and probably most enigmatic is the increased viscosity of morphologically normal sickle cells, which is due to mild to moderate decrease in red cell deformability. This decrease in deformability is apparently due to a decrease in oxygen tension with changes in the hemoglobin molecule that raise intracellular viscosity without altering the morphology of the cells. The decreased deformability of these cells contributes to more sluggish flow, greater oxygen extraction, and progression to the second phase, that of the morphologically altered sickle cell. Significant numbers of fully sickled cells result in marked disruption of flow. Biochemical events such as low pH and high osmolarity accelerate the formation of intracellular tactoids and exaggerate the increase in intracellular viscosity to levels greater than those due to mild deoxygenation alone.

Therapies which either reduce the proportion of sickled cells or prevent the biochemical events which exaggerate sickling seem equally effective in reducing both thrombotic episodes and whole blood viscosity.

Erythrocytosis, whether primary or secondary, is associated with increased blood viscosity, the mechanism of which has been well studied and is felt to be clearly related to the increased hematocrit. While the primary form of erythrocytosis is associated with increases in other formed elements, the leukocytes and platelets seldom reach levels at which they can contribute significantly to the viscosity of whole blood. However, there is a marked propensity toward thrombosis and thrombophlebitis. While it is tempting to attribute this propensity to thrombosis to the increaed numbers of platelets, there may be more than one component. First, the platelets in polycythemia have been shown to be defective in ADP release, aggregation, and adhesiveness, which neutralizes to some extent the effect of their presence in greatly increased numbers. Secondly, patients with platelet counts elevated to similar levels due to thrombocytosis following splenectomy have a thrombotic tendency but not of the same degree as those with polycythemia. Finally, patients with the various forms of secondary erythrocytosis whose platelet count and function are normal have greater than normal incidence of thrombosis and vaso-occlusive disease. This observation suggests that the elevation of viscosity in patients with significant erythrocytosis is an important part of the pathogenesis of thrombosis in these conditions.

Patients with leukemia of any cell type have hyperviscosity if the leukocytosis exceeds $100,000/\mu l$. When leukocyte counts exceed this figure, patients with chronic or acute granulocytic leukemia may develop the "leukostasis syndrome" of progressive respiratory failure, peripheral vascular thrombosis, and neurologic changes with decreasing mental acuity. This may progress to coma or stroke and is associated with intravascular leukocyte thrombi and increased blood viscosity.[17] This syndrome can be reversed by leukapheresis. While it is tempting to ascribe this syndrome to the increased blood viscosity, it is not valid to do since patients with chronic lymphocytic leukemia having comparable leukocyte counts and elevated viscosity do not develop the leukostasis syndrome.

There are a number of conditions in which thrombotic or vaso-occulsive disease is associated with a moderate increase of blood viscosity, which is generally due to decreased red cell deformity. The relationship between the two is not at all clear and much work both in physiology and epidemiology remains to be done before the relationship can be understood.

SUMMARY

The role of blood viscosity in the genesis of disease is only beginning to be clarified. In some cases the alterations in blood rheology are clearly the result of increased viscosity. In others the increased blood viscosity may be an epiphenomenon.

It is clear that rheologic factors enter into the physiology or pathophysiology of coagulation and thrombosis by producing the cellular or macromolecular changes that result in the activation of platelets and/or coagulation proteins, but becuase of the wide variation in the rheologic characteristics of the vascular space, both in normal and pathologic states, it is difficult to determine whether they are of primary or secondary imporatance in thrombosis and coagulation. It is likely that as the rheologic disturbances that accompany blood vessel pathology are more fully understood, the role of blood hyperviscosity as etiological factor or epiphenomenon in disease, will be clarified.

The purpose of this chapter has been to provide readers with an awareness of the basic aspects of hemorheology so that they may more objectively assess new information in this area and its relationship to disease processes, especially the pathogenesis of coagulation or thrombosis.

REFERENCES

1. Merrill EW: Rheology of blood. *Physiol Rev* 1969;49:863–888.
2. Goldsmith HL, Mason SG: The microrheology of dispersions, in Eirich FR (ed): *Rheology Theory and Applications.* New York, Academic Press, 1967, vol 4, pp 86–250.
3. Meiselman HJ: Measures of blood rheology and erythrocyte mechanics, in Cokelet GR, Meiselman HJ, Brooks DR (eds): *Erythrocyte Mechanics and Blood Flow.* New York, Alan R Liss, 1980, pp 75–118.
4. Whorlow RW: *Rheologic Techniques.* New York, John Wiley & Sons, 1980.
5. Schramm G: *Introduction to Practical Viscometry.* Karlsruhe, Gebruder HAAKE GmbH, 1981.
6. Anderson L, Lundén R: The composition of human plasma, in Blombäck B, Hánson LA (eds): *Plasma Proteins.* New York, John Wiley & Sons, 1979, pp 17–24.
7. Hardwicke J, Squire JR: The basis of the erythrocyte sedimentation rate. *Clin Sci* 1952;11:333–355.
8. Chien S: Biophysical behavior of red cells in suspensions, in Surgenor DM (ed): *The Red Blood Cell.* New York, Academic Press, 1975, vol 2, pp 1032–1135.
9. Fahraeus R: The influence of rouleau formation on the rheology of blood. *Acta Med Scand* 1958;161:151–165.
10. Dintenfass L: *Blood Microrheology.* New York, Appleton-Century-Crofts, 1971.
11. Begg TB, Hearns JB: Components in blood viscosity: The relative contribution of haematocrit, plasma fibrinogen and other proteins. *Clin Sci* 1966;31: 87–93.
12. Clivati A, Marazzini L, Agosti R, et al: Effect of hematocrit on the blood viscosity of patients with chronic respiratory disease and secondary polycythemia. *Respiration* 1980;40:201–207.
13. Turitto VT, Weiss HJ, Baumgartner HR: The effect of shear rate on platelet interaction with subendothelium exposed to citrated human blood. *Microvasc Res* 1980;19:352–365.
14. Moritz MW, Reimers RC, Baker RK, et al: Role of cytoplasmic and releasable ADP in platelet aggregation induced by laminar shear stress. *J Lab Clin Med* 1983;101:537–544.
15. Dintenfass L: The clinical impact of the newer research in blood rheology: An overview. *Angiology* 1981;32:217–229.
16. Bygdeman S, Wells R: Studies of platelet adhesiveness, blood viscosity, and the microcirculation in patients with thrombolic disease. *J Atherosclerosis Res* 1969;10:33–39.
17. McKee Jr. L, Collins RD: Intravascular leukocyte thrombi and aggregates as a cause of morbidity in leukemia. *Medicine* 1974;53:463–478.

6 Principles of Antithrombotic Therapy

Edmond Cole

Elizabeth R. Hall

Kenneth K. Wu

The development of thrombosis in man is a consequence of an insidious process arising from an imbalance of the otherwise integrated system of checks and balances which are a vital part of hemostatic processes. Despite the recent advances in the prevention, diagnosis, and treatment of thrombotic episodes, they remain the most common cause of mortality and morbidity among the middle-aged and elderly population of the Western world. In fact, the incidence of thrombotic events may be increasing, not only due to improved methods of detection but also due to inappropriate nutrition, a more sedentary life style, and the use of agents that may alter hemostatic balance (oral contraceptive drugs, tobacco). Therefore, thrombosis in the younger population is not an uncommon occurrence.

In this chapter, we will discuss the agents available to the physician for the prevention and treatment of thrombotic episodes. These agents are primarily those that affect the interactions of the procoagulant and fibrinolytic components of the fluid phase of blood, and drugs that inhibit platelet function.

ORAL ANTICOAGULANTS

Historical Perspectives

In the 1930s, Henrik Dam, a Danish investigator, introduced the term vitamin K to identify the fat-soluble compound which was necessary to prevent a hemorrhagic condition in chicks fed an organic solvent-extracted diet.[1] The structures of the naturally occurring K vitamins are shown in Figure 6-1. The essential feature of the K vitamins is the 2-methyl-1,4-naphthoquinone structure. The K vitamin of plants is 2-methyl-3-phytyl-1,4 naphthoquinone or vitamin $K_{1[20]}$. The vitamins of the K_2 series found in microorganisms and in animals are synthesized from menodione (vitamin K_3). The aliphatic side chain of the K_2 vitamins synthesized by microorganisms may range from 30 to 50 carbons in length, but animals have the ability to substitute a 20-carbon side chain to produce vitamin $K_{2[20]}$.

"

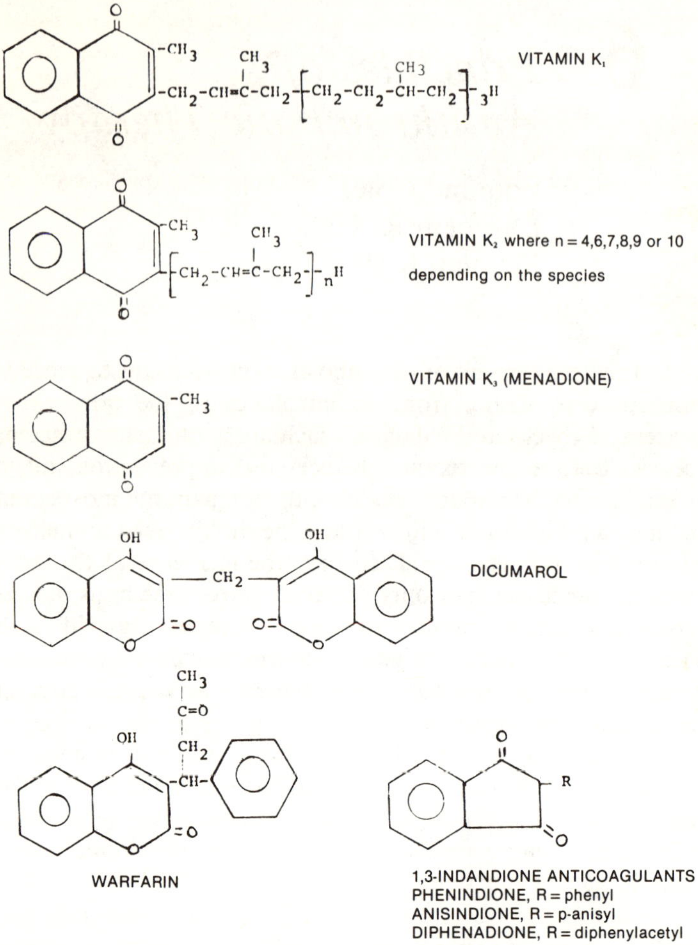

Figure 6-1 Structures of the K vitamins and some common oral anticoagulant drugs.

1941, the anticoagulant responsible for the hemorrhagic disease of cattle caused by spoiled sweet clover had been isolated[2] and characterized.[3] This compound, 3,3′-methylene-bis(4-hydroxycoumarin), or dicumarol, is antagonist of vitamin K action. Coumarins are common constituents of certain plants; microbial-mediated substitution of a hydroxyl group at carbon 4 of coumarin and bridging of two such substituted coumarins with a methylene group results in a compound with anticoagulant properties. The similarity in structure between 4-hydroxy-coumarin and 1,4 naphthoquinone is readily apparent. The oral anticoagulant drugs employed in antithrombotic therapy are derivatives of either 4-hydroxy-coumarin or indan-1,3 dione. Because of its greater absorption from the gastrointestinal tract, warfarin, a 4-hydroxycoumarin derivative, is more commonly used than bishydroxycoumarin in the United States while the indandione derivatives are commonly used in the United Kingdom.

The elucidation of the structure of dicumarol and its synthesis and the development of the one-stage prothrombin time test by Quick in 1935 led to clinical trials of dicumarol for anticoagulant therapy in 1941. At that time it was known that dicumarol depressed the prothrombin level of animals and of man; we now know that synthesis of other vitamin K–dependent coagulation factors (VII, IX, X) are also depressed and contribute to the elevation of the one-stage prothrombin time.

Our understanding of the biochemical and pharmacologic actions of vitamin K and the vitamin K–antagonist drugs has been greatly improved in recent years. Originally Dam et al[4] believed that vitamin K was a component of prothrombin[4] but this has never been confirmed. Martius and Nitz-Litzow[5] suggested that the primary role of the vitamin was in the uncoupling of oxidative phosphorylation. Olson[6] suggested that the rate of prothrombin synthesis was due to the effect of the vitamin on genetic transcription. In the past, most investigators assumed that coumarin derivatives act as direct antagonists of the active site of the vitamin and that this was also their site of action. However, in 1947 Wooley[7] suggested that the mechanism was noncompetitive and that the site of action was different from that of vitamin K. It was also suggested that coumarin anticoagulants interfere with a specific transport site for vitamin K.[8] Bell and Matschiner[9] in 1972 postulated that the anticoagulant effect was mediated through or by build-up of vitamin K oxide, which interferes with the vitamin. By 1973, Suttie[10] suggested that vitamin K activates and vitamin K antagonists inhibit an enzyme required to convert a prothrombin precursor to prothrombin.

During the 1960s, studies indicated that active prothrombin was converted from a liver precursor protein and that the conversion of this protein to prothrombin was the vitamin K–dependent step in prothrombin synthesis. A number of investigators have reported the presence of an inactive prothrombin molecule in humans and cows treated with vitamin K antagonists such as dicumarol.[11-15] These data suggested that prothrombin was synthesized in the absence of vitamin K, but had little biologic activity. Hemker et al called this prothrombin precursor PIVKA (protein in vitamin K absence) and showed that it was a competitive inhibitor in a modified one-stage prothrombin time test.[11] It is now known that there are precursors for each of the vitamin K–dependent factors ($PIVKA_{II}$, $PIVKA_{VII}$, $PIVKA_{IX}$, $PIVKA_X$).

These studies culminated in 1974 with the demonstration that biologically active prothrombin contained a number of residues of a previously unidentified amino acid, gamma-carboxyglutamic acid.[16,17] The molecular role of vitamin K is to serve as a cofactor for an enzyme that carboxylates peptide-bound glutamyl residues near the N-terminal end of the prothrombin molecule, converting them to gamma-carboxyglutamic acid residues. The formation of gamma-carboxyglutamic acid allows prothrombin (and other vitamin K–dependent factors) to bind calcium ions and in turn to be bound to a phospholipid surface, both of which are necessary in the cascade of events leading to clot formation.

Elucidation of the biochemical pathways of vitamin K–mediated synthesis of the biologically active form of prothrombin has also clarified the pharmacologic action of the oral anticoagulant agents. This is illustrated in Figure 6-2. It now appears that the active form of vitamin K is the hydroquinone form, which is the cofactor for carboxylation of glutamyl residues in the N-terminal region of prothrombin precursor protein. In this reaction, the glutamyl residues are converted to gamma-carboxyl glutamyl residues and reduced vitamin K is converted to vitamin K epoxide. Conversion of the epoxide to vitamin K by vitamin K epoxide reductase is inhibited by warfarin and the other oral anticoagulants. In humans receiving therapeutic doses of warfarin, three of the possible ten glutamic acid residues are not carboxylated, resulting in a prothrombin molecule which is more slowly converted to thrombin.[18]

Laboratory Control of Oral Anticoagulant Therapy

Reliable laboratory tests are a prime requisite for proper monitoring of the pharmacologic effects of the oral anticoagulants. This is commonly done by the use of the prothrombin time test (Quick one-stage prothrombin time test), which is sensitive to vitamin K–dependent factors II, VII, and X and to factor V and fibrinogen. Although the test is not sensitive to the vitamin K–dependent factor, factor IX, it reliably reflects the depression of the other three vitamin K–dependent factors provided that factor V and fibrinogen are at normal levels. The test is performed by mixing citrated plasma with calcium and standardized commercially prepared thromboplastin and observing the time required for the formation of a fibrin clot. The patient's prothrombin time is compared to that of normal plasma.

The prothrombin time test appears simple and straightforward, but there are some intrinsic problems that must be considered. The various thromboplastins used in the laboratories throughout the world vary in their sensitivity to detect changes in the levels of coagulation factors involved in the prothrombin time tests. Standardization of laboratory control of oral anticoagulant therapy is a problem that has been considered by groups in Great Britain[19] and in the United States.[20] Human brain thromboplastin is far more sensitive to factor VII than is rabbit brain thromboplastin. This is a prime consideration when the half-life of the vitamin K–dependent factors are taken into account. On induction of

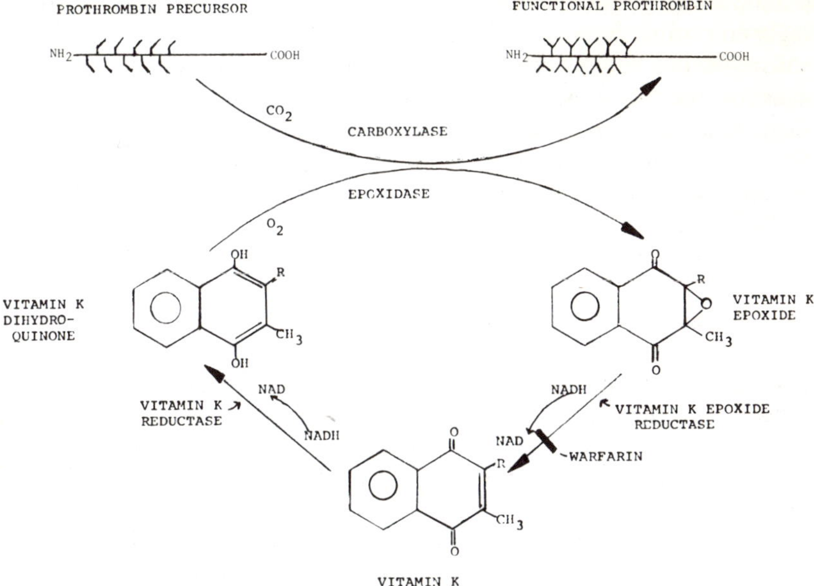

Figure 6-2 The vitamin K cycle leading to postribosomal synthesis of γ-carboxy glutamic acid residues in the N-terminal region of prothrombin.

oral anticoagulant therapy, factor VII with a half-life of 5 hours is the first factor to be depressed followed by factor IX, factor X, and prothrombin, which have half-lives of 25 hours, 40 hours, and 72 hours, respectively. Termination of oral anticoagulant therapy results in a return of these factors to normal levels in the same order. Therefore, the prothrombin time of such patients depends on the choice of thromboplastin. Also, thromboplastins vary in their sensitivity to PIVKA levels, human brain thromboplastin being more sensitive than the animal-derived thromboplastins.

Ideally, adoption of a uniform thromboplastin reagent and a uniform reporting method would solve many problems in the standardization of laboratory control of oral anticoagulant therapy. Until this happens, if ever, it has been suggested that prothrombin time ratios (patient prothrombin time/control prothrombin time) obtained by the individual laboratory using a particular set of conditions — thromboplastin, instrument, etc — be compared to the prothrombin ratio obtained with a reference thromboplastin under the same conditions to give a corrected prothrombin time ratio. This correction has been employed in Great Britain using the British Comparative Thromboplastin, but is not in general use in the United States.

Before induction of oral anticoagulant therapy it is important to detect any abnormality that might potentiate the oral anticoagulant effect (vitamin K deficiency, heptocellular disease, etc). If a nonloading dose regimen is to be followed, the prothrombin time test should be repeated before the third daily dose and then repeated daily until the maintenance dose has been established. Thereafter, the prothrombin time of the patient should be determined twice monthly to insure that the prothrombin time remains in the recommended therapeutic range of 1½ to 2½ times the control value. A value of two times the control value is considered to be the value which insures a proper antithrombotic effect without occurrence of serious spontaneous bleeding.[21]

Oral Anticoagulant Administration

Table 6-1 lists the common oral anticoagulant drugs and maintenance doses used for effective anticoagulation. The average daily dose of warfarin required to maintain patients in the therapeutic range is 6.8 ± 5.6 mg (mean ±2 SD).[22] A loading dose for the induction of therapy is no longer recommended. Therapy with warfarin is initiated with 10 to 15 mg given once daily for two consecutive days. Before the third dose is given, a prothrombin time test is performed, and this is used as a guide for adjusting the subsequent daily doses. It is at this point that the relative sensitivity of the thromboplastin to factor VII must be taken into account. In our institution many physicians prefer to include specific assays of factors II and VII as a guide to establishing the therapeutic maintenance dose of warfarin. As a general rule the maintenance dose is not subject to any great variation unless there is a change in dietary habits, the intake of alcohol, the presence of a febrile illness, or the intake of drugs which may either inhibit or potentiate the pharmacologic effect of warfarin.

Sigell and Flessa[23] and separately Koch-Weser and Sellers[24] have summarized the drug interactions with the coumarin anticoagulants, as

Table 6-1
Oral Anticoagulant Drugs

Drug	Trade Name	Usual Daily Maintenance Dose (mg)
Coumarin Derivatives		
Warfarin sodium	Coumadin, Panwarfarin	2.5–10
Warfarin potasium	Athrombin -K	2.5–10
Bishydroxycoumarin	Dicumarol	25–200
Acenocoumarin	Sintrom	2–10
Phenprocoumon	Liquamar	2–5
Indandione Derivatives		
Phenindione	Hedulin, Danilone	50–150
Anisindione	Miradon	25–250
Diphenadione	Dipaxin	3–6

listed in Table 6-2. Many of these interactions are well established, others are tentative, and the list is almost certainly incomplete, if one considers the number of new drugs marketed since 1971. However, it should make physicians who prescribe oral anticoagulants for their patients mindful of the fact that the maintenance dose required for long-term oral anticoagulant therapy may change upon induction, termination, or change in dosage of another drug. Those drugs which inhibit platelet aggregation

Table 6-2
Drug Interactions with Coumarin Anticoagulants

Potentiates Anticoagulant Effect	*Decreases Anticoagulant Effect*
Displaces Anticoagulant from Plasma Binding Sites	
Indomethacin	
Tolbutamide*	
Hydrochlorothiazide	
Oxyphenylbutazone	
Mefenamic acid	
Nalidixic acid	
Sulfinpyrazone	
Sulfonamides (long-acting)	
Ethacrynic acid	
Phenylbutazone	
Affects Vitamin K Availability in Gut	
Broad-spectrum antibiotics	Oral vitamin K
Cholestyramine	
Affects Degradation of Warfarin	
Allopurinol	Barbiturates
Chloramphenicol	Chloral hydrate
Disulfiram	Ethchloroynol
Mercaptopurine	Glutethimide
Nortriptyline	Phenobarbitol*
Phenyramidol	Griseofulvin
Affects Hepatic Synthesis of Vitamin K–Dependent Factors	
Alcohol	Corticosteroids
Salicylates	Oral contraceptives
Affects Vitamin K–Dependent Factor Catabolism	
Thyroid drugs	
Unknown Mechanism(s)	
Anabolic steroids	
Dextrothyroxine	
Glucagon	
Monoamine oxidase inhibitors	
Quinine	
Quinidine	
Cinchopen	

*Bishydroxycoumarin prolongs the half-life of these drugs and of chloropropamide and diphenylhydantoin.

98

(ie, aspirin, phenylbutazone, oxyphenbutazone, indomethacin) are contraindicated in patients on oral anticoagulant therapy since both primary hemostasis and coagulation would be affected, leading to serious bleeding episodes.

Complications of Oral Anticoagulant Therapy

The most common side-effect of anticoagulant therapy is bleeding, especially from the genitourinary tract, but this can be minimized by maintaining the prothrombin time near two times the control. If, despite proper control, bleeding from the gastrointestinal tract or from any other site occurs, an undetected benign or malignant lesion may be suspected. Other complications that have been reported are: skin necrosis associated with warfarin sodium,[25-27] dermatitis,[28] intramural hematoma of the bowel,[29-32] ovarian hemorrhage,[33] "purple toes" syndrome,[34] and warfarin embryopathy. In regard to the latter complication, there have been several reports of chondrodysplasia punctata (nasal hypoplasia and stippled epiphyses) in infants whose mothers took warfarin during pregnancy.[35-38] Because of these congenital defects and the increased risk of hemorrhage in the fetus and in the mother at delivery, anticoagulant therapy is contraindicated during pregnancy. A serious complication of anticoagulant therapy is soft tissue necrosis and gangrene. Over 150 cases have been reported in the literature, most associated with bishydroxycoumarin administration, but warfarin administration has also been implicated.[39] As pointed out by these authors, this complication is more characteristically associated with females between the first and tenth day of treatment with coumarin derivatives.

Other contraindications   In addition to those contraindications for oral anticoagulant therapy described above, uncontrolled hypertension (diastolic blood pressure over 110 mmHg), severe liver or renal disease, hemorrhagic disorders (congenital or acquired), evidence of severe gastrointestinal or genitourinary bleeding or bleeding into the brain, spine, or eye should be regarded as absolute contraindications.

Management of Bleeding   Vitamin K_1 is the treatment of choice for severe bleeding episodes due to oral anticoagulants. However, it is important to note that the plasma half-life of warfarin is 48 ± 4 hours.[40,41] Plasma half-lives of other commonly used anticoagulants are: ethyl biscoumacetate (1 to 2 hours), phenindione (5 hours), acenocoumarin (24 hours), dicumarol (24 to 96 hours), phenprocoumon (156 hours).[42] Therefore, the time required to reverse the hypoprothrombinemic effect depends on the plasma half-life and plasma concentration of the anticoagulant involved. In nonemergency situations the intravenous administration of 10 mg vitamin K_1 will generally correct the prothrombin time of warfarin-treated patients in one to two days. More rapid correction of the prothrombin time can be achieved by transfusion of 250 to

500 ml of blood bank plasma and administration of vitamin K_1. In cases of massive overdose due to accidental or surreptitious ingestion, plasmapheresis with replacement by normal plasma may be of value, or the treatment regimen may include oral administration of phenobarbital to increase the rate of warfarin metabolism and excretion.[41] At any rate, intervention by vitamin K administration will render the patient refractory to further anticoagulant therapy for one to two weeks.

Termination of Anticoagulant Therapy

Abrupt cessation of long-term anticoagulant therapy should be avoided as there is some evidence for rebound thrombosis in such patients. In one study,[43] four of 60 patients experienced a thromboembotic event 21–28 days after warfarin intake was abruptly terminated. Several investigators have reported this rebound phenomenon while others have found no increased risk. However, at many centers the customary practice is to withdraw anticoagulant therapy gradually over a one- to two-month period.

HEPARIN THERAPY

Historical Perspectives

In 1916, McLean, a student at Johns Hopkins, discovered heparin while looking, not for anticoagulants, but for procoagulants. His discovery was announced by Howell and Holt two years later and despite suggestions to call the new discovery McLean factor, the term heparin was chosen because of its great abundance in the liver. Heparin originates in the mast cells of connective tissue and is most abundant in the mast cells of the liver, lung, and gastrointestinal tract. Heparin of sufficient purity to be used in clinical studies was first prepared by Scott and Charles in 1933.[44] By the late 1930s it was introduced into clinical medicine and surgery in Toronto[45] and Stockholm.[46] Much of the credit for the experimental work on the efficacy of heparin in the treatment of thrombosis and its use in vascular surgery must go to Jaques and his coworkers.[47]

Chemical nature of heparin Biochemically, heparin belongs to the class of compounds known as the mucopolysaccharides, which also includes hyaluronic acid, chondroitin, the chondroitin sulfates, dermatan sulfate, the keratan sulfates, and heparin sulfate. All of these are acidic because of the carboxyl group or sulfate groups. Heparin has the highest negative charge density of any known natural substance and its anticoagulant effect stems from its sulfuric acid content as well as its molecular size. It is important to understand that heparin is polydispersed and molecular weights ranging from 6000 to 50,000 have been reported. The

100

exact chemical structure of heparin is not known. The probable basic unit synthesized is an alternating copolymer of N-acetyl glucosamine and glucuronic acid which undergoes varying degrees of modification. N-acetyl glucosamine may be N-deacetylated and N-sulfated, whereas glucuronic acid may be epimerized to iduronic acid and O-sulfated. A representative tetrasaccharide sequence unit of heparin suggested by Rosenberg[48] is shown in Figure 6-3.

Commercial sources of heparin for clinical use are beef lung and hog intestine. Despite the claims of commercial producers, there is little objective evidence for recommending one source over another. Heparin is usually prepared as the sodium salt and most preparations contain about 12% sodium. Occasionally the potassium, ammonium, calcium, and barium salts are also made available. The potency of heparin preparations are expressed in international units (IU), with one international unit equivalent to 1/130 mg of a standard heparin preparation held by the World Health Organization. Since commercial preparations of heparin vary greatly in their anticoagulant potency, the international unit is ultimately based on a strictly defined assay which measures the anticoagulant effect.

Pharmacodynamics of Heparin

Unlike the coumarin- and indandione-type of oral anticoagulants, heparin has no effect on coagulation factor synthesis. Its action is immediate when given intravenously and is dose-dependent. The elimination of heparin from the body of the recipient is an apparent first-order exponential decay whose half-life ($t\frac{1}{2}$) increases with dose. The papers of Estes and coworkers[49-53] have been useful in understanding the pharmacokinetics of heparin. In one study[49] the plasma $t\frac{1}{2}$ varied from 0.687 to 2.478 hours as the heparin dose varied from 47 IU/kg to 600 IU/kg. As pointed out by McAvory,[54] the $t\frac{1}{2}$ may vary depending on methods used for analyzing the data; different results will be obtained when the $t\frac{1}{2}$ is expressed as bioassayed plasma heparin concentration, as extension of the clotting time, or as clotting time.

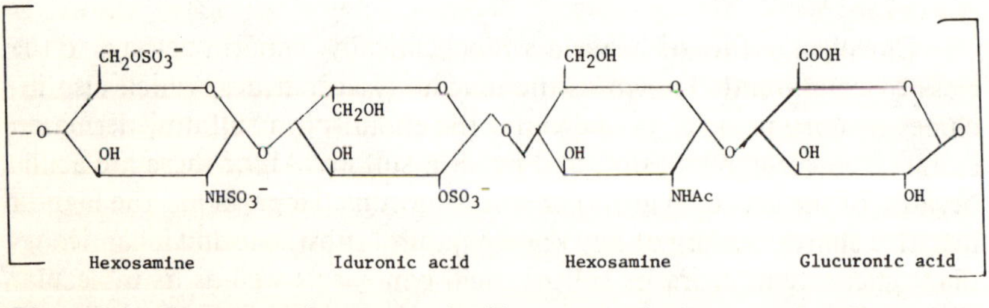

Figure 6-3 Representative tetrasaccharide sequence in the structure of heparin.[48]

Clearance of heparin is principally through the reticuloendothelial system. There is also in vitro evidence that there is heparin uptake on endothelium,[55] and neutralization of heparin by platelets.[56] In the latter report erythrocytes added to platelet-rich plasma containing heparin accelerated the neutralization of heparin but did not affect the extent of neutralization. About 20% of administered heparin appears in the urine. Therefore, both hepatic disease and renal disease would be expected to affect the pharmacokinetics and may necessitate a change in the dose regimen for these types of patients. Exogenous heparin is apparently not taken up by the mast cells of the recipient since there is no increase in heparin concentration in lung mast cells after intrapulmonary ingestion of commercial heparin.[57] The reticuloendothelial system is generally considered to be the storage pool site of injected commercial heparin.

Anticoagulant Effects of Heparin

The addition of heparin to clotting systems composed of highly purified fibrinogen and thrombin does not retard the coagulation time. The anticoagulant properties of heparin are not apparent in the absence of the heparin cofactor, antithrombin III. Although antithrombin III does inhibit the enzymatic activity of thrombin in a slow and progressive manner, the addition of heparin to antithrombin III greatly increases the rate of thrombin inhibition (see chapter 4). This antithrombin III–heparin complex is required for rapid neutralization of the procoagulant properties of not only thrombin but the other serine proteases of the coagulation pathways as well—activated factors X, IX, XI, and XII. Since the rate of activation of prothrombin to thrombin is dependent on a biologic amplifier effect, it is readily appreciated that inhibition of these activated factors will limit the production of thrombin. In addition, the direct inhibition of thrombin will also limit the role of thrombin in the fibrinogen-fibrin transition, in the activation of factor XIII, in the potentiation of the cofactor activities of factors V and VIII, and in platelet aggregation and release of platelet factor 3.

When the polydispersity of heparin in commercial preparations intended for clinical use in antithrombotic therapy is considered, ie, variation of molecular weight, degree of ester sulfation, degree of N-acetylation, and ratio of glucuronic acid to iduronic acid, the question arises as to whether the various molecular species may also vary in their anticoagulant properties. Recent investigations indicate that there are considerable variations in biologic effect of low- and high-molecular weight fractions of heparin preparations. Fractionation of commercial heparin by chromatography[58] and by affinity to antithrombin III[59,60] have shown that only one third of the heparin material accounts for 85% of the total anticoagulant activity.[48] However, even the heparin species which have affinity for antithrombin can be further separated into high- and low-molecular weight fractions which have different biologic effects.[61,62] Low molecular weight heparin (3000–5000 daltons) is more active than high molecular weight heparin (10,000–50,000 daltons) in factor Xa inhibition (with antithrombin III present), in binding to endothelium, and mobilization from subcutaneous injection sites. The high molecular weight fractions produce greater prolongation of the activated partial thromboplastin time and thrombin time, are more active in inducing platelet aggregation, are neutralized more readily by protamine sulfate, and induce a greater lipoprotein lipase response.[63]

Despite the heterogeneity of commercial preparations of heparin and the differences in anticoagulant and other biologic effects among the subfractions, heparin has been used clinically for more than 48 years, and it remains today the only agent available for the prevention and treatment of thrombosis that is rapidly acting, relatively free of toxicity, and rapidly reversible.

Modes of Administration

Heparin is not effective when given orally. The most common routes of administration are intravenous and subcutaneous. Because of the high risk of hematoma formation at the puncture site, heparin should never be given intramuscularly. Commercial preparations of heparin for clinical use are supplied in aqueous solutions in vials containing 1000 to 40,000 IU/ml which may require further dilution in sterile aqueous media suitable for intravenous administration dependent on the route of administration and amount to be given. Heparin must be prescribed on a unit basis and not by weight since commercial heparin preparations vary in their unit/weight ratio, and even the United States Pharmacopeia standards for beef lung and hog mucosa heparin have different unit/weight ratios.

A common mode of administration of heparin by the intravenous route is into a forearm vein. The infusion may be intermittent or continuous. Intermittent infusion, ie, 5000 to 10,000 IU every four hours, has been subject to criticism because of the relatively short t½ of heparin resulting in overanticoagulation almost immediately after infusion and undercoagulation before the next dose. It has been calculated that this mode of administration results in a patient being ineffectively anticoagulated for one third of the four-hour period. Recently the use of continuous infusion has replaced the intermittent method. The continuous versus intermittent modes were evaluated even in the early clinical trials in Toronto and Stockholm with the conclusion that clinical effectiveness was the same for both methods, despite the fluctuations in coagulation times with the intermittent method. More recent investigations[64,65] also have shown no differences in clinical efficacy, but the continuous method was associated with a lower incidence of major bleeding episodes.

The third mode of heparin administration is by subcutaneous injection. Injection of 25,000 to 30,000 IU in a volume of about 1 to 2 ml is made under a fold of skin of the abdominal wall or the iliac crest. To minimize hematoma formation at the injection site a fine needle wiped free of heparin should be used and the angle of entry and withdrawal of the needle should be the same. Subcutaneous injection produces a sustained anticoagulant response for 10 to 14 hours. Refn et al[66] have reported that when the same 30,000-IU dose was administered to patients by the intermittent intravenous, subcutaneous, or intramuscular routes, the anticoagulant effect was the same as that achieved by continuous infusion—an elevation of the clotting time of two to three times normal.

The biologic amplifier system known as the intrinsic coagulation pathway (see Figure 4-2, chapter 4) suggests that inhibition of one or more of the activated coagulation factors participating in the early stages of the pathway would limit the production of thrombin. Although the concept of an amplifier or cascade sequence of reactions was not introduced until 1964,[67,68] DeTakats[69] in 1950 suggested that smaller amounts of heparin are required to prevent a thrombotic episode than to treat it. DeTakats's concept is the basis for today's minidose or low-dose heparin regimen for the prophylaxis of patients who have a high risk for development of thrombosis, ie, patients undergoing joint replacement, abdominal or pelvic surgery, patients with previous history of thrombosis, etc. A common treatment regimen involves subcutaneous injection of 5000 IU of heparin every 12 hours, with the first dose given just prior to surgery. This produces a plasma level of heparin which is not sufficient to appreciably affect the coagulation time. This treatment schedule is usually continued for seven to ten days after surgery or until the patient is ambulatory.

Clinical Indications for Heparin Therapy

Specific heparin treatment modalities for each thromboembolic disorder will be discussed in detail elsewhere in this volume.

Contraindications for Heparin Therapy

The induction of an in vivo anticoagulated state always involves the risk of bleeding, and in patients with pre existing lesions or other particular disease syndromes the risk is exacerbated. Heparin therapy is generally contraindicated in patients with congenital or acquired bleeding diathesis, severe malignant hypertension, bleeding ulcer, or any inaccessible ulcerated lesion of the gastrointestinal or urogenital tracts, cerebral hemorrhage, jaundice, purpura, acute bacterial endocarditis, or any recent surgery where anticoagulation may result in catastrophic bleeding into the organ, ie, eye, brain, or spinal cord. Patients with continuous tube drainage of the stomach or small intestine should not receive heparin therapy.

Complications of Heparin Therapy

Spontaneous bleeding is by far the most common side-effect of heparin therapy. When patients who have clinical syndromes which contraindicate its use are excluded, bleeding is often but not always the consequence of over-anticoagulation. This can be largely prevented by adequate laboratory monitoring of the anticoagulant effects, a subject which will be discussed later. In a prospective study[65] of 100 consecutive patients receiving therapeutic heparin therapy, a 21% incidence of major bleeding and a 16% incidence of minor bleeding occurred. In this study, the bleeding incidence was independent of whether or not the therapy was monitored by the whole blood clotting time. However, these studies were carried out at two major medical centers by individuals with wide experience in the management of thromboembolic disorders and it should not be assumed that monitoring of heparin therapy is not essential. The usual frequency of bleeding complications is about 5% to 10%.[70,71] An incidence of 21% major bleeding episodes found in the study cited above[65] could be due to the large number of patients (60% to 64% in the three patient study groups) who had one or more risk factors for heparin therapy. One of the risk factors was prior administration of antiplatelet drugs (which include aspirin, phenylbutazone, and indomethacin). Since these drugs will interfere with platelet aggregation, their concomitant use with heparin compromises both primary hemostasis and coagulation. It is not always possible to eliminate all risk factors in selecting patients for heparin therapy; the benefits therapy in thrombotic episodes may exceed the risk of bleeding.

Heparin has a direct effect[72] in increasing platelet aggregation, which is apparently due to release of platelet adenosine diphosphate (ADP).[73] However, a more serious side-effect of profound thrombocytopenia has been reported in some patients,[74-80] with the frequency of thrombocytopenia higher for heparin preparations from beef lung than from porcine mucosa.[77,78,81] An immunologic basis for the thrombocytopenia has been shown[74] where the platelet is an innocent bystander of a heparin-induced antibody-heparin reaction. Differences in the degree of sulfation, molecular weight, concentrations of tissue thromboplastin, and von Willebrand's factor[82] and preservatives have been suggested as reasons for the high incidence of heparin-induced thrombocytopenia of beef lung heparin.[63]

Osteoporosis may be an adverse effect of long-term heparin therapy. Two reports[82,83] have indicated that administration of heparin in amounts of 10,000 IU or more daily for six months or longer may produce osteoporosis. This has been confirmed in an experimental osteoporosis model using rats,[84] which revealed decreases in the breaking strength of the humerus, in the cross-sectional area of the humeral cortex, and in the amount of collagen synthesis in bone.

Other side-effects, reported by Lomax,[85] include hypersensitivity, anaphylactoid reactions, acute adrenal hemorrhage, fever, and transient alopecia. The possibility of inhibition of aldosterone synthesis by the adrenal cortex and dysesthesis pedia (itching of the soles of the feet) have been mentioned by Rodman.[82]

Monitoring of Heparin Therapy

Heparin therapy requires some type of monitoring test not only to minimize bleeding episodes but also to insure that sufficient heparin is being administered. As mentioned above, anticoagulant properties vary with the heparin preparation and the type of monitoring test used. In addition, there are differences in response to heparin therapy among individuals. Women tend to have a higher frequency of hemorrhagic complications then men and women over the age of 60 are at high risk.[86] Anticoagulant response will vary according to antithrombin-III levels and with the antiheparin levels present in plasma,[87] erythrocytes,[88] and platelets[89] (ie, heparin-neutralizing factor, platelet factor 4). Therefore, high platelet counts would tend to decrease anticoagulant response to heparin. Unfortunately, there is no single monitoring test that is ideal in all situations; the choice of test is frequently a compromise between sensitivity, reliability, economics (especially the cost of technician time), and the time for reporting results back to the physician.

Until the advent of the activated partial thromboplastin time (aPTT), the Lee-White whole blood clotting time (WBCT)[90] was the method most often used for monitoring of heparin therapy. Although a simple test, the WBCT is time-consuming and subject to considerable variations and poor precision. Its only advantages are that it can be performed at bedside at room temperature and the test material contains all the elements of blood.

A newer modification of the WBCT is the automated whole blood coagulation time, which automatically measures the coagulation time. The coagulation time of 2.5 ml of blood in a special saline-rinsed tube at 37°C is determined. Although this method eliminates observer bias in endpoint detection, the advantages and disadvantages are much the same as for the WBCT.

In addition to the WBCT and aPTT, three heparin-monitoring tests have been proposed for use at the bedside; the activated whole blood clotting time (ACT),[91] the heparin assay rapid easy method (HAREM),[92] and the BaSon test.[93] The ACT, sometimes referred to as the celite test, is a whole blood clotting method carried out in tubes containing celite, a contact activator of the coagulation intrinsic system. The HAREM test involves preparing tubes with precise mixtures of partial thromboplastin and kaolin on a daily basis. The BaSon test is a simplification of the HAREM in that tubes are filled with a commercially available mixture of contact activator and partial thromboplastin (aPTT reagent). In a study comparing the BaSon, HAREM, aPTT, and WBCT,[94] a high degree of correlation between the BaSon and HAREM tests and between the BaSon and WBCT over a wide range of heparin levels was reported, but relatively poorer correlation between the BaSon and the aPTT. The ACT, BaSon, and HAREM tests have been criticized because contact activation may mask the anticoagulant effect of heparin. Other disadvantages of these tests are the need for a temperature control unit at the bedside, the difficulty in maintaining quality control, and the technician time involved. Mean normal clotting times for the BaSon (80 seconds) and the ACT (92 seconds) are longer than for the aPTT (29 seconds)[95] and the recommended therapeutic ranges for each test are 160 to 300 seconds, 140 to 200 seconds, and 60 to 100 seconds, respectively.[95] Lee-White WBCT normal range is generally seven to 14 minutes and the recommended therapeutic range is 2 to 2½ times base line.

The other clotting tests used for monitoring heparin therapy are performed in the laboratory and involve collection of citrated blood. The activated citrated blood recalcification time,[96] whole blood accelerated recalcification time (BART),[97] and platelet-rich plasma recalcification time[98] include platelets as part of the test system, thus measuring the anticoagulant effect of heparin on the overall coagulation system. This implies, however, that variations in platelet concentrations among samples could give inconsistent results.

The most widely employed test for monitoring the anticoagulant effect of heparin is the aPTT, despite considerable differences in sensitivity to in vivo heparin among the commercial aPTT reagents available. Ideally, the aPTT reagent should be sensitive to heparin and show a linear response to in vivo heparin throughout the therapeutic range. That some aPTT reagents lack these desired characteristics has been shown in several recent studies.[99-101] The use of oxalate instead of citrate as the in vitro anticoagulant is associated with reduced heparin sensitivity of the aPTT,[102] and the photoelectric detection systems of some automated instruments preclude the use of oxalate salts due to formation of insoluble calcium oxalate upon recalcification of the plasma sample. The use of calcium salts of heparin administered subcutaneously not only results in lower blood levels of heparin than when given as the sodium salt,[103] but also the aPTT response is lower for calcium heparin than for sodium heparin.[104] Considerable variations in response to calcium heparin by different aPTT reagents have been reported.[105] Nevertheless, the aPTT has proven to be very useful for monitoring heparin therapy. The cardinal principles are that each laboratory must evaluate reagents, instruments, and personnel in establishing its own therapeutic range. In general a therapeutic range of 1½ to 2½ times the mean aPTT of the range for normal individuals is suggested. However, some patients for whom heparin therapy is indicated may have base-line aPTT which fall outside the normal range, and their base-line aPTT may change during the course of therapy. Under these circumstances, a heparin neutralization tablet (Heparsorb, General Diagnostics) could be used to determine the heparin effect before and after heparin neutralization and heparin administration adjusted accordingly.

The thrombin time test theoretically can be used as a heparin therapy monitor, but it has been our experience that the thrombin time is a much more sensitive indicator of heparin than the aPTT; so sensitive, in fact, that a linear response curve is not easily obtained. Conversely, the prothrombin time (PT) is not adversely affected except at heparin levels much higher than those desired for therapeutic anticoagulation with heparin. Monitoring of heparin therapy by inhibition of factor Xa has been proposed by Yin et al.[106] Although very sensitive to heparin (0.01 IU), it has the disadvantages of not measuring other phases of the coagulation system affected by heparin, it is biased toward the low molecular weight fractions of heparin,[107] and the commercial preparations of factor Xa are costly and of poor quality.

Determination of heparin by neutralization with protamine sulfate or hexadimethrine bromide and the more recently introduced methods using chromogenic or fluorogenic substrates to measure heparin levels have a common failing: they measure heparin rather than the overall in vivo anticoagulant effect. Their high reagent cost, instrument cost, and/or technician time cost are additional disadvantages.

Other laboratory tests Because heparin administration can cause thrombocytopenia in a few patients, it is generally recommended that platelet counts be conducted periodically. Hemoglobin levels should also be evaluated periodically to detect any unobserved hemorrhage.

In Vivo Neutralization of Heparin

In view of the very high negative-charge density of heparin, it is not surprising that heparin reacts with many proteins as well as several smaller molecular weight organic and inorganic compounds, including protamine sulfate, polybrene, polylysine, and toluidine blue as well as hexavalent complexes of cobalt and chromium, phosphate, ADP, ATP, and myosin.[108] Protamine sulfate is the drug of choice for clinical use and is employed regularly for neutralization of administered heparin after extracorporeal circulation. Its use for in vivo neutralization of heparin administered for thromboembolic disease occurs less often. Heparin levels greatly above the recommended therapeutic range are generally tolerated for short periods of time and when the relatively short t½ of in vivo heparin is considered, heparin levels of such patients may decrease to within the therapeutic range or below it by the time the results of a monitoring test are available and protamine sulfate treatment can be initiated. When treatment with protamine sulfate is indicated, it is given slowly as a dilute solution. An approximate equivalancy ratio is 1 mg protamine sulfate per 100 IU of heparin to be neutralized. Once the anticoagulant activity of heparin is neutralized, heparin rebound can occur. This phenomenon is characterized by a return of heparin-induced anticoagulant effect and is common following hemodialysis,[109] open heart surgery,[110,111] and in healthy human volunteers.[111] The rebound effect is apparently due to a more rapid clearance of protamine sulfate than heparin from the blood. Ellison et al[111] have suggested that sufficient protamine sulfate be given to insure adequate neutralization to prevent heparin rebound, but administration of additional protamine sulfate after occurrence of heparin rebound is clearly dependent on the magnitude of the anticoagulant effect.

Termination of Heparin Therapy

It should be the goal of heparin therapy in the thromboembolic patient to prevent further extension of the thrombus and allow the fibrinolytic system to lyse the thrombus, or for endothelialization of the thrombotic area to occur. Heparin therapy for seven to ten days will normally cover the period of time for these lytic and reparative processes to occur. For long-term anticoagulation, it is customary to begin treatment with vitamin K antagonists after the seven- to ten-day period, but to allow an overlap of treatment with heparin and establishment of the desired oral anticoagulant effect. During the initiation of oral anticoagulant therapy, administration of heparin should be temporarily delayed to achieve a minimum heparin effect and allow for blood to be drawn for a prothrombin time test. Once the proper therapeutic range for oral anticoagulant therapy is achieved (three to five days), heparin therapy may be discontinued.

THROMBOLYTIC THERAPY

Historical Perspectives

In 1948, Mole[112] reported his observation on the fluidity of blood in cadavers afters sudden traumatic death (an observation also reported earlier by Morawitz in 1906) and postulated a vascular origin for the fibrinolytic activity. Shortly before Mole's report, the first evidence of the presence of plasminogen activators in animal tissues was presented by Astrup and Permin,[113] and in 1958 Todd,[114] using a histochemical fibrin autographic technic, was able to localize plasminogen activator in the walls of veins and venules of many animal tissues. Several investigators have contributed information on the content of plasminogen activators in tissues,[115-118] evidence for a vascular origin,[119,120] and release of activators from vessel walls by vasoactive agents,[121-123] after venous occlusion,[119-124] exercise,[125-128] and mental stress.[129] Much of the information about the biochemical and biophysical properties of the tissue (vascular) activator has come about by purification methods developed by a number of researchers.[130-136] It is a direct activator of plasminogen, has high affinity for fibrin, and is a molecule of about 60,000 to 70,000 daltons. The higher affinity of tissue plasminogen activator (TPA) compared to urokinase[136] makes it a potentially effective agent for clinical thrombolytic therapy, with the fibrinolytic effect largely localized to the thrombus and less likely to induce systemic proteolysis. There is every expectation that such an agent will be available in the future. Human melanoma cell lines in culture produce large quantities of the TPA-type activator and work is now being carried out to produce TPA by DNA recombinant technics.

Another direct activator of plasminogen which has already been used in clinical thrombolytic therapy is human urokinase. It was first discovered in urine by Williams in 1951[137] and its purification from very large quantities of urine by the pharmaceutical industry has resulted in urokinase preparations suitable for clinical use. Through the efforts of Bernik and Kwaan,[138,139] it was discovered that cultures of human kidney produced a plasminogen activator which was later shown by Barlow and Lazer[140] to be immunologically identical to urinary urokinase. This cell culture–derived urokinase is initially synthesized by the cell as an inactive proactivator,[141] which by proteolytic action is converted to active urokinase forms of about 50,000 and 34,000 daltons. Purification and separation of the two principal urokinase forms has resulted in a clinical agent for thrombolytic treatment (Abbokinase, Abbott Laboratories, North Chicago, Ill) which contains primarily the low molecular weight species. High and low molecular weight species are also found in urine-derived urokinase as a result of proteolytic degradation of the native 54,000-dalton urokinase molecule.[141-143]

In 1933 Tillett and Garner[144] observed that filtrates of β-hemolytic streptococci cultures induced lysis of a human clot. The lytic principle, later called streptokinase, has been shown to activate human plasminogen to plasmin.[145,146] The choice of a human clot by Tillett and Garner to observe the fibrinolytic activity of streptokinase was fortuitous since streptokinase activates plasminogen only from the blood of some primates, the cat, dog, and rabbit.[147,148] The latter authors found the plasminogen of man was most rapidly activated, baboon the least, while chimpanzee plasminogen was intermediate in its reactivity with streptokinase. If trace amounts of human plasminogen or plasmin are added to streptokinase, a stoichiometric 1:1 molar complex is formed which then is able to activate all mammalian plasminogens.[147] Streptokinase then is an indirect human plasminogen activator, requiring the formation of a complex between human plasminogen or plasmin for activator activity to be evident. Streptokinase itself has never been demonstrated to possess enzymatic activity.

Streptokinase is a single-chain protein of 48,000 daltons which fragments into several 10,000- to 44,000-dalton polypeptide species, apparently by plasmin action.[149,150] All major fragments are complexed to plasmin and the plasminogen activator activity of each complex is related to the molecular size of the streptokinase fragment with the longest complexes having the highest plasminogen activator activity.[150,151] Although Taylor and Beisswenger[152] reported that the activator activity of a streptokinase fragment–plasmin complex resided in the streptokinase fragment moiety, Brockway and Castellino[153] later reported evidence to show that the activator activity of such complexes resides solely in the plasmin moiety of the complex. This view is supported by Summaria et al[154] who dissociated streptokinase fragments from the complex and showed that the fragments did not have activator activity nor were they capable of forming activator when human plasminogen and the isolated fragment were recombined.

The efficacy of streptokinase as a thrombolytic agent was demonstrated by Johnson and McCarty[155] in 1959, when it was used to lyse thrombi that had been experimentally induced into the forearm veins of human volunteers. Streptokinase as a thrombolytic agent in man has a disadvantage not shared by urokinase: streptokinase is a foreign protein and elicits an immunologic response. Urokinase, on the other hand, is an enzyme synthesized in the human kidney and is secreted into the urine and therefore is not antigenic. The antistreptokinase antibodies present in almost all individuals from prior streptokinase infections must be neutralized at the beginning of therapy by administering streptokinase in excess of that required for a lytic effect. Although this is not a problem with urokinase, its high cost compared to streptokinase is a disadvantage. The cost of a 12-hour infusion has been estimated[156] at $150 and $1500 for streptokinase and urokinase, respectively.

There are many reports in the medical literature which document the beneficial effects of clinical thrombolytic therapy with streptokinase and urokinase; the reader is directed to reviews on the subject by Verstraete,[157] Duckert,[158] Marder,[159] Fratantoni,[160] and Paoletti and Sherry.[161] In 1967, the National Heart, Lung and Blood Insititute organized a controlled clinical trial[162] to evaluate the thrombolytic capability of urokinase and to compare it with heparin in patients with pulmonary embolism. This was later followed by a clinical trial[163] comparing urokinase and streptokinase. Despite the fact that these studies did not show any statistical differences in mortality between patient groups receiving heparin or lytic agents, the patients receiving lytic therapy showed greater resolution of their pulmonary emboli, better reperfusion of the embolized area, and greater improvement of right heart and pulmonary circulation hemodynamics than those patients receiving heparin.

Thrombolytic Agents Available for Clinical Therapy

In the United States, two preparations of streptokinase have been approved for use: Kabikinase (Kabi Group, Greenwich, Conn) and Streptase (Hoechst-Roussel Pharmaceuticals, Inc., Somerville, NJ) are licensed for use in patients with pulmonary embolism, deep vein thrombosis, arterial thrombosis and embolism, and for clotted arteriovenous cannulae. Urokinase, available as Abbokinase (Abbott Laboratories, North Chicago, Ill) or Breokinase (Breon Laboratories, New York, NY), is licensed for use in patients with pulmonary embolism. Abbokinase is derived from human embryo kidney cell cultures; Breokinase is from human urine. Activities of streptokinase and urokinase are expressed in terms of CTA (Committee on Thrombolytic Agents) units[164] or international units[165] which are of about equal equivalence. In Europe and Japan urokinase preparations may be labeled in Ploug units; 1 Ploug unit is equal to 1.35 CTA units.

General Principles of Thrombolytic Therapy

The basic mechanisms of thrombolysis are complex and even today three principal theories have been proposed for the dissolution of thrombi by thrombolytic agents.[166-168] Relatively large amounts of antiplasmins are present in plasma and the question of how a localized lytic effect is achieved has not been fully answered. Ambrus and Marcus[166] have proposed that fibrin has a higher affinity for plasmin than does antiplasmin, leading to the dissociation of the plasmin-antiplasmin complex and localization of plasmin at the thrombus site. The second theory[167] takes into account the affinity of partially degraded plasminogen for fibrin. The loss of the preactivation peptide from native plasminogen by plasmin-catalyzed proteolysis may insure adsorption of the Lys-(Met, Val)-plasminogen molecule onto the thrombus surface where it is then fully activated to plasmin by streptokinase or urokinase diffusing into the thrombus. Another attractive theory[168] involves the adsorption of streptokinase or urokinase onto the fibrin network; perfusion of the thrombus with plasminogen results in plasmin formation and lysis of the thrombus. However, it is evident that streptokinase and urokinase induce both localized and systemic proteolytic effects since fibrinolysis, fibrinogenolysis, degradation of plasmin-sensitive coagulation factors (factors V and VIII), and protolysis of other plasma proteins can be observed. These nonspecific effects may be minimized in the future if tissue-type plasminogen activators become available for clinical use. Intravenously administered TPA was found to be very effective in the lysis of experimental pulmonary emboli in rabbits[169] and in the lysis of iliofemoral vein thrombi in man[170] without accompanying systemic plasminogen activation or production of coagulation system deficits.

The standard dose regimen of 250,000 units of streptokinase or 2000 U/lb body weight of urokinase administered by continuous intravenous infusion over a 30-minute or 10-minute period, respectively, is the recommended loading dose for thrombolytic therapy. This is followed by maintenance infusion of 100,000 U/h of streptokinase or 2000 U/lb/h of urokinase. This standard regimen has been found to induce a lytic state in 95% of patients, regardless of the antistreptokinase antibody titer. As demonstrated by the Urokinase-Streptokinase Pulmonary Embolism Trial,[163] infusion with urokinase for 12 to 24 hours or with streptokinase for 24 hours is recommended for pulmonary embolism, while treatment of deep vein thrombosis with streptokinase is usually continued for 72 hours.

Thrombolytic therapy is commonly an adjunct to heparin therapy, which is employed prior to and after thrombolytic therapy. Its use prior to thrombolytic therapy allows time to establish a definite diagnosis of thromboembolism and to screen the patient for serious hemostatic deficits which may preclude thrombolytic therapy. Heparin administration is interrupted to allow blood heparin levels to decline out of the therapeutic range. At the end of thrombolytic therapy, heparin therapy is again initiated for a period sufficient to allow re-endothelialization of the lesion, since re-thrombosis may recur. It is especially important to initiate thrombolytic therapy as quickly as possible after the thrombotic event, since fresh thrombi are more easily lysed than old ones. Thrombolytic therapy should not be started more than five days (urokinase) or seven days (streptokinase) after the thrombotic event.

Contraindications for Thrombolytic Therapy

Patient selection is one of the most important considerations in minimizing complications of thrombolytic therapy. Since thrombolytic agents do not discriminate between pathologic thrombi and hemostatic plugs, the benefits of thrombolytic therapy have to be carefully weighed against the risks of bleeding in patients with lesions due to recent surgery or biopsy or in those patients with mild coagulation or platelet deficits. Absolute contraindications to thrombolytic therapy are those conditions where bleeding may be catastrophic: cerebrovascular accident, intracranial neoplasm, malignant hypertension, or current severe gastrointestinal or genitourinary bleeding. In addition, thrombolytic therapy should not be employed within ten days after the event in patients undergoing major surgery, cardiopulmonary resuscitation, biopsy of an inaccessible area, or patients in the postpartum state. Invasive procedures and treatment with oral anticoagulants and/or antiplatelet therapy should be avoided immediately before and during thrombolytic therapy.

Complications of Thrombolytic Therapy

Bleeding is by far the most frequent and serious complication of thrombolytic therapy. The National Institutes of Health (NIH) clinical trials[162,163] revealed that serious bleeding was infrequent at sites that had not been invaded, with most bleeding occurring at sites of blood vessel punctures and cutdowns. Therefore, careful selection of patients as candidates for therapy and minimizing of invasive procedures, concurrent anticoagulant and antiplatelet drug administration, and physical manipulation of the patient are important considerations in reducing the bleeding risks. Some bleeding episodes may be expected when heparin therapy is reinstituted one hour after termination of thrombolytic therapy. After five to ten days of heparin administration, oral anticoagulant therapy is instituted for long-term antithrombotic treatment. Minor bleeding from invaded sites is controlled by the use of compression bandages. More serious hemorrhage, especially into a vital organ, may necessitate termination of thrombolytic therapy and transfusion with erythrocytes and a fibrinogen source, either plasma or cryoprecipitate.

Other side-effects of thrombolytic therapy are usually minor. Temperature elevation and pruritis have been encountered in the use of both urokinase and streptokinase with the frequency of occurrence of skin rash, nausea, vomiting, headaches, flushing, muscle pain, urticaria, and (rarely) anaphylaxis more closely associated with streptokinase as the thrombolytic agent. The use of antihistamines, acetaminophen, and intravenous hydrocortisone are sometimes used to alleviate these side-effects.[171]

Laboratory Monitoring of Thrombolytic Therapy

The objective of thrombolytic therapy is to achieve a systemic lytic state. The use of laboratory tests to adjust thrombolytic agent dosages is not essential when the standard dose regimen is followed. For the relatively small percentage of patients receiving streptokinase who fail to achieve a lytic state due to high titers of streptococcal antibodies, the use of urokinase is recommended. A number of laboratory tests have been employed to insure that a lytic state is achieved and maintained during thrombolytic therapy. The thrombin time is a simple and rapid method which is sensitive to concentrations of fibrinogen and fibrin (fibrinogen) degradation products. Quantification of plasma fibrinogen by suitable clotting time method or estimation of fibrin (fibrinogen) degradation products also are reasonably rapid and effective methods of monitoring for a lytic state. The whole blood euglobulin time is the method that has been used in most clinical trials. In our laboratory we found the plasma euglobulin lysis time and the factor V assay to be unpredictable as indicators of a lytic state.

ANTIPLATELET AGENTS

Commonly Used Agents

The use of compounds that inhibit platelet function in the prevention and treatment of arterial thromboembolic disorders, and to a lesser extent recurrent venous thrombosis, is based on the concept that platelet thrombus formation plays a crucial role in the pathogenesis of human arterial occlusive diseases. Although many compounds have been used, only a very few have been investigated adequately: (1) aspirin, (2) sulfinpyrazone, and (3) dipyridamole. Readers are referred to an excellent and detailed review by Fuster and Chesebro of all the clinical trials that have utilized these compounds in various clinical disorders.[172] The purpose of this section is to summarize the efficacy of each of the three drugs and to delineate their pharmacologic mechanisms as well as discuss the new compounds that are being developed.

Aspirin is an ancient drug which among its many pharmacologic properties inhibits platelet aggregation. As will be discussed in more detail below, its mechanism of action on platelet aggregation is mediated by its inhibition of cyclooxygenase, whereby thromboxane A_2 synthesis in platelets is blocked.[173] Many clinical trials have been conducted to evaluated the efficacy of aspirin. In three large-scale randomized trials, aspirin was shown to be efficacious in preventing transient ischemic attacks and/or ischemic stroke in men, but had no demonstrable effect in women.[172] There have been many trials to evaluate the efficacy of aspirin in preventing recurrent myocardial infarction. Except for the AMIS (Aspirin Myocardial Infarction Study), which showed no effect, there was a tendency in favor of the aspirin-treated group, but the difference was statistically insignificant.[172] Hence, the efficacy of aspirin in preventing myocardial infarction at the dosage used, ie, 960 ~ 1300 mg daily, was uncertain. Aspirin at a lower dose (160 mg daily) was shown to be efficacious in preventing thrombosis in arteriovenous shunt.[174] Clinical trials have been conducted to determine the efficacy of aspirin in hip replacement-induced deep vein thrombosis and arterial thrombosis following carotid endarterectomy, but the results remain controversial.[172]

In summary, the efficacy of aspirin in most arterial thromboembolic disorders has not been established and requires further investigation. The therapeutic dosage of aspirin cannot be recommended at the present time because of the following pharmacologic dilemma. Cyclooxygenase is one of the enzymes in the arachidonate pathway that is important for synthesis of thromboxane A_2 (TXA_2) and prostacyclin (PGI_2).[175] Cyclooxygenase inhibitors such as aspirin inhibit not only the production of TXB_2 but also PGI_2 production. Since PGI_2 is a potent inhibitor of platelet aggregation and is considered to play an important role in defense against thrombosis, blocking of its production by aspirin represents an undesirable effect. Experimental studies have indicated that platelet cyclooxygenase is more sensitive to aspirin than endothelial cell cyclooxygenase and it has been theorized that "low" doses of aspirin may differentially block platelet cyclooxygenase and spare the endothelial cell enzyme activity.[176] Several experimental studies have yielded conflicting results concerning the optimal dosage of aspirin. The problem is compounded further by the lack of understanding with respect to the capacity of platelets and endothelium to synthesize TXA_2 and PGI_2 in various disease conditions. The side-effects of aspirin are primarily gastrointestinal. It may occasionally cause hepatitis, allergic reactions, and elevation of blood urea and uric acid levels.

Sulfinpyrazone is a weaker inhibitor of cyclooxygenase. It does not prolong bleeding time and has little effect on platelet aggregation. It exhibits an inhibitory effect on platelet adhesion to the damaged vessel wall. Its clinical efficacy in preventing ischemic stroke was evaluated by the Canadian stroke study and the results were disappointing. In the Anturane Reinfarction Trial, sulfinpyrazone reduced sudden death within the first seven months following myocardial infarction.[178] This effect was attributed to its direct antiarrhythmic effect rather than to its antithrombotic effect. Sulfinpyrazone appears to reduce recurrent deep vein thrombosis accompanied by normalization of shortened platelet survival time. The common dose used is 200 mg every six hours. Sulfinpyrazone produces few side-effects, which are generally mild. It causes minimal gastric side-effects. Recently it has been noted that it may potentiate the anticoagulant effect of warfarin and the hypoglycemic effect of sulfonylurea agents. It is a uricosuric agent and may cause uric acid stone precipitation.

Dipyridamole exerts its antiplatelet effect by inhibiting phosphodiesterase whereby cyclic AMP (cAMP) degradation is retarded. Increased platelet cAMP leads to inhibition of platelet aggregation. Relatively high doses (>400 mg daily) are required to achieve its pharmacologic action when used alone. Since dipyridamole at large doses frequently causes headache, it is commonly used in combination with other antithrombotic drugs such as aspirin or warfarin. In the PARIS (Persantine-Aspirin Reinfarction Study) in which a combination of aspirin (972 mg daily) and dipyridamole (225 mg daily) was compared with aspirin (972 mg daily) alone and placebo in preventing myocardial reinfarction, a favorable trend was noted with the combination drug therapy but the data were inconclusive.[179] Thromboembolism is a common complication

116

of mechanical prosthetic heart valves. Several randomized double-blind studies have been carried out to compare the efficacy of a combination of warfarin and dipyridamole (400 mg daily) with warfarin alone and/or placebo. A significant reduction of thromboembolic occurrences was observed with the combination therapy.[172] Hence, patients should receive warfarin and dipyridamole following prosthetic valve replacement.[172] The adverse effects of dipyridamole include gastric irritation, headache and, infrequently, allergic reactions.

A number of drugs such as clofibrate, propranolol, tricyclic antidepressant compounds, ticlopidine, vitamin E, etc are recognized to possess an inhibitory effect on platelet function, but their use as antithrombotic agents has not been carefully evaluated, and at the present time cannot be recommended for clinical therapeutic use.

Despite costly multicenter trials to evaluate the efficacy of sulfinpyrazone and dipyridamole, the therapeutic efficacy of these drugs is at best marginal. The reasons are severalfold: (1) multiple pathogenetic mechanisms of arterial thromboembolic disorders, (2) lack of complete understanding of platelet physiology, and (3) lack of specific platelet inhibitors. Tremendous advances have been made in the field of platelet physiology and pharmacology in the past decade. New concepts in the development of more selective and potent platelet inhibitors have emerged. We feel that it is valuable for the readers to grasp this field at the state of the art, although it should be emphasized that the discussions that follow are theoretical and certain compounds are still in the early phases of development.

Pharmacologic Considerations

The adhesion and aggregation of platelets is an essential function of normal hemostasis and yet is a cause of clinically important thromboembolic disorders. Extensive work has been devoted to the elucidation of the mechanisms involved in these platelet reactions under physiologic and pathologic conditions. The aim of such investigations is to provide a rational basis for the design and production of new, specific, and potent platelet inhibitors. The involvement of a remarkable variety of agents which can trigger and consolidate platelet aggregation provides a safeguard for sustaining an adequate hemostatic function, but poses some difficulties for developing effective drugs for inhibiting thrombus formation. However, there appear to be certain common intracellular events leading to platelet activation and aggregation. Therefore, even though platelet activation and aggregation are still inadequately understood, an extremely active search has been underway for acceptable "antiplatelet" compounds. The mechanism of formation of platelet thrombi suggests four general areas of platelet function that could be inhibited: (1) platelet adherence, (2) primary aggregation, (3) the release reaction and secondary aggregation, and (4) common intracellular events leading to platelet inactivation (eg, calcium mobilization).

Inhibition of platelet adherence Conceptually, a specific inhibitor of platelet adhesion might obviate the need for inhibitors of release or aggregation, at least for thrombi initiated by damaged vascular surfaces. Yet relatively little has been reported on inhibitors of platelet adhesion. One of the major problems has been the difficulty of specifically measuring platelet adherence. Although several compounds have been implicated as inhibitors of platelet adhesion onto the subendothelial matrix, eg, epoprostenol sodium, sulfinpyrazone, and dipyridamole, all of these compounds inhibit other platelet functions as well, at lower dosages than required to inhibit platelet adhesion.

Primary aggregation There are several compounds that inhibit platelet aggregation by antagonizing the platelet response to a specific stimulus by blocking the interaction of the stimulant with its receptor. Examples of these compounds are: dihydroergotamine, which block adrenaline-induced aggregation; methylsergide, which blocks action of serotonin; and 2-methylthio-AMP, which inhibits ADP-induced aggregation. To date none of these compounds has proved suitable for clinical use, except ergotamine, which may have therapeutic value when combined with anticoagulants.

Inhibition of release reaction and secondary aggregation The majority of available drugs and indeed many of those under development are compounds that inhibit the platelet release reaction. Thromboxane A_2 (TXA_2) is a key mediator of platelet aggregation and release.[175,180] In resting platelets, its biosynthesis is insignificant. However, when platelets are activated, TXA_2 is rapidly synthesized. Compounds that block TXA_2 synthesis or inhibit its action inhibit arachidonic acid and prostaglandin endoperoxide–induced aggregation, sharply reduce the aggregation response to collagen, and inhibit the second wave of ADP- and epinephrine-induced aggregation. The biosynthesis of TXA_2 is a multistep process involving several enzymatic steps (see Figure 6-4). Its biosynthesis involves the liberation of arachidonic acid by platelet phospholipases and the metabolism of arachidonate by prostaglandin endoperoxide synthase (commonly called cyclooxygenase) and thromboxane synthase. Inhibitors of any of these enzymes will result in reduced TXA_2 formation and therefore reduced platelet function.

Phospholipase inhibitors Since virtually all arachidonic acid in quiescent platelets is present in esterified form, a prerequisite and rate-limiting step in thromboxane production is the release of arachidonate from complex lipids. Platelet arachidonate is liberated either directly by phospholipase A_2[181] or by the sequential actions of phospholipase C and diglyceride lipase[182-183] as described in previous chapters. Platelet phospholipases have an absolute requirement for calcium, such that the

118

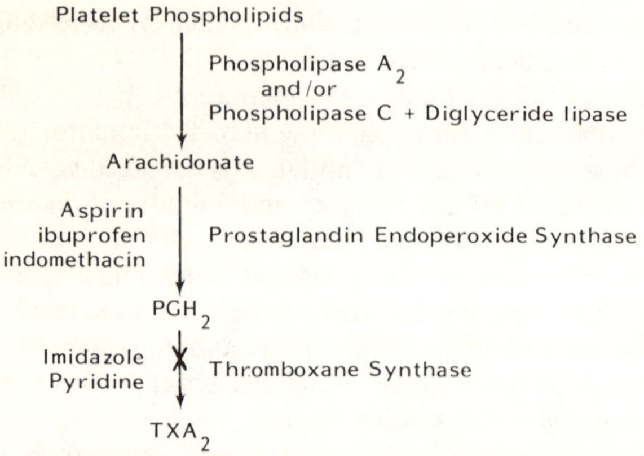

Figure 6-4 Inhibitors of arachidonic acid metabolism.

effects of several phospholipase inhibitors appear to reflect their effects on calcium. TMB-8, an amphiphilic compound that has been reported to block calcium flux associated with platelet secretion,[184] also inhibits phospholipid hydrolysis.[185] Inhibition by TMB-8 is similar to that of other compounds which displace Ca^{++} from critical sites or prevent its release from the dense tubular system, such as quinacrine hydrochloride,[186,187] propranolol[188] and chlorpromazine.[188] Alkylating reagents such as bromophenacyl bromide[186,189] have also been reported to inhibit platelet phospholipases. Finally, the possibility that serine esterases are involved in the activation of the lipases or are themselves lipases has been investigated.[190,191]

The TXA_2 pathway, although pivotal for aggregation by arachidonate, is not the only pathway for platelet activation. Lysophospholipids and platelet-activating factor are also capable of aggregating platelets that are inhibited to various degrees by phospholipase inhibitors. Thus, phospholipase inhibitors may interfere with platelet function to a greater extent than just the inhibition of cyclooxygenase alone. It should be noted, however, that similar (or identical) phospholipases exist in other cells in the body, including endothelial cells. Therefore, unless specific inhibitors of platelet phospholipases are found, phospholipase inhibitors may also inhibit the production of prostacyclin, which is an important defense factor against thrombus formation.

Once released from the membrane phospholipids, arachidonic acid undergoes oxygenation and cyclization to form the prostaglandin endoperoxides, PGG_2 and PGH_2. These reactions are catalyzed by the enzyme known as cyclooxygenase. Its activity is inhibited by numerous nonsteroidal anti-inflammatory drugs such as acetylsalicylic acid (aspirin, ibuprofen, indomethacin, phenylbutazone, and naproxen, as well as the uricosuric agent sulfinpyrazone.[172] The mechanisms by which these drugs inhibit cyclooxygenase differ. Aspirin selectively acetylates the serine at the amino terminus of the cyclooxygenase. This enzyme modification inactivates the enzyme in a permanent and irreversible manner.[173] Since platelets lack the intracellular machinery to synthesize new enzyme molecules to replace those that have been acetylated, the effects of aspirin persist for the life of the platelet. Consequently, the ingestion of a single aspirin tablet can inhibit platelet function for over a week, or until the affected platelets have been replaced by new ones.[192] Aspirin also inhibits the endothelial cell cyclooxygenase which may lead to a potentially harmful reduction in prostacyclin production. However, platelet cyclooxygenase appears to be more sensitive to aspirin than is the endothelial cell cyclooxygenase.[176] One reason for this may be that, in contrast to platelets, endothelial cells can resynthesize cyclooxygenase and therefore the inhibitory effects of an aspirin tablet probably only last for 24 hours.[193]

Although aspirin ingestion normally produces a slight prolongation of the bleeding time, high doses of aspirin may have no effect on or even shorten the bleeding time.[194] These results were interpreted as indicating that low-dose (0.3 to 1 g) aspirin inhibits only TXA_2 formation by platelets, whereas high-dose aspirin inhibits both TXA_2 formation and blood vessel PGI_2 synthesis. Although this interpretation has been questioned, several animal experiments have arrived at similar conclusions.[195,196] The relevance of these experimental findings in a clinical setting is unclear but must be investigated.

Sulfinpyrazone, like the other nonsteroidal anti-inflammatory drugs, is a reversible inhibitor of platelet function. In fact, its effects do not outlast the time of its effective circulatory concentration.[197] Sulfinpyrazone is a weak inhibitor of cyclooxygenase and its metabolites may be as potent as the parent compound.[198] It is unclear whether there exists a differential sensitivity of the platelet and endothelial cell cyclooxygenase to sulfinpyrazone as is seen with aspirin.

Thromboxane synthase inhibitors   Concern that primary inhibitors of cyclooxygenase, such as aspirin, may inhibit not only the platelet production of TXA_2 but also the vessel wall synthesis of PGI_2 has prompted an intensive search for inhibitors of thromboxane synthase. The rationale for this kind of inhibitor is that it would prevent the formation of TXA_2 while leaving intact the PGI_2 pathway. Several inhibitors of thromboxane synthase have been developed. Benzydamine[199] and a phenyl phosphonate derivative of phloretin-phosphate (N-0164)[200] do inhibit the enzyme in microsomal preparations, but neither compound is very selective since at slightly higher concentrations they also inhibit cyclooxygenase. Imidazole and several of its derivatives are much more selective inhibitors of thromboxane synthase.[201-204] Other compounds include pyridine and its derivatives[205,206] and 9,11-azaprosta-5,13 dienoate (azo analog I).[207] The majority of these compounds exhibit an in vitro inhibition of platelet aggregation and several have an inhibitory effect in vivo as well.[208-210] However, the assumption that the inhibition of TXA_2 will result in the prevention of platelet aggregation has proved too simplistic. When thromboxane synthesis is blocked, most of the PGH_2 is converted to PGE_2, and under these conditions the combination of the weak aggregator PGH_2 with PGE_2, which markedly potentiates the effects of PGH_2, can cause aggregation.[211] Therefore, inhibition of thromboxane synthase may not prove as effective as was initially hoped. On the other hand, the inhibition of thromboxane synthase may allow for an increased accumulation and even secretion of PGH_2, which could be utilized by the endothelial cells for the synthesis of PGI_2.[212,213] Clearly, more work is needed to clarify the properties of the compounds and their antiaggregatory properties in vivo.

TXA_2 receptor antagonists   Another area being actively pursued by synthetic organic chemists is the synthesis of TXA_2 and PGH_2 receptor antagonists. Recently, several of these compounds have been reported. These compounds do not interfere with arachidonate metabolism in platelets or in vascular cells; instead, they appear to block the binding of TXA_2 to its membrane receptors and inhibit the platelet release reaction and secondary aggregation in vitro. The currently available receptor antagonists are prostanoic acid derivatives that are structurally related to PGH_2 and TXA_2. As such, they most likely act as competitive inhibitors. This imples that their concentration at the receptor level must be kept constant—a challenging task in clinical practice. Such compounds include 9,11-epoxyamino-prosta-5,13-dienoic acid,[214] carbocyclic TXA_2,[215] pinane TXA_2,[216] 9,11-aza-13-oxa-15-hydroxyprostanoic acid,[217] 13-azaprostanoic acid,[218] etc. Among these antagonists, 13-azaprostanoic acid appears to possess the most specific properties in that it inhibits vasoconstriction and platelet aggregation but does not interfere with arachidonate metabolism. Its inhibitory properties are reversible and stereospecific. However, to date none of these compounds has been evaluated for their in vivo effectiveness.

Inhibitors of common intracellular events   A triggering of calcium mobilization may be the ultimate biochemical mechanism by which platelet stimulants initiate platelet activation. An elevation of cyclic adenosine 5′-monophosphate (cAMP) enhances Ca^{++} sequestration and is invariably associated with the inhibition of platelet function. Likewise, compounds which can displace calcium from its binding sites or prevent the efflux of intracellular Ca^{++} are also associated with decreased platelet function. However, since cAMP and Ca^{++} are ubiquitous intracellular messengers, drugs that would affect them would not be restricted to platelets and may therefore have limited clinical value.

Increased cAMP   Increased cAMP levels may be achieved either by stimulating its production or by preventing its breakdown. Adenylate cyclase stimulants (PGI_2, PGE_1, 6-keto-PGE_1, and PGD_2) exert their inhibitory effects on platelets by elevating cAMP levels.[219-221] When these compounds are tested for their ability to block ADP-induced aggregation, PGI_2 is the most potent inhibitor with 6-keto-PGE_1 > PGD_2 > PGE_1. This rank order of potency is directly related to their ability to stimulate platelet adenylate cyclase. Human platelets contain at least two receptors for the inhibitory prostaglandins. Since the effects of PGI_2 parallel those of PGE_1, it has been suggested that PGE_1 and PGI_2 share a receptor distinct from that acted on by PGD_2, and that PGI_2 is the endogenous ligand for the putative PGE_1 receptor.[222,223]

In view of the therapeutic potential of a prostanoid inhibitor of platelet aggregation, numerous PGE_1 analogs have been synthesized and tested for their effects on platelet aggregation.[224] Likewise, a plethora of chemical modifications of PGI_2 have been made, generally removing its vinyl ether moiety in an effort to increase its stability.[224] The effects of PGD_2 analogs have not been studied in as great detail as those of PGE_1 and PGI_2. However, none of these compounds is available as yet for an evaluation in vivo.

Augmentation of endogenous PGI_2 production represents a new mechanism to explain the antiaggregatory and vasodilating effects of certain drugs which are used for coronary artery disease. Recent studies have revealed that one of the effects of nitroglycerin, commonly prescribed for the relief of angina pectoris, may be due to its stimulation of prostacyclin production.[225] Several other compounds have been reported to have similar effects.[226]

Compounds which suppress platelet phosphodiesterase activity (such as dipyridamole and theophylline) and thus prevent the breakdown of cAMP can also lead to an elevation of platelet cAMP. Dipyridamole is classified by the Food and Drug Administration as a coronary vasodilator, possibly effective in long-term therapy of chronic angina pectoris. Recent interest, however, has focused on its antithrombotic activity. Dipyridamole is often used in conjunction with an adenylate cyclase stimulator and has been shown to potentiate the effectiveness of PGI_2.[227] However, dipyridamole possesses other pharmacologic actions and must be investigated further.

Blockers of calcium mobilization   Local anesthetics and other drugs with similar structures (verapamil, chlorpromazine, diphenhydramine, hydrochloride, etc) have been widely used to study the influence of Ca^{++} in platelets. These compounds prevent the efflux of calcium from intracellular stores and displace calcium from critical binding sites.[228,229] Verapamil, for instance, has been reported to inhibit platelet aggregation and secretion and to potentiate the antiaggregating activity of PGI_2 at

122

relatively low concentrations.[230] The antithrombotic effects of these drugs should be evaluated.

COMMENTS

Currently available antithrombotic drugs such as heparin and warfarin are effective in controlling venous thrombosis and pulmonary embolism. Fibrinolytic agents (urokinase and streptokinase) add a new dimension for treating these disorders. These drugs are, however, accompanied by significant bleeding complications because of their interference with normal coagulation function. Several approaches are now being taken to alleviate this problem. Preliminary results from experimental studies are promising, but their practical application awaits further evaluation. Nevertheless, it is worth mentioning here that one approach is to purify the active ingredients of the heparin preparations which contain more than 20 molecules with diversified biologic activities. It is hoped that the active ingredients will have more specific anticoagulants without an adverse effect on platelet function. The second approach is to utilize tissue-type plasminogen activators for local dissolution of fibrin thrombi without causing lysis of coagulation proteins such as fibrinogen and factor VIII. The third approach is to inject the fibrinolytic agents directly into a thrombotic artery, such as the coronary artery. This approach allows the fibrinolytic agents to dissolve the clots with less influence on normal coagulation function as would result from systemic administration. Extensive experiences are being accumulated and the results are promising.

It is apparent that the currently available antiplatelet drugs are far from ideal. Their clinical efficacy remains controversial. New agents based on their more selective pharmacologic actions represent an interesting area of development. Moreover, combinations of drugs with different biochemical mechanisms should be evaluated as well, because they may potentiate each other, thus enhancing the antithrombotic efficacy and attenuating the adverse effects. This approach was tested experimentally in rabbits. As discussed previously, dipyridamole potentiated the antiplatelet aggregatory actions of PGI_2 alone.[227] The theoretical explanation is that PGI_2 increases platelet cAMP levels by stimulating adenylate cyclase, whereas dipyridamole reduces degradation of cAMP by inhibiting phosphodiesterase. Hence, the platelet cAMP levels are built up whereby the platelet function is greatly inhibited. The other potential combination strategies include: (1) the combination of PGI_2 with thromboxane synthase inhibitors, (2) PGI_2 with thromboxane receptor antagonists, and (3) thromboxane synthase inhibitors and thromboxane receptor antagonists. Thromboxane synthase inhibitors may exert a synergistic effect on PGI_2 because inhibition of platelet thromboxane synthase leads to the accumulation of the endoperoxide PGH_2, which shunts into endothelium as a substrate for synthesis of PGI_2 (the so-called steal hypothesis).

Angioplasty represents a potentially efficacious way of treating acute arterial thromboembolism. Revascularization by an intra-arterial balloon catheter has received a good deal of attention since Grüntzig first introduced the technic for relief of coronary artery stenosis. Although its long-term value has not been established, this procedure is considered to be effective in relieving anginal pain in patients with angiographically documented single coronary artery disease. The procedure may be extended for use in arterial occlusive lesions of other vessels. It thus represents a new antithrombotic strategy without use of chemicals or drugs.

REFERENCES

1. Dam H: The antihemorrhagic vitamin of the chick. *Nature* 1935;135:652.
2. Campbell HA, Link KP: Studies on the hemorrhagic sweet clover disease. IV. The isolation and crystallization of the hemorrhagic agent. *J Biol Chem* 1941;138:21–33.
3. Stahmann MA, Huebner CF, Link KP: Studies on the hemorrhagic sweet clover disease. V. Identification and synthesis of the hemorrhagic agent. *J Biol Chem* 1941;138:513–527.
4. Dam H, Schonheyder F, Tage-Hansen E: Studies on the mode of action of vitamin K. *Biochem J* 1936;30:1075–1079.
5. Martius C, Nitz-Litzow D: Oxydative Phosphorylierung und Vitamin K Mangel. *Biochim Biophys Acta* 1954;13:152–153.
6. Olsen RE: Vitamin K induced prothrombin formation: antagonism by actinomycin D. *Science* 1964;145:926–928.
7. Wooley DW: Recent advances in study of biological competition between structurally related compounds. *Physiol Rev* 1947;27:308–333.
8. Lowenthal J, Birnbaum H: Vitamin K and coumarin anticoagulants: dependence of anticoagulant effect on inhibition of vitamin K transport. *Science* 1969;164:181–183.
9. Bell RG, Matschiner JR: Warfarin and the inhibition of vitamin K activity by an oxide metabolite. *Nature* 1972;237:32–33.
10. Suttie JW: Mechanism of action of vitamin K: demonstration of a liver precursor of prothrombin. *Science* 1973;179:192–194.
11. Hemker HC, Veltkamp JJ, Hensen A, et al: Nature of prothrombin bioxynthesis: preprothrombinemia in vitamin K deficiency. *Nature* 1963;200:589–590.
12. Neisestuen GL, Suttie JW: The purification and properties of an abnormal prothrombin protein produced by dicumarol-treated cows. *J Biol Chem* 1972;247:8176–8182.
13. Ganrot PO, Niléhn JE: Plasma prothrombin during treatment with Dicumarol. II. Demonstration of an abnormal prothrombin fraction. *Scand J Clin Lab Invest* 1968;22:23–28.
14. Stenflo J: Dicumarol-induced prothrombin in bovine plasma. *Acta Chem Scand* 1970;24:3762–3765.

15. Reekers PPM, Lindout MJ, Kop-Klassen BM, et al: Demonstration of three anomalous plasma proteins induced by a vitamin K antagonist. *Biochim Biophys Acta* 1973;317:559–562.
16. Stenflo J, Fernlund P, Egan W, et al: Vitamin K dependent modifications of glutamic acid residues in prothrombin. *Proc Natl Acad Sci USA* 1974;71:2730–2733.
17. Nelsestuen GL, Zytkovicz TH, Howard JB: The mode of action of vitamin K: identification of γ-carboxyglutamic acid as a component of prothrombin. *J Biol Chem* 1974;249:6347–6350.
18. Esnouf MP, Prowse CV: The gamma-carboxy glutamic acid content of human and bovine prothrombin following warfarin treatment. *Biochim Biophys Acta* 1977;490:471–476.
19. Control of anticoagulant treatment, editorial. *Lancet* 1969;2:990.
20. Miale JB, Kent JW: Standardization of the therapeutic range for oral anticoagulants based on standard reference plasmas. *Am J Clin Pathol* 1972;57:80–88.
21. Sevitt B, Innes D: Prothrombin-time and thrombo test in injured patients on prophylactic anticoagulant therapy. *Lancet* 1964;1:124–129.
22. O'Reilly RA, Aggeler PM, Hoag MS, et al: Hereditary transmission of exceptional resistance to coumarin anticoagulant drugs. *N Engl J Med* 1964;271:809–815.
23. Sigell LT, Flessa HC: Drug interactions with anticoagulants. *JAMA* 1970;214:2035–2038.
24. Koch-Weser J, Sellers EM: Drug interactions with coumarin anticoagulants. *N Engl J Med* 1971;285:547–558.
25. Martin CM, Engstrom PF, Chandor SB: Skin necrosis associated with warfarin sodium. *Calif Med* 1970;113:78–80.
26. Moses RG, Warren JR: Coumarin necrosis. *Med J Aust* 1973;2:76–77.
27. Nalbandion RM, Beller FK, Kamp AK, et al: Coumarin necrosis of skin treated with heparin. *Obstet Gynecol* 1971;38:395–399.
28. Kwong P, Roberts P, Prescott SM: Dermatitis induced by warfarin. *JAMA* 1978;239:1884–1885.
29. Culver GJ, Pirson HS, Milch E, et al: Intramural hematoma of the jejunum. *Radiology* 1961;76:785–789.
30. Sears AD, Hawkins J, Kilgore BB, et al: Plain roentgenographic findings in drug induced intramural hematoma of the small bowel. *Am J Roentgen* 1964;91:808–813.
31. Cocks JR: Anticoagulants and the acute abdomen. *Med J Aust* 1970;1:1138–1141.
32. Hacker NF: Spontaneous bowel hematoma with anticoagulant therapy. *Med J Aust* 1973;2:220–223.
33. Manny J, Merin G, Rozin RR, et al: Ovarian hemorrhage complicating anticoagulant therapy. *Obstet Gynecol* 1973;41:512–514.
34. Di Cato M-A: "Purple toes" syndrome: an uncommon complication of oral anticoagulant therapy. *Postgrad Med* 1975;58:133–134.
35. Pauli RM, Madden JD, Kranzler KJ, et al: Warfarin therapy initiated during pregnancy and phenotypic chondrodysplasia punctata. *J Pediatr* 1976;88:506–508.
36. Becker MH, Genieser NB, Finegold M, et al: Chondrodysplasia punctata. Is maternal warfarin therapy a factor? *Am J Dis Child* 1975;129:356–359.
37. Shaul WL: Chondrodysplasia punctata and maternal warfarin use during pregnancy. *Am J Dis Child* 1975;129:360–362.
38. Richman EM, Lahman JE: Fetal abnormalities associated with warfarin

therapy initiated shortly prior to conception. *J Pediatr* 1976;88:509–510.

39. Bahadir I, James EC, Feddie CW: Soft tissue necrosis and gangrene complicating treatment with the coumarin derivatives. *Surg Gynecol Obstet* 1977;145:497–500.

40. Nagashima R, O'Reilly RA, Levy G: Kinetics of pharmacologic effects in man: the anticoagulant action of warfarin. *Clin Pharmacol Ther* 1969;10:22–35.

41. Levy G, O'Reilly RA, Aggeler PM, et al: Pharmacokinetic analysis of the effect of barbiturate on the anticoagulant action of warfarin in man. *Clin Pharmacol Ther* 1970;11:372–377.

42. O'Reilly RA: The pharmacodynamics of the oral anticoagulant drugs, in Spaet TH (ed); *Progress in Hemostasis and Thrombosis*, New York, Grune & Stratton, 1974, vol 2, pp 175–213.

43. Evans RW, O'Rourke RA: Thromboembolic complications after anticoagulant withdrawal. *Milit Med* 1970;135:1157–1160.

44. Scott D, Charles AE: Studies on heparin. III. The purification of heparin. *J Biol Chem* 1933;102:437–448.

45. Jorpes JE: *Heparin, Its Chemistry, Physiology and Application in Medicine*, ed 1. London, Oxford University Press, 1939.

46. Murray DWG, Best CH: The use of heparin in thrombosis. *Ann Surg* 1938;108:163–173.

47. Murray DWG, Jaques LB, Perret TS, et al: Heparin and the thrombosis of veins following injury. *Surgery* 1937;2:163–187.

48. Rosenberg RD: Biologic actions of heparin. *Semin Hematol* 1977;14:427–440.

49. Estes JW, Pelikan EW, Kruger-Thiemer E: A retrospective study of the pharmacokinetics of heparin. *Clin Pharmacol Ther* 1969;10:329–337.

50. Estes JW: Kinetics of the anticoagulant effect of heparin. *JAMA* 1970;212:1492–1495.

51. Estes JW: The kinetics of heparin. *NY Acad Sci* 1971;179:187–204.

52. Estes JW: The heterogeneity of the anticoagulant response to heparin. *J Clin Pathol* 1972;25:45–48.

53. Estes JW, Paulin PF: Pharmacokinetics of heparin: Distribution and elimination. *Thromb Diath Haemorrh* 1974;33:26–37.

54. McAvoy TJ: The biological half-life of heparin. *Clin Pharmacol Ther* 1979;25:372–379.

55. Hiebert LM, Jaques LB: Heparin uptake on endothelium. *Artery* 1976;2:26–37.

56. Zuckerman L, Ramstack JM, Vagher JP, et al: Neutralization of heparin by cellular blood elements. *Thromb Res* 1975;7:149–159.

57. Kavanagh LM, Jaques LB: A new route of heparin administration—the lung. *Arzneimittel Forsch* 1976;26:389–392.

58. Lam LH, Silbert JE, Rosenberg RD: The separation of active and inactive forms of heparin. *Biochem Biophys Res Commun* 1976;69:570–577.

59. Danishefsky I, Tzeng F, Ahrens M, et al: Synthesis of heparin-Sepharoses and their binding with thrombin and antithrombin-heparin cofactor. *Thromb Res* 1976;8:131–140.

60. Höök M, Bjork I, Hopwood J, et al: Anticoagulant activity of heparin: separation of high activity and low activity heparin species by affinity chromatography on immobilized antithrombin. *FEBS Lett* 1976;66:90–93.

61. Laurent TC, Tengblad A, Thunberg L, et al: The molecular weight-dependence of the anticoagulant activity of heparin. *Biochem J* 1978;175:691–701.

62. Jordan R, Beeler D, Rosenberg R: Fractionation of low-molecular weight heparin species and their interaction with antithrombin. *J Biol Chem* 1979; 254:2902–2913.

63. Triplett DA: Heparin-clinical use and laboratory monitoring, in Triplett DA (ed); *Laboratory Evaluation of Coagulation*, Chicago, American Society of Clinical Pathologists Press, 1982, pp. 272–313.

64. Glazier RL, Crowell EB: Randomized prospective trial of continuous vs. intermittent therapy. *JAMA* 1976;236:1365–1367.

65. Salzman E, Deykin D, Shapiro RM, et al: Management of heparin therapy. Controlled prospective trial. *N Engl J Med* 1977;292:1046–1050.

66. Refn I, Raasch F, Vestergaard L: Subcutaneous application of heparin, in Koller T, Merz WR (eds); *Thrombosis and Embolism*, Proc 1st Int Conf Thromb Embolism, Basel, Schwabl, 1955, pp. 758–762.

67. Macfarlane RG: An enzyme cascade in the blood clotting mechanism and the function of a biochemical amplifier. *Nature* 1964;202:498–499.

68. Davie EW, Ratnoff OD: Waterfall sequence for intrinsic blood clotting. *Science* 1964;145:1310–1312.

69. DeTakats G: Anticoagulants in surgery. *JAMA* 1950;142:527–537.

70. Walker AM, Jick H: Predictors of bleeding during heparin therapy. *JAMA* 1980;244:1209–1212.

71. Hattersly PG, Mitsuoka JC, King JH: Sources of error in heparin therapy of thromboembolic disease. *Arch Intern Med* 1980;140:1173–1175.

72. Eika C: Anticoagulant and platelet aggregating activities of heparin. *Thromb Res* 1973;2:349–360.

73. Eika C: On the mechanism of platelet aggregation induced by heparin, protamine and polybrene. *Scand J Haematol* 1972;9:248–257.

74. Rhodes GR, Dixon RH, Silver S: Heparin induced thrombocytopenia with thrombotic and hemorrhagic manifestations. *Surg Gynecol Obstet* 1973; 136:409–416.

75. Mishler JM: Adverse reactions associated with heparin therapy for ischemic heart disease and thrombophlebitis. *Am J Hosp Pharm* 1973;30:1158–1161.

76. Bell W, Tomasulo PA, Alving BM, et al: Thrombocytopenia occurring during the administration of heparin: A prospective study in 52 patients. *Ann Intern Med* 1976;85:155–160.

77. Malcolm ID, Wigmore TA, Steinbrecher UP: Heparin-associated thrombocytopenia low frequency in 104 patients treated with heparin of intestinal origin. *Can Med Assoc J* 1979;120:1086–1088.

78. Hrushesky WJ: Subcutaneous heparin induced thrombocytopenia. *Arch Intern Med* 1978;138:1489–1491.

79. Holm HA, Eika C, Laake K: Thrombocytes and treatment with heparin from porcine mucosa. *Scand J Haematol* 1980;25(suppl 36):81–84.

80. Eika C, Golal HC, Laake K, et al: Low incidence of thrombocytopenia during treatment with hog mucosa and beef lung heparin. *Scand J Haematol* 1980;25:19–24.

81. Bell WR, Royall RM: Heparin-associated thrombocytopenia. A comparison of three heparin preparations. *N Engl J Med* 1980;303:902–907.

82. Rodman T: in Rabinowitz JS, Meyerson RM (eds); *Topics of Medicinal Chemistry*, New York, Interscience, 1968, vol. 2, pp. 113–153.

83. Griffin GE, Nichols G, Asher JD, et al: Heparin osteoporosis. *JAMA* 1965; 193:91–94.

84. Thompson RC Jr: Heparin osteoporosis. An experimental model using rats. *J Bone Joint Surg* 1973;55-A:606–612.

85. Lomax P: in Bevan JA (ed); *Essentials of Pharmacology*. New York,

Harper & Row, 1969, pp. 337–342.
86. Jick H, Stone D, Borda I: Efficacy and toxicity of heparin in relation to age and sex. *N Engl J Med* 1968;279:284–286.
87. Dewhurst F, Poller L: Antiheparin activity of some human blood protein fractions and their possible relationship to thrombosis. *J Clin Pathol* 1965; 18:339–344.
88. Rapaport SI, Ames SB: Antiheparin activity of erythrocyte hemolysate. *Proc Soc Exp Biol Med* 1957;95:158–160.
89. Conley CL, Hartmann RC, Lalley JS: The relationship of heparin activity to platelet concentration. *Proc Soc Exp Biol Med* 1948;69:284–286.
90. Lee RI, White PD: A clinical study of the coagulation of blood. *Am J Med Sci* 1913;145:495–503.
91. Hattersly P: Activated coagulation time of whole blood. *JAMA* 1966;196: 436–440.
92. Blakeley JA: A rapid bedside method for the control of heparin therapy. *Can Med Assoc J* 1968;99:1072–1076.
93. Baden JP, Sonnenfield M: The BaSon test: a rapid bedside test for control of heparin therapy. *Surg Forum* 1971;22:172–174.
94. Baden JP, Sonnenfield M, Ferlie RM, et al: The precise management of heparin therapy. *Am J Surg* 1972;124:777–779.
95. Congdon JE, Kardinil CG, Wallin JD: Monitoring heparin therapy in hemodialysis. A report on the activated coagulation time tests. *JAMA* 1973; 226:1529–1533.
96. Ray PK, Harper TA: Comparison of activated recalcification time and partial thromboplastin tests as controls of heparin in therapy. *J Lab Clin Med* 1971;77:901–907.
97. Reno WJ, Rotman M, Grumbine FC, et al: Evaluation of the BART test (a modification of the whole blood activated recalcification time test) as a means of monitoring heparin therapy. *Am J Clin Pathol* 1974;61:78–84.
98. Miale JB: *Laboratory Medicine: Hematology*, St. Louis, C V Mosby Co, 1972, p. 1270.
99. Shapiro GA, Huntzinger SW, Wilson JE: Variation among commercial activated partial thromboplastin time reagents in response to heparin. *Am J Clin Pathol* 1977;67:477–480.
100. Soloway HB, Cornett MB, Grayson JW: Comparison of various activated partial thromboplastin reagents in the laboratory control of heparin therapy. *Am J Clin Pathol* 1973;59:587–590.
101. Poller L, Thompson JM, Yee KF: Heparin and partial thromboplastin time: An international survey. *Br J Haematol* 1980;44:161–165.
102. Soloway HB, Cox SP, Donahoo JV: Sensitivity of the activated partial thromboplastin time to heparin. *Am J Clin Pathol* 1973;59:760–762.
103. Thomas DP, Sagar S, Stamatakis JD, Maffei FNA, Erdi A, Kakkar VV: Plasma heparin levels after administration of calcium and sodium salts of heparin. *Thromb Res* 1976;9:241–248.
104. Low J, Biggs JC: Comparative plasma heparin levels after subcutaneous sodium and calcium heparin. *Thromb Haemost* 1978;40:397–406.
105. Banez EI, Triplett DA, Koepke J: Laboratory monitoring of heparin therapy: The effect of different salts of heparin on the activated partial thromboplastin time: An analysis of the 1978 and 1979 CAP hematology survey. *Am J Clin Pathol* 1980;74:569–574.
106. Yin ET, Wessler S, Butler JV: Plasma heparin: a unique practical, submicrogram-sensitive assay. *J Lab Clin Med* 1973;81:298–310.
107. Holmer E: Anticoagulant properties of heparin and heparin fractions.

128

Scand J Haematol 1980;25(suppl 36):25–39.

108. Ehrlich J, Stivala SS: Chemistry and pharmacology of heparin. *J Pharm Sci* 1973;62:517–544.

109. Hampers CL, Blaufox MD, Merrill JP: Anticoagulation rebound after hemodialysis. *N Engl J Med* 1966;275:776–778.

110. Gollub S: Heparin rebound in open heart surgery. *Surg Gynecol Obstet* 1967;124:337–346.

111. Ellison N, Beatty P, Blake DR, et al: Heparin rebound. Studies in patients and volunteers. *J Thorac Cardiovasc Surg* 1974;67:723–729.

112. Mole RH: Fibrinolysin and the fluidity of blood post mortem. *J Pathol Bact* 1948;60:413–427.

113. Astrup T, Permin PM: Fibrinolysis in the animal organism. *Nature* 1947; 159:681–682.

114. Todd AS: Fibrinolysis autographs. *Nature* 1958;181:495–496.

115. Albrechtsen OK: The fibrinolytic activity of human tissues. *Br J Haematol* 1957;3:284–291.

116. Albrechtsen OK: Fibrinolytic activity of animal tissues. *Acta Physiol Scand* 1957;39:284–290.

117. Albrechtsen OK: Fibrinolytic activity in the organism. *Acta Physiol Scand* 1959;47(suppl 165):13–111.

118. Astrup T, Sterndorff I: The plasminogen activator in animal tissues. *Acta Physiol Scand* 1956;36:250–255.

119. Kwaan HC, McFadzean AJS: On fibrinolytic activity induced by ischemia. *Clin Sci* 1957;15:245–257.

120. Chakrabarti R, Birks PM, Fearnley GR: Origin of blood fibrinolytic activity from veins and its bearing on the fate of venous thrombi. *Lancet* 1963;1: 1288–1290.

121. Holemans R, Langdell RD: Histamine-induced increase of fibrinolytic activity. *Proc Soc Exp Biol Med* 1964;115:584–587.

122. Holemans R: Enhancing the fibrinolytic activity of the blood by vasoactive drugs. *Med Exptl* 1963;9:5–12.

123. Markwardt F, Klocking HP: Studies on the release of plasminogen activator. *Thromb Res* 1976;8:217–223.

124. Holemans R: Increase in fibrinolytic activity by venous occlusion. *J Appl Physiol* 1963;18:1123–1129.

125. Keber D, Stengmar M, Keber I, et al: Influence of moderate and strenuous daily physical activity on fibrinolytic activity of blood: Possibility of plasminogen activator stores depletion. *Thromb Haemost* 1979;41:745–755.

126. Biggs R, MacFarlane RC, Pilling J: Observations on fibrinolysis. *Lancet* 1947;1:402–405.

127. Iatridis SG, Ferguson JH: Effect of physical exercise on blood clotting and fibrinolysis. *J Appl Physiol* 1963;18:337–344.

128. Cash JD, Allan AGE: The fibrinolytic response to moderate exercise and intravenous adrenaline in the same subjects. *Br J Haematol* 1967;13:376–383.

129. Cash JD, Allan AGE: Effect of mental stress on the fibrinolytic reactivity to exercise. *Br Med J Clin Res* 1967;2:545–548.

130. Bachmann F, Fletcher AP, Alkjaersig N, et al: Partial purification and properties of the plasminogen activator from pig heart. *Biochemistry* 1964;3: 1578–1585.

131. Kok P, Astrup T: Isolation and purification of a tissue plasminogen activator and its comparison with urokinase. *Biochemistry* 1969;8:79–86.

132. Rickli EE, Zaugg H: Isolation and purification of highly enriched tissue

plasminogen activator from pig heart. *Thromb Diath Haemorrh* 1970;23: 64–76.

133. Cole ER, Bachmann F: Purification and properties of a plasminogen activator from pig heart. *J Biol Chem* 1977;252:3729–3737.

134. Radcliffe R, Heinze T: Isolation of plasminogen activator from human plasma by chromatography on lysine-Sepharose. *Arch Biochem Biophys* 1978;189:185–194.

135. Rijken DC: *Plasminogen Activator from Human Tissue*, thesis, State University of Leiden, 1980.

136. Thorsen S, Astrup T: Differences in the reactivities of human urokinase and the porcine tissue plasminogen activator. *Haemostasis* 1976;5:295–305.

137. Williams JRB: The fibrinolytic activity of urine. *Br J Exp Pathol* 1951;32: 530–537.

138. Bernik MB, Kwaan HC: Origin of fibrinolytic activity in cultures of human kidney. *J Lab Clin Med* 1967;70:650–661.

139. Bernik MB, Kwaan HC: Plasminogen activator activity in cultures from human tissue: An immunological and histochemical study. *J Clin Invest* 1969;48:1740–1753.

140. Barlow GH, Lazer L: Characterization of the plasminogen activator from human embryo kidney cells. Comparison with urokinase. *Thromb Res* 1972;1:201–208.

141. White WF, Barlow GH, Mozen MM: The isolation and characterization of plasminogen activators (urokinase) from human urine. *Biochemistry* 1966; 5:2160–2169.

142. Lesuk A, Terminiello L, Traver JH, et al: Biochemical and biophysical studies on human urokinase, abstracted. 15th Symposium on Blood, Detroit, 1967.

143. Soberano ME, Ong EB, Johnson AJ: The effect of inhibitor on the catalytic conversion of urokinase. *Thromb Res* 1976;9:675–681.

144. Tillett WS, Garner R: The fibrinolytic activity of hemolytic streptococci. *J Exp Med* 1933;58:485–502.

145. Christensen LR: Streptococcal fibrinolysis: A proteolytic reaction due to a serum enzyme activated by streptococcal fibrinolysin. *J Gen Physiol* 1945; 28:363–383.

146. Sherry S: The fibrinolytic activity of streptokinase-activated human plasmin. *J Clin Invest* 1954;33:1054–1063.

147. Wulf RJ, Mertz ET: Studies on plasminogen. VIII. Species specificity of streptokinase. *Can J Biochem* 1969;47:927–931.

148. McKee PA, Lemmon WB, Hampton JW: Streptokinase and urokinase activation of human, chimpanzee and baboon plasminogen. *Thromb Diath Haemorrh* 1971;26:512–522.

149. Siefring GE, Castellino FJ: Interaction of streptokinase with plasminogen. Isolation and characterization of streptokinase degradation product. *J Biol Chem* 1976;251:3913–3920.

150. Markus G, Evers JL, Hobika GH: Activator activities of the transient forms of the human plasminogen-streptokinase complex during its proteolytic conversion to the stable activator complexes. *J Biol Chem* 1976;251: 6495–6504.

151. Robbins KC, Markus G: The interaction of human plasminogen with streptokinase, in Gaffney PJ, Balkuv-Ulritin S (eds): *Fibrinolysis: Current Fundamental and Clinical Concepts*, London, Academic Press, 1978, p.61.

152. Tayor FB Jr, Beisswenger JG: Identification of modified streptokinase as

the activator of bovine and human plasminogen. *J Biol Chem* 1973;248: 1127–1134.

153. Brockway WJ, Castellino FJ: A characterization of native streptokinase and altered streptokinase isolated from a human plasminogen activator complex. *Biochemistry* 1974;13:2063–2070.

154. Summaria L, Robbins KC, Barlow G: Dissociation of the equimolar human plasmin-streptokinase complex. *J Biol Chem* 1971;246:2136–2142.

155. Johnson AJ, McCarty WR: The lysis of artificially induced intravascular clots in man by intravenous infusion of streptokinase. *J Clin Invest* 1959; 38:1627–1643.

156. Marder VJ, Bell WR: Fibrinolytic therapy, in Colman RW, Hirsh J, Marder VJ, Salzman EW (eds): *Thrombosis and Hemostasis: Basic Principles and Clinical Practice*, Philadelphia, Lippencott Co., 1982, p. 1038.

157. Verstraete M: Biochemical and clinical aspects of thrombolysis. *Semin Hematol* 1978;15:35–54.

158. Duckert F: Thrombolytic therapy in myocardial infarction. *Prog Cardiovasc Dis* 1979;21:342–349.

159. Marder VJ: The use of thrombolytic agents: Choice of patient, drug administration, laboratory monitoring. *Ann Intern Med* 1979;90:802–808.

160. Fratantoni JC: Thrombolytic therapy: current status. *N Engl J Med* 1975; 293:1073–1078.

161. Paoletti R, Sherry S (eds): *Thrombosis and Urokinase*, New York, Academic Press, 1977.

162. Sasahara AA, Hyers TM, Cole CM, Ederer F, Murray JA, Wenger NK, Sherry S, Stengle JM: The urokinase pulmonary embolism trial. A national cooperative study. *Circulation* 1973;47(suppl 2):1–108.

163. Sasahara AA, Bell WR, Simon TL, et al: The phase II urokinase-streptokinase pulmonary embolism trial. *Thromb Diath Haemorrh* 1975;33: 464–476.

164. Johnson AJ, Kline DL, Alkjaersig N: Assay methods and standard preparations for plasma, plasminogen and urokinase in purified systems. *Thromb Diath Haemorrh* 1969;21:259–272.

165. World Health Organization (WHO) 26th Expert Committee on Biological Standardization (ECBS). *WHO Tech Rep. Ser* 413,1968

166. Ambrus CM, Markus G: Plasmin-antiplasmin complex as a reservoir of fibrinolytic enzyme. *Am J Physiol* 1960;199:491–494.

167. Alkjaersig N, Fletcher AP, Sherry S: The mechanism of clot dissolution by plasmin. *J Clin Invest* 1959;38:1086–1095.

168. Chesterman CN, Allington MJ, Shart AA: Relationship of plasminogen activator to fibrin. *Nature* 1972;238:15–17.

169. Matsuo O, Rijken DC, Collen D: Thrombolysis of human tissue plasminogen activator and urokinase in rabbits with experimental pulmonary embolus. *Nature* 1981;291:590–591.

170. Weimar W, Stibbe J, Van Sayen AJ, et al: Specific lysis of an iliofemural thrombus by administration of extrinsic (tissue-type) plasminogen activator. *Lancet* 1981;2:1018–1020.

171. Sharma GVRK, Cella G, Parsi AF, et al: Thrombolytic therapy. *N Engl J Med* 1982;306:1268–1276.

172. Fuster V, Chesebro JH: Antithrombotic therapy: role of platelet-inhibitor drugs. II. Pharmacologic effects of platelet-inhibitor drugs. *Mayo Clin Proc* 1981;56:102–112,185–195,265–273.

173. Roth GJ, Majerus PW: The mechanism of the effect of aspirin on human

platelets. 1. Acetylation of a particulate fraction protein. *J Clin Invest* 1975; 56:624–632.

174. Harter HR, Burch JW, Majerus PW, et al: Prevention of thrombosis in patients on hemodialysis by low-dose aspirin. *N Engl J Med* 1979;301:577–579.

175. Marcus AJ: The role of lipids in platelet function with particular reference to the arachidonic acid pathway. *J Lipid Res* 1978;19:793–826.

176. Burch JW, Baenziger NL, Stanford N, et al: Sensitivity of fatty acid cyclo-oxygenase from human aorta to acetylation by aspirin. *Proc Natl Acad Sci USA* 1978;75:5181–5184.

177. The Canadian Cooperative Study Group: A randomized trial of aspirin and sulfinpyrazone in threatened stroke. *N Engl J Med* 1978;299:53–59.

178. The Anturane Reinfarction Trial Research Group: Sulfinpyrazone in the prevention of sudden death after myocardial infarction. *N Engl J Med* 1980; 302:250–256.

179. The Persantine-Aspirin Reinfarction Study Research Group: Persantine and aspirin in coronary heart disease. *Circulation* 1980;62:449–461.

180. Hamberg M, Svensson J, Samuelsson B: Thromboxanes: a new group of biologically active compounds derived from prostaglandin endoperoxides. *Proc Natl Acad Sci USA* 1975;72:2994–2998.

181. Bills TK, Smith JB, Silver MJ: Selective release of arachidonic acid from the phospholipids of human platelets in response to thrombin. *J Clin Invest* 1977;60:1–6.

182. Rittenhouse-Simmons S, Russell FA, Deykin D: Production of diglyceride from phosphatidylinositol in activated human platelets. *J Clin Invest* 1979;63:580–587.

183. Bell RL, Kennerly DA, Standrod N, Majerus PW: Diglyceride lipase: a pathway for arachidonate release from human platelets. *Proc Natl Acad Sci USA* 1979;76:3238–3241.

184. Le Breton GC, Dinerstein RJ: Effect of the Ca^{++} antagonist TMB-8 on intracellular calcium redistribution associated with platelet shape change. *Thromb Res* 1977;10:521–523.

185. Rittenhouse-Simmons S, Deykin D: The activation by Ca^{++} of phospholipase A$_2$: effects of dibutyryl cyclic adenosine monophosphate and 8-(N,N-diethylamino)-octyl-3,4,5-trimethoxybenzoate. *Biochim Biophys Acta* 1978;543:409–422.

186. Vallee E, Gougat J, Navarro J, et al: Anti-inflammatory and platelet anti-aggregant activity of phospholipase-A$_2$ inhibitors. *J Pharm Pharmacol* 1979;31:588–592.

187. Blackwell GJ: Phospholipase A$_2$ and platelet aggregation. *Adv Prostaglandin Thromboxane Res* 1978;3:137–142.

188. Vanderhoek JY, Feinstein MB: Local anesthetics, chlorpromazine and propranolol inhibit stimulus-activation of phospholipase A$_2$ in human platelets. *Mol Pharmacol* 1979;16:171–180.

189. Vargaftig BB, Fouque F, Chignard M: Interference of bromophenacyl bromide with platelet phospholipase A$_2$ activity induced by thrombin and by the ionophore A23187. *Thromb Res* 1980;17:91–102.

190. Aoki N, Naito K, Yoshida N: Inhibition of platelet aggregation by protease inhibitors. Possible involvement by proteases in platelet aggregation. *Blood* 1978;52:1–12.

191. Feinstein MB, Vanderhoek JY, Walenga R: Serine-esterase (protease) inhibitors block stimulus-induced mobilization of arachidonate in platelets. *Adv Prostaglandin Thromboxane Res* 1980;6:321–325.

192. Kocsis JJ, Hernandovick J, Silver MJ, et al: Duration of inhibition of platelet prostaglandin formation and aggregation by ingested aspirin or indomethacin. *Prostaglandins* 1973;3:141.
193. Jaffe E, Weksler BB: Recovery of endothelial cell prostacyclin production after inhibition by low doses of aspirin. *J Clin Invest* 1979;63:532–535.
194. O'Grady J, Moncada S: Aspirin: a paradoxical effect on bleeding time. *Lancet* 1978;2:780.
195. Kelton JG, Hirsh J, Carter CJ, et al: Thrombogenic effect of high-dose aspirin in rabbits: relationship to inhibition of vessel wall synthesis of prostaglandin-I_2-like activity. *J Clin Invest* 1978;62:892–895.
196. Wu KK, Chen Y-C, Fordham E, et al: Differential effect of two doses of aspirin on platelet vessel-wall interaction in vivo. *J Clin Invest* 1981;68:382–387.
197. Ali M, McDonald JWD: Reversible and irreversible inhibition of platelet cyclooxygenase and serotonin release by nonsteroidal antiinflammatory drugs. *Thromb Res* 1978;13:1057.
198. Buchan MR, Rosenfeld J, Hirsh J: The prolonged effect of sulfinpyrazone on collagen-induced platelet aggregation in vivo. *Thromb Res* 1978;13:883–892.
199. Moncada S, Needleman P, Bunting S, et al: Prostaglandin endoperoxide and thromboxane generating systems and their selective inhibition. *Prostaglandins* 1976;12:323–325.
200. Kulkarni PS, Eakin KE: N-0164 inhibits generation of thromboxane A_2-like from prostaglandin endoperoxides by human platelet microsomes. *Prostaglandins* 1976;12:465–469.
201. Needleman P, Raz A, Ferrendelli JA, et al: Application of imidazole as a selective inhibitor of thromboxane synthetase in human platelets. *Proc Natl Acad Sci USA* 1977;74:1716–1720.
202. Moncada S, Bunting S, Mullane K, et al: Imidazole: a selective inhibitor of thromboxane synthetase. *Prostaglandins* 1977;13:611–618.
203. Tai HH, Yuan B: On the inhibitory potency of imidazole and its derivatives and thromboxane synthetase. *Biochem Biophys Res Commun* 1978;80:236–242.
204. Yoshimoto T, Yamamoto S, Hayaishi O: Selective inhibition of prostaglandin endoperoxide thromboxane isomerase by 1-carboxy-alkylimidazole. *Prostaglandins* 1978;16:529–540.
205. Gryglewski RJ, Zmuda A, Korbut R, et al: Selective inhibition of thromboxane A_2 biosynthesis in blood platelets. *Nature* 1977;267:627–628.
206. Tai HH, Lee N, Tai CL: Inhibition of thromboxane synthetase and platelet aggregation by pyridine and its derivatives. *Adv Prostaglandin Thromboxane Res* 1980;6:447–452.
207. Gorman RR, Bundy GL, Peterson DC, et al: Inhibition of human platelet thromboxane synthetase by 9,11-azoprosta-5,13-dienoic acid. *Proc Natl Acad Sci USA* 1977;74:4007–4011.
208. Harris RH, Fitzpatrick T, Schmeling J, et al: Inhibition of dog platelet reactivity following 1-benzylimidazole administration. *Adv Prostaglandin Thromboxane Res* 1980;6:457–461.
209. Hall ER, Chen Y-C, Ho T, et al: The reduction of platelet thrombi on damaged vessel wall by thromboxane synthetase inhibitor in rabbits. *Thromb Res* 1982;27:501–511.
210. Thler HM, Saxton CAPO, Parry MJ: Administration to man of UK-37,248-01

a selective inhibitor of thromboxane synthetase. *Lancet* 1981;1:629.
211. Smith JB, Araki H, Lefer AM: Thromboxane A_2, prostacyclin and aspirin: effects on vascular tone and platelet aggregation. *Circulation* 1980;62 (suppl 5):19–25.
212. Marcus AJ, Weksler BB, Jaffe EA, et al: Synthesis of prostacyclin from platelet-derived endoperoxides by cultured human endothelial cell. *J Clin Invest* 1980;66:979–986.
213. Needleman P, Wyche A, Raz A: Platelet and blood vessel arachidonate metabolism and interactions. *J Clin Invest* 1979;63:345–349.
214. Fitzpatrick FA, Bundy GL, Gorman RR, et al: 9,11 epoxyaminoprosta-5,13 dienoic acid is a thromboxane A_2 antagonist in human platelets. *Nature* 1978;275:764–766.
215. Lefer AM, Smith EF III, Araki H, et al: Dissociation of vasoconstrictor and platelet aggregatory activities of thromboxane by carbocyclic thromboxane A_2, a stable analog of thromboxane A_2. *Proc Natl Acad Sci USA* 1980;77: 1706–1710.
216. Nicholau KC, Magolda RL, Smith JB, et al: Synthesis and biological properties of pinane-thromboxane A_2, a selective inhibitor of coronary artery constriction, platelet aggregation, and thromboxane formation. *Biochemistry* 1979;76:2566–2570.
217. Kam ST, Portoghese PS, Dunham DW, et al: 9-11-aza-13-oxa-15-hydroxy-prostanoic acid: a potent thromboxane synthetase inhibitor and a PGH_2/TXA_2 receptor antagonist. *Prostaglandins Med* 1979;3:279–290.
218. Le Breton GC, Venton DL, Enke SE, et al: 13-azaprostanoic acid: a specific antagonist of the human blood platelet thromboxane/endoperoxide receptor. *Proc Natl Acad Sci USA* 1979;76:4097–4101.
219. Gorman RR, Bunting S, Miller OV: Modulation of human platelet adenylate cyclase by prostacyclin (PGX). *Prostaglandins* 1977;13:377–388.
220. Tateson JE, Moncada S, Vane JR: Effects on prostacyclin (PGX) on cyclic AMP concentrations in human platelets. *Prostaglandins* 1977;13:389.
221. Vigdahl RL, Marquis NR, Tavormina PA: Platelet aggregation. II. Adenyl cyclase, prostaglandin E_1 and calcium. *Biochem Biophys Res Commun* 1969;37:309.
222. Whittle BJR, Moncada S, Vane JR: Comparison of the effects of prostacyclin (PGI$_2$), prostaglandin E_1 and D_2 on platelet aggregation in different species. *Prostaglandins* 1978;16:373–388.
223. Shafer AI, Cooper B, O'Hara D: Identification of platelet receptors for prostacyclin I_2 and D_2. *J Biol Chem* 1979;254:2914–2917.
224. MacIntyre DE: Platelet prostaglandin receptors, in Gordon JL (ed); Platelets in Biology and Pathology, ed 2. New York, Elsevier/North Holland Biomedical Press, 1981, pp 211–247.
225. Levin RI, Jaffe EA, Weksler BB, et al: Nitroglycerin stimulates synthesis of prostacyclin by cultured human endothelial cells. *J Clin Invest* 1981;67: 762–769.
226. Vermylen J, Chamone DAF, Verstraet M: Stimulation of prostacyclin release from vessel wall by BAYf 6575, an antithrombotic compound. *Lancet* 1979;1:518–520.
227. Moncada S, Korbut R: Dipyridamole and other phosphodiesterase inhibitors act as antithrombotic agents by potentiating endogenous prostacyclin. *Lancet* 1978;1:1286–1289.
228. Feinstein MB, Fiekers J, Fraser C: An analysis of the mechanism of local

anaesthetic inhibition of platelet aggregation and secretion. *J Pharmacol Exp Ther* 1976;197:215–228.
229. Low PS, Lloyd DH, Stein TM, et al: Calcium displacement by local anesthetics: dependence of pH and anesthetic charge. *J Biol Chem* 1979;254: 4119–4125.
230. Ikeda Y, Kikuchi M, Toyama K, et al: Inhibition of human platelet functions by verapamil. *Thromb Haemos* 1981;45:158–161.

7 *Thrombosis and Embolism in Peripheral Vascular Disease*

Bruce J. Pardy

Numerous disorders of the heart, arterial system, and blood may manifest as thrombosis and embolism, which in turn can initiate or complicate vascular disease.

DEFINITIONS

Peripheral Vascular Disease

The term peripheral vascular disease is restricted in this chapter to disorders involving the infrarenal abdominal aorta, and the arteries supplying blood to the limbs. Peripheral vascular disease has many forms, but the commonest are occlusive disease, aneurysm, and arteriosclerotic plaque formation.

Arterial occlusive disease　Aortic and arterial narrowing or complete occlusion is most commonly the result of arteriosclerotic occlusive disease (arteriosclerosis obliterans). Males over 50 years of age who smoke cigarettes are particularly at risk, while the nonsmoking, nondiabetic, premenstrual female is relatively immune. The lower limbs are affected much more frequently than the upper, and curiously, there is a threefold preponderance of left arm involvement over the right. Arterial flow to the lower limbs may be disturbed by arteriosclerosis at one or more sites between the infrarenal abdominal aorta above, and the proximal foot below, while upper limb arteriosclerosis shows a predilection for the subclavian arteries, particularly the origin of that on the left.

Arteriosclerosis tends to be a widespread disorder, and limb artery involvement is frequently associated with disease in the coronary, carotid, and mesenteric arteries. There is a particularly strong association between ateriosclerotic occlusion of the "trifurcation" of the popliteal artery, where it divides into the anterior tibial, posterior tibial, and peroneal arteries, and severe coronary artery disease. Arteriosclerosis also tends to be a progressive disorder, although the rate is very variable. Rapid progress in a few patients leads to early limb loss, while in others there is minimal deterioration over a number of years.

Less common causes of arterial occlusion are arterial embolism, thromboangiitis obliterans (Buerger's disease), arteritis, vasospastic disorders, arterial injury, cystic adventitial disease, and thrombosis secondary to hematologic abnormalities.

Aneurysmal disease   The great majority of aneurysms are arteriosclerotic, and the sites most frequently involved are the infrarenal abdominal aorta, and the popliteal and common femoral arteries. In recent years, the common femoral artery has displaced the popliteal artery as the second commonest site of acquired aneurysm because vascular reconstructive procedures in the groin, particularly those involving prosthetic material, predispose to aneurysm formation. Furthermore, an increasing number of these operations is being performed. The etiology of aneurysms occurring after vascular reconstruction is uncertain, but an important factor is almost certainly compliance mismatches between native artery, suture material, and graft.

Aneurysms are true or false. The wall of a true aneurysm is formed by native artery, while the wall of a false aneurysm is formed by surrounding tissues. The aneurysm that forms at the site of a previous reconstructive procedure is false when dehiscence of the suture line or rupture of the wall has occurred, and true when the wall is formed by artery. A convenient all-embracing term is anastomotic aneurysm.

Further types of aneurysms are poststenotic and mycotic aneurysms. The former develops distal to a site of stenosis such as that caused by compression of the subclavian artery by a cervical rib or band, while mycotic aneurysm commonly occurs at the site of arrest of an infected embolus.

Arterial ulceration   Atheroma of the larger arteries often results in the formation of an intimal plaque, which is prone to ulceration. This complication causes the underlying collagen, a potent platelet proaggregatory substance, to be exposed to the circulating blood.

Thrombosis

Thrombosis (Greek, curdling) is defined as the formation in the living heart of vessels of a solid mass or plug from constituents of the blood. In the arterial circulation, two types of thrombus are seen. Composed mainly of platelets, white thrombus forms when blood passes over diseased or artificial surfaces such as the walls of aneurysms, ulcerated surfaces of atheromatous plaques, and the lumens of prosthetic grafts (Figure 7-1). Red thrombus, which is essentially blood clot and therefore contains many red blood cells, forms in conditions of marked stasis, eg, after complete arterial occlusion. Thrombosis complicates most arterial disorders to a greater or lesser degree, but may occur de novo in certain hematologic abnormalities.

Embolism

Arterial embolism (Greek, plug) is the distal passage and eventual arrest of material, usually thrombus, in the arterial tree. Large emboli

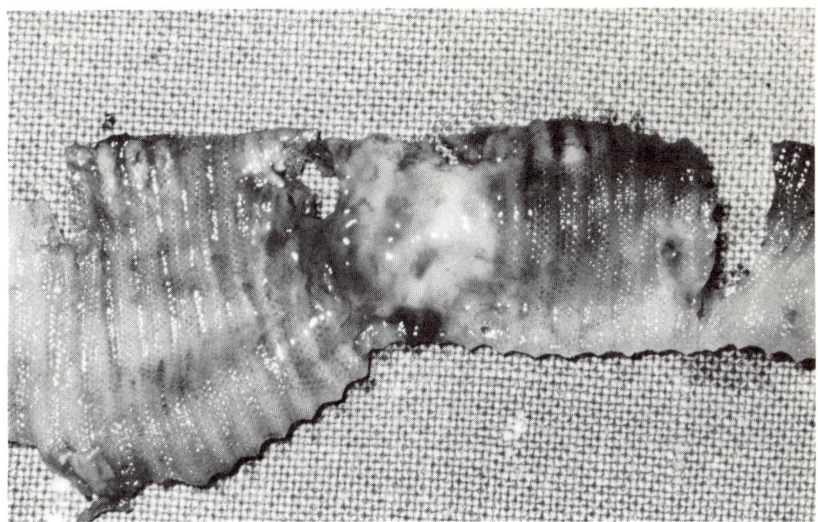

Figure 7-1 Platelet thrombus formed in a woven Dacron femoro-femoral crossover graft removed from an adult female patient.

tend to arrest at the origin of a large branch or at a bifurcation because the axial artery diameter is reduced at these sites. In contrast, small emboli often reach the extremity end-arteries. Embolism affects lower blood flow ten times more commonly than upper limb flow.[1]

ETIOLOGY AND PATHOGENESIS

Thrombosis

Platelet thrombus forms on diseased and prosthetic surfaces that are in contact with flowing arterial blood, and red thrombus forms when there is severe stasis. Although complete arterial occlusion may cause an artery to become filled with red thrombus, the distal microcirculation initially remains patent. However, when stasis is severe and prolonged, the microcirculation often becomes occluded although the exact mechanism is unclear. The extent of red thrombus formation after arterial occlusion is determined by the site of the next large arterial branch or collateral.

Factors that promote arterial thrombosis include a thrombogenic surface, reduced or turbulent blood flow, and blood hypercoagulability, and these variables may operate singly or in combination. Arterial occlusion secondary to thrombosis is usually permanent, but recanalization of the radial artery that has thrombosed after insertion of a monitoring cannula has been reported in all subjects studied.[2] Recanalization is also the rule in venous thrombosis, albeit the valves remain incompetent.

It is of considerable interest that although platelet adherence and aggregation are the mechanisms by which white platelet thrombus forms, and that platelet activity is increased in 50% of patients with arteriosclerotic disease,[3] antiplatelet therapy does not prevent thrombosis in diseased limb arteries.[4] The conditions in which arterial thrombosis is seen are now described.

Arterial occlusive disease   Platelet thrombus tends to form at any site of severe arterial narrowing, because the normal laminar flow of blood is disrupted and flow becomes turbulent. The result is the production of vortices, eddy currents, and zones of stasis and back flow. Turbulent blood flow may also cause endothelial injury, and the zones of stasis predispose to thrombus formation.

Not only do endothelial disease and turbulent blood flow predispose to thrombosis in arteriosclerosis, but blood hypercoagulability may also be important because certain coagulation factors are increased in patients with coronary artery disease.[5] Another factor may be raised blood viscosity secondary to increases in hematocrit[6] and plasma fibrinogen,[7] and to reduced red cell deformability.[8] Arteriosclerotic narrowing may occur at any level in the lower limb, and there may be intervening areas of relatively unaffected artery. In contrast, thromboangiitis obliterans usually progresses centripetally from the foot as a continuous occlusive process, while arteritis tends to be confined to the extremities. Cystic adventitial disease causes localized narrowing and thrombosis of the popliteal artery.

Cardiac failure   Cardiac failure associated with a reduction of peripheral blood flow may cause limb arterial thrombosis,[9] particularly in the presence of pre-existing occlusive disease.

Aneurysm   Aneurysms often contain a large amount of platelet thrombus. Blood flow is turbulent within an aneurysm, and the tendency for this to occur is a function of the ratio of the aneurysm diameter to the entrance and exit diameters. The higher the ratio, the lower the flow velocity required to produce turbulence. The flow of blood through an aneurysm is in the form of a cylindrical core that has a diameter equal to the entrance and exit tubes; in the hemispherical area surrounding the core, blood flows as closed vortex rings. Increased shear stress on the diseased aneurysm wall, increased platelet–vessel wall interaction, and turbulent flow all contribute to thrombus formation.

Although an aortic aneurysm often contains a vast quantity of thrombus, blood flow is rarely obstructed. In contrast, smaller aneurysms, eg, of the popliteal artery, not uncommonly thrombose completely, an event that causes severe acute ischemia. Aneurysm thrombus, particularly that formed in the poststenotic subclavian and popliteal aneurysms, is an important source of arterial emboli.

Ulcerated plaque   When ulceration of an atheromatous plaque exposes subendothelial collagen to the circulating blood, platelets adhere and aggregate, and thrombus formation is likely.

Arterial injury   Traumatic injury to the arterial wall may be induced by catheters that are introduced into arteries for diagnostic, monitoring or therapeutic purposes.

Investigational procedures: Cardiac catheterization and arteriography are associated with a low but important incidence of injury to the aorta and limb arteries. The brachial artery is relatively small and prone to spasm, and when used for access, thrombosis may be precipitated by endothelial injury, obstruction to blood flow by the catheter, arterial narrowing following inexpert suturing after the procedure, and spasm. The femoral artery is larger and less prone to spasm, but involvement by atheromatous disease is frequent and passage of a catheter may raise an intimal flap that causes obstruction and thrombosis. At any site, accidental injection of contrast material into the wall of an artery may produce a dissection, with subsequent obstruction and thrombosis of the lumen.

Monitoring procedures: Increasing use is being made of radial artery cannulation for continuous recording of arterial pressure, and for serial sampling of arterial blood for gas and pH measurement. Should hand blood flow be markedly dependent on the radial artery, ischemia during and after cannulation may result. Although the radial artery is dominant in 55% of patients,[10] severe complications are unusual. In a prospective study, the radial artery thrombosed after cannulation in 38% of cases, but recanalization subsequently occurred in all those who were followed up.[2]

Therapeutic procedures: Aortic balloon counterpulsation in cardiogenic shock is associated with a high incidence of arterial thrombosis and lower limb ischemia. The technic requires the passage of a large balloon catheter via the femoral artery to the thoracic aorta, where the catheter remains for several days. The iliac and femoral arteries in these patients are usually atheromatous, and elevation of an intimal plaque during catheter insertion, and partial arterial occlusion by the catheter, explain the high incidence of complications.

The Fogarty balloon catheter, introduced in 1963,[11] revoluationized the removal of arterial embolic material and thrombus. During embolectomy, the catheter tip or balloon may also raise an intimal flap and precipitate thrombosis. Percutaneous transluminal angioplasty is another procedure that involves the passage of a special balloon catheter, in this case to the site of an arterial stenosis which is dilated by inflation of the balloon. The technic is mainly employed to dilate a localized atheromatous stenosis in the iliac artery. After dilatation, early thrombosis may occur secondary to a dissection or intimal flap.

Accidental injury: Blunt injury, gunshot injury, and a displaced bone fracture or joint dislocation may result in arterial compression, crushing, stretching, penetration, laceration, or complete severance. Laceration may also be caused by broken glass or a knife. Penetrating injury, often with associated sepsis, is seen in the femoral and brachial arteries of drug addicts. The passage of a high-velocity bullet some distance from an artery sets up shearing forces that disrupt the intima. The end results of accidental trauma include endothelial damage, an intimal flap, vasospasm, and thrombosis.

Chronic compression: Long-standing arterial compression may result in arterial injury and thrombosis. Examples are subclavian artery compression by surrounding bone and muscle in the thoracic outlet syndrome, and popliteal artery compression by the medial head of the gastrocnemius muscle, when that muscle passes lateral to the artery. Prolonged incorrect use of a crutch severely damages the axillary artery, which may eventually thrombose.

Chemical injury: This commonly occurs when a therapeutic agent intended for intravenous administration is inadvertently injected into a nearby artery. Particularly at risk from this misadventure is the patient with a high bifurcation of the brachial artery, in which case the ulnar artery tends to run a superficial course. Thrombosis proceeding to ischemic muscle contracture and skin gangrene after the intra-arterial injection of thiopental sodium 10% and 5% is well documented, but is fortunately very rare when the 2.5% solution is used. Thiopental causes production of large amounts of catecholamines in the arterial and arteriolar walls, and there may be intra-arterial deposition of thiopental crystals. Intra-arterial injection of diazepam[12] and floxacillin[13] also causes severe ischemia, as does sodium tetradecyl sulphate (STD), which is employed for sclerotherapy of varicose veins. STD does not appear to cause direct arterial injury, but denatures the blood-causing formation of a sludge that obstructs the microcirculation.[14]

Cold injury: The thermal injury caused by exposure to freezing causes the subcutaneous vessels to become packed with sludged and agglutinated red blood cells, and thrombosis frequently follows.

Compression Prolonged external arterial compression reduces blood flow and leads to thrombosis. One cause is severe muscle swelling within a fascial compartment after unaccustomed exercise, muscle ischemia or trauma, or venous injury. The increased pressure within the compartment impairs venous return, and may also be sufficient to cause arterial thrombosis. Prolonged application of a limb tourniquet, particularly in a patient with sickle cell anemia, is a further example.

Vascular grafts Grafts employed in the treatment of peripheral vascular disease usually comprise autologous vein or prosthetic material, which is implanted as a patch, or as a tube to bypass diseased native vessels. Following the insertion of a prosthetic graft, healing occurs on the inner graft surface with the formation of a neointima (or pseudo-intima) that is initially composed of thrombus. After compression by blood flowing through the graft, this thrombus is replaced by a less thrombogenic lining of fibrin.

Platelets adhere to a newly inserted graft,[15] and are intimately concerned in graft thrombus formation.[16] At this time, platelet survival is markedly shortened, and may not have returned to normal nine months later.[16] Nonthrombogenic endothelial linings in grafts develop as a pannus ingrowth from the anastomosed vessel or from blood stream sources, but rarely, if ever, does this ingrowth completely coat grafts in humans.[17] Accordingly, nonendothelialized neointima is a persistent feature of prosthetic grafts in humans.

The choice of graft material and diameter are two important considerations in graft thrombosis, particularly in low blood flow situations such as pertain below the knee. Regarding thrombogenicity, Dacron is only satisfactory where there is a high flow, and therefore its use is usually confined to reconstructions above and including the common femoral artery. Below this level, saphenous vein, the least thrombogenic graft, is employed when possible. Commonly used substitutes for saphenous vein are expanded polytetrafluoroethylene and gluteraldehyde-stabilized umbilical vein. These materials are almost as satisfactory as vein when placed above the knee, but are definitely more prone to thrombosis when used below the knee.

The relationship between graft diameter and thrombosis is not entirely clear. The graft must be wide enough to carry the required blood flow, but narrow enough for blood flow velocity to exceed the critical value that allows thrombus to form. Allowance must be made for the reduction in graft luminal area and increased hemodynamic resistance caused by the layer of pseudointima which may be up to 1.5 mm thick. Turbulence is more likely in small grafts (0 to 5 mm diameter), and this factor seems to counteract the benefit of increased velocity. Prosthetic grafts less than 6 mm diameter and vein grafts less than 4 mm diameter are infrequently used because of the greater tendency to thrombosis.

Graft thrombosis may occur early after insertion, and the usual causes are reduction of graft blood flow by impaired cardiac output during anesthesia or hypovolemia, inadequate inflow pressure related to proximal arterial disease, inadequate "run off" because of severe distal disease, graft twisting or kinking, and a technical error such as an intimal flap or narrowing at one of the anastomoses. In contrast, late graft occlusion is strongly associated with smoking, the incidence of occlusion being three to four times higher in smokers than nonsmokers.[18] Further causes are progress of arterial disease, graft compression such as that caused by sleeping on the side of an axillo-femoral graft, and graft kinking. Prolonged couching may kink a graft that crosses the knee.

Late graft thrombosis is also caused by excessive thickening of the neointima, a disorder termed neointimal fibrous hyperplasia. Platelets contribute to this lesion, which forms a circumferential deposit of fibrous tissue, usually at the site of an arterial-prosthetic graft anastomosis.[19] Vein graft stricture at the site of a valve or where injury by a clamp has occurred during surgery, and arteriosclerotic stenosis in the vein are also causes of late thrombosis.

Vasospasm Raynaud's syndrome is the commonest of the vasospastic disorders, and the severe form, Raynaud's phenomenon, is most frequently associated with scleroderma, in which there may be thrombosis of the distal ulnar artery, superficial palmar arch, and digital arteries.[20] Prolonged ingestion of excessive amounts of ergot-containing drugs by migraine sufferers induces extremity arterial spasm, which in severe cases progresses proximally and leads to extensive thrombosis and gangrene. The treatment of cardiogenic shock by prolonged administration of a high dose of an inotropic drug that has alpha-adrenergic activity, may also result in extremity vasoconstriction of sufficient severity to cause arterial thrombosis. Beta-blocker drugs impair the peripheral circulation and aggravate the effects of arterial occlusive and vasospastic disease,[21] even to the extent of causing gangrene.[22]

Embolism Embolism causes occlusion and stasis thrombosis in healthy and diseased arteries.

Vascular surgery The use of an aortic or aterial clamp during vascular surgery results in distal stasis, and red thrombus often forms in the arterial tree. Technical faults such as excessive arterial narrowing during repair of an arteriotomy, or failure to secure an intimal flap after endarterectomy may result in impaired blood flow and thrombosis. Stasis during surgery is also promoted by hypovolemia, hypotension, and limb cooling; and in the brachial, radial, and ulnar arteries, by severe spasm.

Venous obstruction Phlegmasia cerulea dolens and arteriovenous fistula are two situations in which venous return may be compromised to the extent that gangrene and arterial thrombosis occur.

Blood disorders Polycythemia, leukemia, sickle cell anemia, and paraproteinemias such as myeloma are associated with increased blood viscosity and resistance to blood flow, while thrombocytosis and thrombocythemia increase blood coagulability. Severe dehydration also increases blood viscosity, and may lead to acute limb ischemia.[23] Circulating cryoglobulins, cryofibrinogens, and cold agglutinins increase the chance of small vessel occlusion during cold exposure. These disorders, together with the previously described increase in hemoglobin and fibrinogen concentration, and reduction of red cell flexibility that occur in peripheral vascular disease, predispose to arterial thrombosis.

Heparin administration is occasionally associated with the development of thrombocytopenia, heparin resistance, and arterial platelet thrombus formation,[24,25] and the mechanism is probably an immune-mediated reaction. Antithrombin III deficiency is inherited as an autosomal dominant trait with incomplete penetrance, or occurs in other conditions such as hepatic insufficiency, and may cause arterial and prosthetic graft thrombosis.[26] Severe disseminated intravascular coagulation may also cause extremity artery thrombosis.

Carbon monoxide poisoning   Carbon monoxide reduces blood pressure and causes tissue asphyxia. These changes, together with prolonged skin pressure in the unconscious patient and pre-existing limb arteriosclerosis, predispose to limb gangrene which probably precedes thrombosis.[27,28]

Advanced carcinoma   Malignant disease is frequently complicated by venous thrombosis, but occasionally large arteries such as the popliteal, and smaller ones such as the digital arteries, thrombose.[29]

Embolism

About 80% of arterial emboli come from the heart, and arteriosclerotic heart disease has replaced rheumatic heart disease as the commonest cause. In about 10% of cases of embolism, no source can be found. Most arterial emboli pass to sites that influence limb blood flow.

Heart   Thrombus formation occurs on damaged and prosthetic heart valves, and on endocardium injured by underlying myocardial infarction. Thrombus also forms where blood flow is stagnant or turbulent, such as in the left atrium in atrial fibrillation and mitral valve disease, and in a left ventricular aneurysm or ventricle affected by cardiomyopathy. Myxoma, a tumor usually found in the left atrium, is a rare cause of systemic embolism.

Aorta and the large arteries   Arteriosclerotic ulcerating,[30-33] occlusive and aneurysmal disease are associated with the formation of platelet thrombus, which, together with atheromatous debris, can become detached and embolize. Proximal arteriosclerotic disease is being increasingly incriminated as a source of small emboli to the limbs. In the upper limb, thrombus often embolizes from the stenosed origin of the left subclavian artery, or from a subclavian poststenotic aneurysm in patients with a cervical rib or band (Figure 7-2). Similarly, thrombus within a popliteal aneurysm commonly embolizes to the foot. In both the upper and lower limb, repeated embolism with progressive occlusion of the distal circulation sometimes necessitates major amputation.

Embolism of atheromatous and thrombotic material occasionally occurs during surgical dissection around the abdominal aorta and iliac arteries or during removal of the left lumbar sympathetic chain, and results in "trash" foot or leg. Another cause of embolism from the aorta and large arteries is dislodgment of atheromatous debris and thrombus by a needle or catheter during arteriography or percutaneous transluminal angioplasty, and by a balloon counterpulsation catheter during insertion.

Drug particles   A not infrequent sight in the vascular surgical ward is the drug addict who has injected a solution containing powdered drug particles into a wrist or groin artery, the outcome being acute hand or foot ischemia.

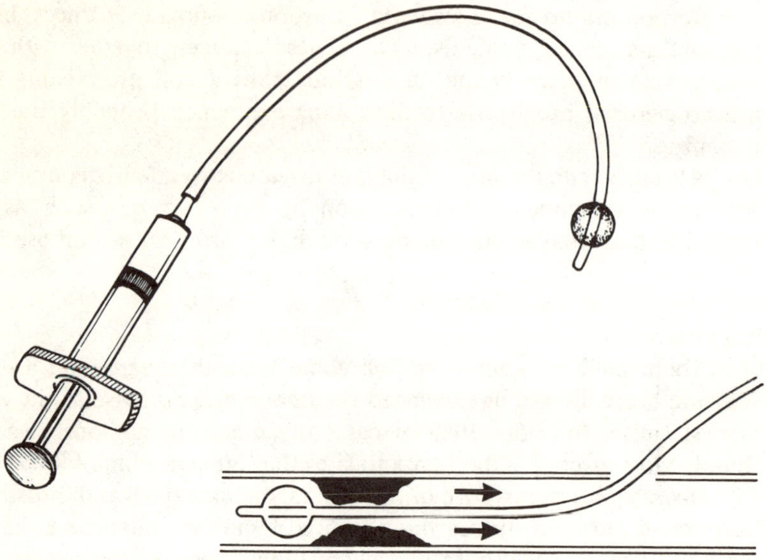

Figure 7-2 Fogarty balloon catheter, and embolectomy technic.

Paradoxical embolism Venous thromboembolism may be associated with arterial embolism when the foramen ovale is patent or when a septal defect is present.

Heparin Heparin administration for more than a few days may result in thrombocytopenia, arterial thrombosis, and systemic embolism.[25]

Prosthetic graft As described previously, thrombus formation in prosthetic grafts is common, and occasionally this thrombus breaks free and embolizes. Unstable graft neointima may also embolize.

Therapeutic embolism Intra-arterial injection of absorbable gelatin sponge, lyophilized human dura mater, plastic or glass beads, or instant-setting polymers is employed to occlude certain types of vascular malformation and benign tumors of vascular origin. Should the material pass into the arterial tree distal to the lesions, vascular occlusion may result.

Outcome

Embolism and thrombosis causing arterial occlusion result in acute ischemia, the severity of which is related to the completeness of arterial obstruction, the level of obstruction, the rapidity with which stasis clot propagates, the existence of previous disease, the status of the collateral circulation, the cardiac output, the duration of the obstruction, and the age of the patient. With regard to age, sudden occlusion of the common femoral artery in the adult is very likely to cause ischemic necrosis, but in the infant or child may cause only impairment of limb growth.[34]

Pallor because of reduced tissue blood content, and anesthesia because nerve tissue is most sensitive to local ischemia, are the first signs of acute severe limb ischemia. Skeletal muscle shows histologic evidence of injury after two hours of severe ischemia, and after six to eight hours, both skin and muscle are markedly damaged. The outcome of septic embolism from bacterial endocarditis may be a mycotic aneurysm.

CLINICAL MANIFESTATIONS

The clinical manifestations of limb thrombosis and emobolism are ischemia and features of the underlying disorder. Thus, the clinician must confirm the presence of ischemia and evaluate its severity, and also make every effort to find the cause.

Ischemia

The symptoms of acute limb ischemia are paresthesia, numbness, pain, and inability to move the part. The history includes a careful account of the time, and the site and suddenness of onset of symptoms, and details of the subsequent course. Symptoms of acute ischemia at more than one site, eg, the abdomen and a limb, suggest multiple emboli. Progressive symptoms point to very severe ischemia with increasing tissue damage, whereas a gradual easing of symptoms indicates that blood flow is sufficient to maintain tissue viability. The history also includes details of recent chest pain, cardiac disease, past limb ischemia, vascular surgical procedures, drug ingestion, arterial trauma, and other pointers to an underlying cause.

Inspection of the limb will show pallor if ischemia is severe and the duration is short; otherwise there may be a bluish mottling. Muscle wasting, atrophic skin, and nail deformities indicate long-standing ischemia. A sinus over the groin or elbow vessels suggests repeated puncture associated with drug abuse. Grooves in the lower limb subcutaneous tissue are caused by spasm of variocose veins in ergot poisoning, and marked extremity skin gangrene is a feature of frostbite. Signs of cardiac failure are frequent in older patients.

The heart rhythm is noted, and all the peripheral pulses are examined, namely the radial, subclavian, carotid, and superficial temporal in the upper half of the body; the abdominal aorta; and the iliac, common femoral, popliteal, and ankle pulses in the lower half. Pulsation should also be sought in any superficial vascular bypass graft. The limb skin temperature gradient is determined by passing the back of the hand distally along the limb. Normally, there is a progressive decrease in temperature, but a sudden fall over an ischemic part is characteristic. The site of the symptoms, the pattern of pulse deficit, and the presence of an abnormal skin temperature gradient are guides to the approximate level of arterial obstruction.

Extremity sensation and movement are tested. Anesthesia of the glove or stocking type indicates severe skin and cutaneous nerve ischemia, and muscle paralysis and tenderness imply severe muscle ischemia. Muscle contracture (rigor) is a sign of ischemia of more than 24 hours duration, and indicates that the condition is irremedial. This sign is most frequently encountered as a fixed plantar flexion of the foot caused by irreversible ischemia of the posterior tibial muscle. Further signs of irremedial ischemia are patchy, fixed skin cyanosis that may become confluent, and skin blistering.

The physical examination also includes a search for signs of the cause of ischemia, as now described.

Thrombosis

Ischemic symptoms and signs may be mild when thrombotic arterial occlusion is superimposed on marked arteriosclerotic stenosis, for two reasons. Firstly, arterial blood pressure and flow are not appreciably impaired until the arterial cross-sectional area is reduced by more than 75% (usually 80% to 95%), corresponding to not less than a 50% reduction in diameter.[35] Secondly, as narrowing of the main artery occurs, any impairment of blood flow is compensated for by an increase in collateral flow. Therefore, quite marked arterial stenosis may occur without causing symptoms, and the onset of superadded thrombosis and complete occlusion in an atheromatous lower limb artery is often associated with nothing more than moderate intermittent claudication. This symptom is characterized by pain which develops in muscle after a constant amount of exercise, and which is relieved by rest. An example is the patient with complete occlusion of the superficial femoral artery who has to stop walking after 100 yards because of pain in the calf muscles. After a brief period of rest, pain is relieved and the patient continues walking.

Should the collateral circulation not be well developed—a situation that applies when the occluded artery was previously healthy, or the collateral vessels are diseased—thrombosis is likely to cause severe acute ischemia. If the limb survives, the outcome may be severe chronic ischemia, and the chief symptom is rest pain. This pain is felt in the foot, particularly at night, and tends to be relieved by hanging the foot out of bed or by standing. Very severe rest pain causes the patient to sleep in a chair, and to flex the limb close to the body such that flexion deformities eventually develop. The foot is tender, and there is pallor on leg elevation, and rubor when the foot is pendent.

Thrombotic occlusion of the arteriosclerotic infrarenal abdominal aorta in the male presents as the Leriche syndrome, in which there is impotence, bilateral buttock claudication, and absence of the lower limb pulses. Restriction of blood flow in both internal iliac arteries is likely to manifest as buttock claudication and vasculogenic impotence. External iliac arterial occlusion is associated with thigh claudication and wasting.

Inadvertent intra-arterial drug injection causes immediate, burning extremity pain, followed within hours by patchy skin cyanosis and limb swelling. Thrombosis of the radial and ulnar arteries characteristically causes Volkmann's ischemic contracture of the forearm muscles, while digital artery thrombosis is likely to lead to black mummification of the digits.

Underlying disorder Whenever thrombosis is diagnosed, the underlying cause must be sought. Arteriosclerotic occlusive disease is indicated by a past history of intermittent claudication or rest pain in one or both legs, evidence of ischemia elsewhere such as angina or stroke, and the presence of risk factors such as smoking and diabetes. Additionally, there may be a past history of vascular reconstructive surgery as evidenced by healed surgical wounds. Inquiry will be made concerning recent accidental trauma, intra-arterial investigative and therapeutic procedures, intra-arterial drug injection, ingestion of ergot-containing drugs, and any known blood disorder.

Examination of the fingers may show nicotine staining, and examination of the abdominal aorta and limb arteries may reveal pulse deficits, bruits, and thrills. Signs of neuropathy such as anesthesia and lack of extremity sweating are found in diabetics. Vascular graft thrombosis is sometimes caused by athero-embolism from a proximal aneurysm or ulcerated atheromatous plaque,[36] and clinical evidence for these possibilities should be sought.

Thrombosis of an aneurysm as the cause of ischemia is diagnosed by the finding of a tender mass at the groin or behind the knee, and in such a patient there may also be a pulsating aneurysm in the abdomen or behind the contralateral knee.

Embolism

Most patients with embolism have a history of cardiac disease and of associated disorders such as peripheral arterial occlusive disease and diabetes mellitus. A small proportion of patients will have suffered a previous embolic episode. Many arterial emboli are clinically silent, and the first sign is often the incidental finding of missing peripheral pulses in a patient with mitral stenosis or atrial fibrillation. In contrast, saddle embolism presents as a life-threatening catastrophe.

Major embolism The arrest of a large embolus in a previously normal arterial tree causes severe ischemia because the collateral circulation is not well-developed. About 15% of emboli that impair lower limb blood flow arrest at the aortic bifurcation, and the result is severe bilateral leg ischemia and loss of all lower limb pulses. One third of emboli lodge at the common femoral artery bifurcation, and in this case there is ischemia from the mid-thigh distally, and loss of knee and ankle pulses although the groin pulse is usually preserved. Most large emboli to the upper limb lodge in the proximal brachial artery at the origin of the deep brachial artery or at the brachial artery bifurcation.

Minor embolism   A small embolus may partially occlude a large artery and cause mild ischemia, or completely occlude a smaller, more distal artery. A very small embolus will often reach the extremity and produce painful cyanosis of one digit.[31] In this case, the subsequent course is either one of improvement, or of progression to well-demarcated digital gangrene. "Trash" foot is diagnosed when there is pain, skin mottling, and coolness despite the presence of normal ankle pulses, during or immediately after arterial surgery. Multiple systemic emboli from thrombus in a mycotic aneurysm may cause diffuse miliary sepsis of the extremity soft tissues.

Multiple embolism   About 10% of lower limb embolic episodes are associated with simultaneous embolism to another site. Therefore, evidence should be sought for acute ischemia at sites other than the limbs, such a the gut, kidneys, and brain. Multiple aneurysms at unusual sites suggest multiple septic emboli.

Septic embolism   A septic embolus may lead to the formation of a mycotic aneurysm, and 80% of cases have this etiology. Mycotic aneurysm comprises some 4% of all aneurysms, and presents as a painful, inflamed pulsating mass, perhaps with evidence of systemic sepsis. Continuing enlargement may result in rupture.

Source of embolism   In acute limb ischemia and suspected embolism, the history and examination must always include a search for an embolic source. Relevant factors in the history will be known atrial fibrillation, recent myocardial infarction with the possibility of a left ventricular mural thrombosis, ischemic heart disease, rheumatic heart disease, prosthetic heart valve insertion, and cardiomyopathy. Subacute bacterial endocarditis affecting the aortic or mitral valves is a likely embolic source in mycotic aneurysm. A known proximal aneurysm, or a history of recent trauma which could produce a false aneurysm may be important, as may heparin administration, or the injection of a powdered drug. The physical examination includes determination of heart rhythm and size, and a search for cardiac murmurs. Aortic and more distal aneurysms and bruits will be sought, not forgetting examination of the popliteal arteries.

INVESTIGATIONS

Certain investigations should be urgently performed in every patient presenting with acute limb ischemia, because these investigations, together with the history and physical examination, enable decisions to be made regarding immediate treatment. Subsequently, more complex studies may be required fully to elucidate the nature of the underlying disorder, and to guide long-term management.

Ischemia Although evaluation of the severity of acute limb ischemia is mainly by clinical assessment, the systolic arterial pressure at the wrist or ankle should be measured using the Doppler ultrasound probe. This pressure is then compared with the pressure in the uninvolved brachial artery. The ankle/brachial systolic arterial pressure index is normally greater than 1.0, but in severe ischemia secondary to major arterial occlusion may be less than 0.25. In the most severe forms of ischemia, no arterial Doppler signal can be detected over the anterior tibial, posterior tibial, or peroneal arteries at the ankle, or over the radial or ulnar arteries at the wrist. Doppler systolic arterial pressure is similarly used as an index of improvement after treatment. Unfortunately, there is no sensitive, easily performed, and reliable means of quantifying extremity ischemia, but skin appearance, sensation, and temperature are guides to changes in extremity blood flow.

Blood tests Routine investigations include the hemoglobin concentration to exclude anemia and polycythemia, the white cell count to exclude infection and leukemia, and the platelet count. A high platelet count may be caused by thrombocythemia, or thrombocytosis associated with underlying malignancy, inflammatory disease, infection, or asplenism. A low platelet count in a patient receiving heparin suggests heparin-induced thrombocytopenia. It is important that the platelets be counted, and that reliance is not solely placed on examination of a blood film. Baseline clotting studies are of value if anticoagulant therapy has been or is likely to be administered. Repeated blood cultures are essential if bacterial endocarditis or mycotic aneurysm is suspected.

The erythrocyte sedimentation rate will be raised in patients with arteritis, bacterial endocarditis, and atrial myxoma. The fasting blood sugar level should always be estimated, because a fifth or more of patients with peripheral vascular disease are diabetic. At a later stage, the fasting blood lipids should also be examined. Cardiac enzymes are of value if it is suspected that mural thrombus overlying a recent myocardial infarct has embolized, and thyroid function tests should be considered in all patients with atrial fibrillation to exclude thryotoxicosis as the cause. The serum proteins are analyzed to exclude paraproteinemia.

The diagnosis of arteritis will be aided by immunologic tests including anti-nuclear antibodies, complement profile, rheumatoid factor, and other autoantibodies. The finding of thrombocytopenia in a patient receiving heparin requires in vitro analysis of the effect of heparin on platelet aggregation. For this test, platelet-poor plasma is prepared and mixed with donor platelets; the result is positive if platelet aggregation occurs on the addition of heparin. Occasionally, this test is negative, but is positive on the addition of heparin to a mixture of the patient's platelet-poor plasma and his own platelets. In the patient with concurrent venous and arterial thrombosis, or in whom recurrent graft thrombosis has occurred without discernible cause, the antithrombin III level should be estimated.

ECG   All patients presenting with acute limb ischemia should have an electrocardiogram to detect disturbance of cardiac rhythm, recent myocardial infarction, long-standing ischemic heart disease, evidence of mitral valve disease, and left ventricular aneurysm. Because rhythm disturbances are often episodic, a 24-hour tape recording of the electrocardiogram should be made if dysrhythmia is strongly suspected.

Radiography   The chest film gives information about the heart and the thoracic aorta, and may show a cervical rib. Left atrial enlargement suggests mitral stenosis, and left ventricular enlargement may indicate myocardial ischemia, a ventricular aneurysm, or cardiomyopathy. A calcified or prosthetic heart valve will be noted. A mediastinal mass may represent a thoracic aortic aneurysm, and a cervical rib indicates the possibility of a poststenotic subclavian artery aneurysm.

The plain abdominal radiograph will detect calcified atheromas in the abdominal aorta and iliac arteries, particularly when these are aneurysmal. A lateral view of the abdomen centered anterior to the spine frequently identifies the anterior and posterior walls of an abdominal aortic aneurysm. In the patient with suspected limb embolism, the presence of bowel fluid levels indicates the need to consider simultaneous visceral embolism.

Limb arteriography is frequently not of value in severe acute ischemia because the procedure is time-consuming and the findings do not usually alter management. When limb ischemia is very severe and embolism is strongly suspected, time should not be wasted performing arteriography. However, when severe ischemia persists for several days in a limb that is still viable, arteriography will indicate whether the cause was thrombosis or embolism, and whether delayed embolectomy or surgical reconstruction is possible. Embolism is suggested by a well-defined transverse or convex upper limit of the obstruction which may be at an unusual site for thrombosis, normal proximal vessels, and lack of a well-developed collateral circulation. An incompletely occluding embolus will be seen as a filling defect. Arteriography is essential when mycotic aneurysm is suspected.

Localization of the source of an embolus may require cardiac angiography as described below, or aortic or peripheral angiography, looking for atheromatous plaques or an aneurysm.

Ultrasound   Doppler ultrasound velocimetry is a very useful method for determining patency of a superficial vascular graft, because failure to detect arterial flow signifies graft occlusion. Initial evaluation of the heart as a source of emboli is best achieved using echocardiography, which shows details of the valves, the size of the heart chambers and thickness of the walls, and the filling defects in the left atrium and ventricle. If further detail is required, cardiac angiography should be performed.

Abdominal ultrasound, computed tomography (CT) of the thoracic and abdominal aorta, and ultrasound of the subclavian and popliteal arteries enable detection of an aneurysm that may be a source of emboli.

DIAGNOSIS AND DIFFERENTIAL DIAGNOSIS

Diagnosis

Thrombosis and embolism may both present as acute limb ischemia, and although the distinction is often difficult, correct diagnosis is important because the management is usually very different. Attempted thrombectomy of a badly diseased artery in the mistaken belief that embolism has occurred is likely to fail, and may even extend the occlusive process. Conversely, not to remove an occluding embolus from a normal major artery is likely to have dire consequences. A frequent difficulty is that most patients with embolism have ischemic heart disease and associated moderate or severe peripheral vascular disease. Also, thrombosis occasionally occurs suddenly without an apparent underlying cause, making differentiation from embolism difficult. Acute ischemia in the patient who is under 40 years of age and who does not have a history of rheumatic heart disease is likely to be caused by thrombosis secondary to a nonvascular disorder.

Severe ischemia Severe limb ischemia is diagnosed by the history and examination. The sudden onset of pain and skin color change is often associated with inability to use the affected part. Examination shows pulse deficiency, and distal coolness and anesthesia. The ischemic part is not swollen and warm as in acute venous occlusion, and the absence of pulses excludes severe extremity vasospasm. When there is neither a history suggestive of previous ischemia, nor signs of arterial occlusion elsewhere, embolism should be strongly suspected.

Saddle embolus is diagnosed when sudden acute ischemia of both legs is associated with the loss of all lower limb pulses. A common femoral embolus is characterized by acute ischemia from the mid-thigh down, and loss of the ipsilateral knee and ankle pulses; the contralateral limb is frequently normal. Acute arm ischemia is usually caused by embolism because atheroma is unusual in the upper limb. Evidence for a source of embolism, such as a heart disease, proximal occlusive or aneurysmal arterial disease, or a proximal vascular graft that is still patent supports a diagnosis of embolism.

In contrast to the above, acute ischemia in association with long-standing vascular disease suggests that the cause is superadded thrombosis of a stenosed artery. This etiology is also likely when the severity of

152

ischemia is much less than would be expected from the pattern of pulse deficiency, indicating that the collateral circulation is well-developed. When acute ischemia occurs in a limb with a vascular graft that is pulseless and without a Doppler arterial signal, the presumptive diagnosis is that the graft has thrombosed. A recently thrombosed artery is often tender for some weeks. and this sign helps to confirm the diagnosis. A tender mass behind the knee in a patient with acute lower leg ischemia strongly suggests a thrombosed popliteal aneurysm.

Mild ischemia   The onset of mild ischemia may be the result of partial arterial occlusion by an embolus in a previously normal limb, or of thrombosis in a limb with diseased arteries and a good collateral circulation. It is important that the possibility of embolism is considered in this situation.

Digital ischemia   Localized, well-demarcated digital ischemia suggests a small embolus, a vasospastic disorder, arteritis, a blood disorder such as thrombocythemia, or an underlying malignancy.

Progressive distal ischemia   Multiple small arterial emboli may present with a clinical picture of chronic extremity ischemia initially affecting the digits alone, but with time, progressing more proximally. Undiagnosed, progress is relentless and eventually necessitates major amputation. A typical example is hand and forearm ischemia secondary to multiple small athero-emboli arising from a poststenotic subclavian aneurysm associated with a cervical rib or band.

Mycotic aneurysm   An aneurysm at an unusual site that has not been traumatized strongly suggests that the lesion is a mycotic aneurysm secondary to an infected embolus, particularly when there is a history of bacterial endocarditis.

Differential Diagnosis

Reduced cardiac output   A prolonged reduction of cardiac output, as in cardiogenic shock, may result in cold mottled limbs and difficulty palpating the pulses. Reassurance that the axial limb arteries are patent is obtained by measuring ankle and wrist systolic pressures with the Doppler ultrasound probe, and comparing these values with the brachial artery pressure.

Vasoconstrictor drugs   Prolonged systemic administration of cardiac inotropic agents that have alpha-adrenergic activity may result in marked extremity cyanosis and coldness, although the wrist and ankle systolic pressures are normal. Ingestion of a high dose of an ergot preparation used for the treatment of migraine causes the well-known condition of ergotism. Initially, the extremities are cold and blue, but there may be centripetal progression if the drug is not withdrawn. Enquiry should always be made about headache and migraine to exclude the possibility of ergotism.

Venous gangrene   Severe limb ischemia secondary to phlegmasia cerulea dolens or arteriovenous fistula is associated with limb swelling, edema, cyanosis, and skin blistering.

Dissecting aneurysm   Chest and abdominal pain in a hypertensive subject may be followed by acute pulseless ischemia in one or more limbs. The chest film may show widening of the thoracic aorta and a double outline at the aortic arch. Computed tomography confirms the diagnosis.

Vasospastic disorders   Certain chronic vasospastic disorders may give the appearance of severe limb ischemia. Acrocyanosis appearing de novo, or in association with limb paralysis secondary to spina bifida of spinal injury, presents as persistently cold, blue extremities. However, the wrist and ankle systolic pressure are usually normal.

Beta-blockers   Beta-blocker therapy in the patient with peripheral vascular disease frequently aggravates limb ischemia, causing increased cold sensitivity, extremity cyanosis, and occasionally, painful digital skin ulcers. Careful enquiry about drug ingestion must always be made in the patient presenting with limb ischemia.

Lumbar spinal canal stenosis   Stenosis of the lumbar spinal canal may cause ischemia of the cauda equina during lower limb exercise, resulting in neurogenic intermittent claudication of the legs. Leg pain tends to come on after standing or a certain amount of exercise, but unlike vascular claudication, takes a long time to resolve on resting and often causes the patient to sit down for ten or 15 minutes. There may be other symptoms related to the lumbosacral plexus such as perineal paresthesias, and urinary sphincter incontinence. Arterial examination is normal in these patients.

Venous claudication   The patient with iliofemoral vein obstruction may develop increased venous pressure in the calf when walking. This ambulatory venous hypertension is manifested as a tight, bursting pain coming on after walking a certain distance, and this symptom may be confused with ischemic claudication.

TREATMENT AND PREVENTION

Immediate management is dictated by the duration, severity, and cause of ischemia.

Ischemia

Severe acute ischemia   Treatment is urgent. As soon as acute severe limb ischemia is diagnosed, pain should be relieved with intravenous morphine given by the titration method. Provided there is no contraindication such as recent trauma or leaking aneurysm, intravenous heparin 10,000 IU is given to limit anterograde and retrograde thrombosis. The limb is kept cool, and limb pressure points are protected. In the lower limb, use of a bed cradle and a skeepskin boot or underblanket will relieve pressure on the heels. Impaired cardiac output associated with hypovolemia, dehydration, and cardiac disease is corrected.

Major embolism   When major lower limb embolism is diagnosed, embolectomy with a balloon catheter (Figure 7-3) should be carried out

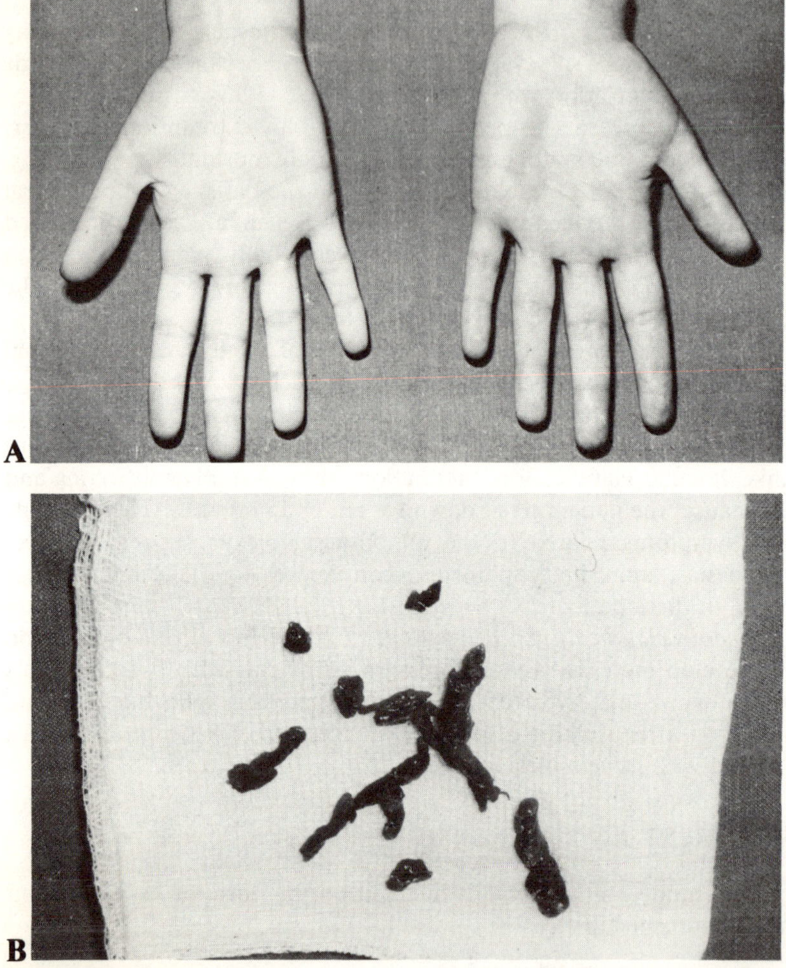

Figure 7-3   A Hands of 22-year-old female with bilateral cervical ribs and athero-embolism to the right arm over a four-week period. Absent right arm pulses and a right subclavian poststenotic aneurysm. Treated by resection of the right cervical rib, cervical sympathectomy, thrombectomy, and repair of the aneurysm, and balloon catheter thrombectomy of the arm as far as the wrist. **B** Athero-embolic material removed from the aneurysm and arm arteries. Microscopic examination showed thrombus, culture sterile. Excellent clinical result.

urgently, usually under local anesthesia. To remove a saddle embolus, the common femoral artery is exposed in both groins and a balloon catheter passed proximally via an arteriotomy in each artery, to the aortic bifurcation. The balloon is inflated and the catheter gently withdrawn, bringing with it the thromboembolic material. This procedure is repeated until a good downflow of blood is achieved. Thrombus in the deep and superficial femoral arteries is similarly removed until good backflow is established.

When a common femoral artery embolus is diagnosed, the ipsilateral artery is opened, and arterial pressure from above often expresses the embolus. All thrombus is removed using the balloon catheter as previously described. It is most important that the embolectomy specimen is both cultured and examined microscopically. Microscopic examination may show cleft-like cholesterol spaces suggestive of athero-embolism, platelet thrombus, or myxoma. The growth of organisms on culture of the embolus will instigate investigation for possible bacterial endocarditis.

When severe leg ischemia has been present for more than six hours, revascularization of the damaged lower leg muscles may be followed by complications. Each of the three lower leg muscle groups is confined within a discrete fascial compartment, and gross swelling of the revascularized muscle causes a compartment compression syndrome with pain and paralysis of the muscles concerned. Should compartment compression be considered likely to occur, division of the deep fascia over the involved compartments is necessary.

Myoglobinemia is another important complication associated with revascularization of the severely ischemic limb. Myoglobinuria causes renal injury and acute renal failure,[37] and efforts should therefore be made to obtain a good diuresis at the time of embolectomy. If myoglobinuria occurs, sodium bicarbonate is given to alkalinize the urine because myoglobin precipitates more readily in the renal tubules in an acid milieu.

The athero-embolism that occurs during vascular surgery and causes "trash" foot and/or leg is not responsive to balloon catheter thrombectomy because the main arteries are patent. However, the author has had good results in two patients treated with prostaglandin E_1 by a central intravenous infusion, 10–15 ng kg^{-1} min^{-1} for 72 hours (Figure 7-4).

Thrombosis Most patients with acute leg ischemia secondary to thrombosis have severe underlying arterial disease, and initial treatment is with intravenous heparin to inhibit clot propagation. There is currently little enthusiasm for treatment of acute thrombosis by thrombolytic therapy with local intra-arterial infusion of streptokinase or urokinase, because the incidence of complications is high. Symptomatic improvement in patients treated conservatively is dependent on an increase in collateral blood flow. Frequently, there is no improvement, and if symp-

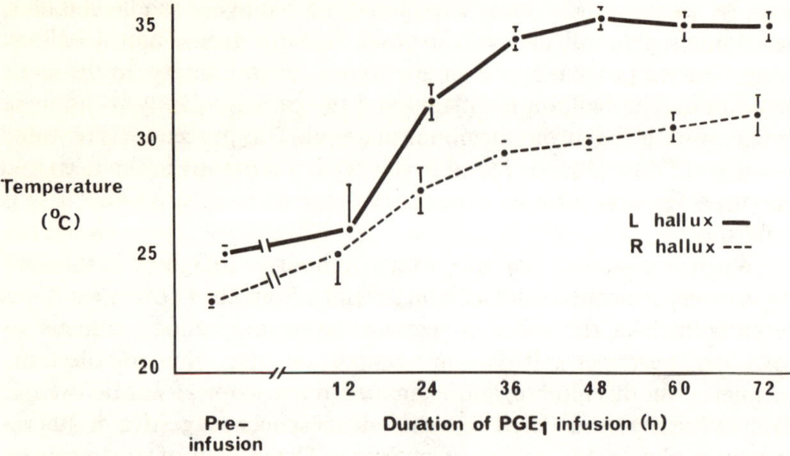

Figure 7-4 Hallux skin temperature changes during prostaglandin E₁ infusion in a 69-year-old man. Severe "trash" feet and legs, worse on the right, occurred after a difficult redo aorto-iliac reconstruction. No response with intravenous dextran 70 and alcohol. Prostaglandin E₁ infusion 3 ng kg⁻¹ min⁻¹ commenced 24 hours after operation, and the dose increased to 10 ng kg⁻¹ min⁻¹. Skin temperature measured in uncontrolled ward conditions. Data shown as mean and SD of hourly recordings during each preceding 12 hours. Clinical response excellent.

toms continue to be severe and arteriography shows that vascular reconstruction is not possible, major amputation must be considered although lumbar sympathectomy occasionally averts this disaster. Sometimes, the patient's general condition at presentation is so poor that only symptomatic treatment is indicated, for death often occurs within several days. Untreatable mid- or high-thigh ischemia is generally fatal.

A number of patients have such severe ischemia at presentation that urgent surgery must be considered, particularly if a vascular graft is thought recently to have thrombosed. However, the surgical procedure in these cases is often complex, and if the limb is clearly viable and not deteriorating, it may be considered advantageous to continue with heparin therapy and to carry out all necessary investigations before performing elective surgery. Surgical reconstruction is most likely to be feasible when the problem is thrombosis of a bypass graft, and this may be managed by graft thrombectomy and correction of the underlying cause, or by insertion of a new graft.

Occlusion of one limb of a Dacron aorto-bifemoral graft is frequently corrected by graft thrombectomy. In the case of an occluded infra-inguinal graft, thrombectomy is often possible when the graft material is polytetrafluoroethylene or woven Dacron, but may be very difficult with knitted Dacron. Thrombectomy of a vein graft is not normally possible. Thrombus in a prosthetic graft is mobilized with balloon catheters and metal strippers. Good arterial downflow and backflow is established, and the cause of the thrombosis is then sought and corrected, often with the aid of on-table arteriography. A frequent cause of failure of one limb of an aorto-bifemoral graft is stenosis of the origin of the sole run-off artery, the deep femoral, and fortunately this can easily be widened. Thrombosis of a more distal graft is often caused by neointimal fibrous hyperplasia in the region of one of the anastomoses, and it is a simple procedure either to widen the anastomosis, or to extend the graft further proximally or distally as required. Should graft be deemed unsuitable for further use, a new graft can be inserted.

Graft redo operations can sometimes be performed many times. The author has experience of a patient, who at approximately yearly intervals, has undergone five such operations for thrombosis of a femoro–below knee popliteal graft with preservation of the ankle pulse. The ability to restore blood flow on each occasion was almost certainly related to the fact that the patient checked his ankle pulse every morning, and when unable to find it, immediately reported to hospital. The chance of success is much higher when a redo operation is performed soon after graft thrombosis.

When a local cause cannot be found to explain graft thrombosis, other factors should be sought. If proximal ulcerating arteriosclerosis or aneurysm is considered to be the source of athero-embolism, bypass grafting of the relevent segment is indicated. Hematologic abnormalities should also be considered, including antithrombin III deficiency.

Acute limb ischemia associated with recent trauma is usually an indication for urgent surgical exploration to prevent ischemic muscle contracture. After inadvertent intra-arterial drug injection, the needle should be left in place and heparin and reserpine 0.5 mg infused. Prostacyclin or prostaglandin E_1 might also be of value, the latter being infused in a dose of about 0.15 ng kg^{-1} min^{-1}, or 10 ng kg^{-1} min^{-1} intravenously.

Delayed presentation   No time limit can be place on surgical intervention to restore limb blood flow after thrombosis or embolism. Rather, it is the degree of ischemic damage that determines treatment policy. Major embolic arterial occlusion in the absence of well-developed collaterals may cause greater ischemic injury in six hours than a small embolus causing partial occlusion for three days. Signs of irreversible ischemia such as skin blistering and fixed mottling, and calf muscle contracture with fixed foot plantar flexion are contraindications to attempts at revascularization, and early amputation should be performed. In less severe ischemia secondary to embolism, arteriography may localize the site of obstruction and indicate the suitability for surgery. Embolectomy by a direct approach over the occluded vessel may be effective even when performed many weeks after the embolic episode.[38]

158

Isolated extremity ischemia Treatment of extremity ischemia associated with normal pulses in the adjacent arteries is nonsurgical, and heparin and possibly low molecular weight dextran may be given. Prostaglandin E_1 or I_2 therapy may also be of value. Digital gangrene usually demarcates well, and if auto-amputation does not occur, surgical debridement will be required.

Mycotic aneurysm Although relatively uncommon, mycotic aneurysm is associated with a high incidence of mortality and morbidity from hemorrhage and overwhelming sepsis. Vessel ligation and excision of the aneurysm without reconstruction of vascular continuity is the procedure of choice. Should reconstruction be essential, but is best done avoiding the use of prosthetic material, although extra-anatomic reconstruction using prosthetic material placed in clean tissue planes is often necessary. The aneurysm wall and contents are cultured and examined histologically, and appropriate antibiotic therapy is continued for at least six weeks.

Prevention of Underlying Diseases

Embolism It goes without saying that every effort must be made to diagnose the source of an embolus and to remove the cause if possible. Correction of the cause may be achieved by antibiotic therapy for subacute bacterial endocarditis, repair or replacement of a stenosed mitral valve, removal of a left ventricular aneurysm or a left atrial myxoma, or repair of an aortic or arterial aneurysm. Embolism from an ulcerated atheromatous plaque may be treated by endarterectomy,[32] or by exclusion and bypass. Antithyroid drugs will be required in the patient with atrial fibrillation secondary to thyrotoxicosis. Embolism from a poststenotic subclavian aneurysm associated with a cervical rib or band will require removal of the constricting lesion, and aneurysm thrombectomy and repair.

"Trash" foot and leg is prevented by the early application of an arterial clamp distal to the proposed site of dissection around an atheromatous artery that contains thrombus. For example, early clamping of the common iliac arteries will prevent athero-embolism from the sac of an aortic aneurysm during dissection of the neck.

The passage of a balloon catheter up one limb of a thrombosed aortic bifurcation graft may cause detached thrombus to spill over and embolize down the patent limb. This is prevented by the passage of a balloon catheter proximally to occlude the entrance into the thrombosed limb, while a metal stripper threaded over the catheter, strips thrombus from the graft wall. Both devices are then withdrawn together, the balloon drawing down the loose thrombus.

When embolism secondary to heparin-induced thrombocytopenia is diagnosed, heparin is withdrawn and circulating heparin reversed with protamine sulphate, and treatment is commenced with low molecular weight dextran and warfarin. Embolism and thrombosis associated with heparin therapy is prevented by early recognition of thrombocytopenia. Platelet counts should be performed on all patients after heparin administration for four days, and on alternate days thereafter. Should the count fall to less than 100,000 μl, the test for heparin-induced platelet aggregation is carried out.

When a diagnosis of venous thrombosis and paradoxical embolism is made, prolonged anticoagulation with warfarin may be indicated. Repeated embolism from a diseased or prosthetic heart valve is prevented by anticoagulation with or without antiplatelet therapy.

If the embolic source cannot be corrected or removed, and provided there are no contraindications, the patient should be anticoagulated for life.[1] Heparin is continued in the postoperative period, and subsequently changed to warfarin sodium, with laboratory control of dosage.

Thrombosis   Total abstention from smoking must be emphasized to all patients with arterial occlusive disease, and particularly to those with a vascular graft. Beta-blocker drugs and oral contraceptives should not be used. Warning is given against sleeping on the same side as an axillo-femoral graft, and against acute knee flexion which will cause kinking of a graft that crosses the knee joint.

During vascular surgery, constant vigilance is required to prevent pre- and postoperative arterial thrombosis. Although routine practice has been the employment of systemic heparinization before aortic and arterial clamping, there is currently a trend toward not using heparin, particularly in straightforward procedures when the distal arterial tree is patent. Bleeding is reduced, and should distal thrombosis occur, a balloon catheter can be passed. To prevent thrombosis during vascular clamping, the distal arterial tree may be filled with heparin-saline solution just before application of the clamp.

Early vascular graft thrombosis is prevented by avoiding errors in judgment regarding selection of operative candidates and the level of significant obstruction, and by ensuring good cardiac output and graft blood flow. Technical errors during graft insertion must also be avoided. Loose intima which may lift as a flap and occlude blood flow is secured by "tacking" sutures. Before completion of the last anastomosis, care is taken to ensure good downflow and backflow, and to flush out all debris. On-table arteriography is being increasingly used as a safeguard to check that blood flow is unobstructed, and measurement of graft blood flow using an electromagnetic flow meter is a further useful technic.

Late thrombosis of a vascular graft may be prevented by the early detection and correction of a developing stenosis. Regular follow-up and the use of noninvasive technics are of value in detecting graft stenosis, which is confirmed by arteriography. Early correction either by transluminal angioplasty or by surgical reconstruction will prevent thrombosis and failure of the graft.

Thrombosis following major artery cannulation requires thrombectomy and correction of the cause. Before insertion of a radial artery cannula for pressure monitoring, the ulnar pulse is checked, and the Allen test employed to exclude marked radial artery dependency of hand blood flow. Treatment of a poststenotic subclavian aneurysm has been described. Acute leg ischemia caused by thrombosis of popliteal aneurysm is prevented by ligation exclusion of the aneurysm and bypass grafting. Thrombosis of the popliteal artery compressed by the medial head of the gastrocnemius is prevented by division of the muscle.

Blood disorders such as polycythemia, leukemia, and thrombocythemia will be treated by the hematologist, and thrombocytosis will initiate a search for underlying malignancy if no other cause is apparent. Antithrombin III deficiency may require prolonged oral anticoagulant therapy.

The place of antiplatelet therapy in the prevention of prosthetic graft thrombosis is currently uncertain, but there is some experimental[39] and human[40] experience to indicate that this therapy may be effective. When a prosthetic graft is placed in the axillo-femoral, femoro-femoral, or infra-inguinal position, the current practice of many clinicians is to give long-term aspirin 300 mg either daily or on alternate days, dipyridamole 25 mg qds and warfarin sodium. Experimental approaches presently being explored to reduce the incidence of graft thrombosis include seeding the graft with endothelial cells before insertion,[41] and heparin binding with a cationic surfactant agent such as tridodecylmethylammonium chloride.[42] Antiplatelet therapy is routinely employed after percutaneous transluminal angioplasty.

The results of antiplatelet therapy in the prevention of arterial thrombosis and embolism have not been dramatic. However, the thromboxane synthetase inhibitor dazoxiben promises to be an exceptionally effective antiplatelet agent,[43] and the results of early studies are awaited with interest. No drug therapy has been shown to prevent thrombosis in diseased peripheral arteries.

CLINICAL COURSE AND PROGNOSIS

Overall, acute lower extremity arterial ischemia caused by embolism or thrombosis has a mortality of more than 25% and the cause of death in 80% is probably cardiopulmonary failure or embolism.[44] Lower limb amputation is required in 30 to 40%.[44]

Embolism

The immediate outcome is usually determined by whether the embolus is single or multiple, the delay between the onset of symptoms and treatment, and the general condition of the patient. Simultaneous limb, visceral, and carotid embolism is usually fatal. However, even after successful treatment of a solitary leg embolus, the death rate in elderly patients is high, and it is likely that peripheral embolism in these patients is the result of a gradual decline in cardiac output during the dying process. It has been argued that survival can be increased by anticoagulation rather than embolectomy,[48] but the cost may be increased limb loss.

In the long term, patients with arterial embolism have a markedly reduced life expectancy, eg, a mean survival of 3.1 years in contrast to that of 17 years in the general population.[1] The prognosis is improved when the embolic source can be identified and eliminated, but even when this is not possible, long-term anticoagulation is associated with an eightfold reduction in 20-year mortality.[1]

Effect of delay in treatment   The results of embolectomy deteriorate as the duration of delay in treatment increases up to one week. Thereafter, there is a reverse trend because of the harvesting effect of time lapse, ie, during the first seven days of observation, those patients with the most severe degrees of ischemia have died or lost their limbs. The limbs that survive the first week have sufficient collateral flow and do well with or without surgical treatment.

Thrombosis

Treatment of severe acute limb ischemia secondary to thrombosis is often less successful than that caused by embolism. If the collateral circulation is well developed, the limb will survive. Unfortunately, this is frequently not the case and the outcome is either rapid deterioration or severe irremedial chronic ischemia, and only major amputation brings relief. When thrombosis of a stenosed atheromatous artery produces only a minor degree of ischemia, the usual trend is for symptoms to improve as the collateral circulation carries an increasing flow of blood. For example, a claudication distance of 50 yards immediately after superficial femoral artery thrombosis may lengthen to 100 yards during the next six months.

The long-term outcome after thrombosis depends on the underlying condition. Patients with arteriosclerotic occlusive disease have a reduced life expectancy because of myocardial infarction, but the outlook for the ischemic limb is usually good and most patients die with their limbs intact. However, the diabetic fares badly both in terms of mortality and limb loss. Patients with thromboangiitis obliterans have a normal life expectancy, and there may be no local progression of their disease if abstention from smoking is complete.

Delay in treatment of arterial trauma may result in severe muscle contracture, and survival of a useless limb. Therapy probably makes little difference to the outcome after inadvertent intra-arterial drug injection, and muscle fibrosis with joint deformities, and extremity mummification are common. The outcome after toe or finger arterial thrombosis in the presence of normal wrist and ankle pressures usually is well-demarcated black mummification. In the long term, the affected digits are often cold-sensitive, and may be the site of neuralgic pain.

REFERENCES

1. Elliott JP, Hageman JH, Szilagyi DE, et al: Arterial embolization: Problems of source, multiplicity, recurrence, and delayed treatment. *Surgery* 1980; 88:833–845.
2. Bedford RF, Wollman H: Complications of percutaneous radial-artery cannulation: an objective prospective study in man. *Anesthesiology* 1973; 38:228–236.
3. Ritchie JL, Harker LA: Platelet and fibrinogen survival in coronary atherosclerosis. Response to medical and surgical therapy. *Am J Cardiol* 1977;39:595–598.
4. Clagett GP, Collins GJ: Platelets, thromboembolism and the clinical utility of antiplatelet drugs. *Surg Gynecol Obstet* 1978;147:255–272.
5. Meade TW, Chakrabarti R, Haines AP, et al: Hemostatic function and cardiovascular death: early results of a prospective study. *Lancet* 1980; 1:1050–1054.
6. Bouhoutsos J, Morris T, Chavatzas D, et al: The influence of haemoglobin and platelet levels on the results of arterial surgery. *Br J Surg* 1974;61: 984–986.
7. Dormandy JA: Clinical significance of blood viscosity. *Ann R Coll Surg Engl* 1970;47:211–228.
8. Reid HL, Dormandy JA, Barnes AJ, et al: Impaired red cell deformability in peripheral vascular disease. *Lancet* 1976;2:666–667.
9. Cotton RT, Bedford DR: Symmetric peripheral gangrene complicating acute myocardial infarction. *Am J Med* 1956;20:301–307.
10. Husum B, Palm T: Arterial dominance in the hand. *Br J Anaesth* 1978; 50:913–916.
11. Fogarty JT, Cranley JJ, Krause RJ, et al: A method for extraction of arterial emboli and thrombi. *Surg Gynecol Obstet* 1963;116:241–244.
12. Gould JDM, Lingam S: Hazards of intra-arterial diazepam. *Br Med J Clin Res* 1977;2:290–299.
13. Zideman DA, Morgan M: Inadvertent intra-arterial injection of flucloxacillin. *Anaesthesia* 1981;36:296–298.
14. Mac Gowan WAL, Holland PDJ, Browne HI, et al: The local effects of intra-arterial injections of sodium tetradecyl sulphate (S.T.D.) 3 percent. *Br J Surg* 1972;59:101–104.
15. McCollum CN, Kester RC, Rajah S, et al: Arterial graft maturation: the duration of thrombotic activity in Dacron aortobifemoral grafts measured by platelet and fibrinogen kinetics. *Br J Surg* 1981;68:61–64.
16. Hanson SR, Harker LA, Ratner BD, et al: In vivo evaluation of artificial surfaces with a non human primate model of arterial thrombosis. *J Lab Clin Med* 1980;95:289–304.
17. Lindenauer SM: The synthetic vascular prosthesis, in Rutherford RB (ed): *Vascular Surgery*. Philadelphia, WB Saunders Co, 1977, pp 367–379.
18. Myers KA, King RB, Scott DF, et al: The effect of smoking on the late patency of arterial reconstructions in the legs. *Br J Surg* 1978;65:267–271.

19. Imperato AM, Bracco A, Kim GE, et al: Intimal and neointimal fibrous proliferation causing failure of arterial reconstructions. *Surgery* 1972; 72:1007-1017.
20. Pardy BJ, Eastcott HHG: Prostaglandin therapy in severe limb ischemia. *World J Surg,* to be published.
21. Zacharias FJ, Gowen KJ, Prestt J, et al: Propanolol in hypertension: A study of long-term therapy. *Am Heart J* 1972;83:775-761.
22. Vale JA, Van de Pette SJ, Price TML: Peripheral gangrene complicating beta blockade. *Lancet* 1977;2:412.
23. Eastcott HHG: *Arterial Surgery*, ed 2. London, Pitnam Medical, 1973, p 24.
24. Rhodes GR, Dixon RH, Silver D: Heparin-induced thrombocytopenia. *Ann Surg* 1977;186:752-758.
25. Baird RA, Convery RF: Arterial thromboembolism in patients receiving systemic heparin therapy. *J Bone Joint Surg* 1977;59:1061-1064.
26. Towne JB, Berhard VM, Hussey C, Garancis JC: Antithrombin deficiency — a cause of unexplained thrombosis in vascular surgery. *Surgery* 1981; 89:735-742.
27. Fowler PBS: Gangrene of the leg, following carbon-monoxide asphyxia. *Lancet* 1954;1:240-241.
28. Enzer N, Spilberg S: Gangrene of lower extremity following carbon monoxide asphysia. *Am J Clin Pathol* 1946;16:111-116.
29. Hawley PR, Johnston AW, Rankin JT: Association between digital ischemia and malignant disease. *Br Med J Clin Res* 1967;3:208-212.
30. Heiskell CA, Conn J: Aortoarterial emboli. *Am J Surg* 1976;132:4-7.
31. Karmody AM, Powers SR, Monaco VJ, et al: "Blue toe" syndrome. *Arch Surg* 1976;111:1263-1268.
32. Wagner RB, Martin AS: Peripheral atheroembolism: Confirmation of a clinical concept, with a case report and review of the literature. *Surgery* 1973; 73:353-359.
33. Haimovici H: Peripheral arterial embolism; study of 330 unselected cases of embolism of extremities. *Angiology* 1950;1:20-45.
34. Bassett FH, Lincoln CR, King TD, et al: Inequality in the size of the lower extremity following cardiac catheterization. *South Med J* 1968;61:1013-1017.
35. May AG, Van de Berg L, DeWeese JA, et al: Critical arterial stenosis. *Surgery* 1963;54:250-259.
36. Flinn WR, Harris JP, Rudo ND, et al: Atheroembolism as cause of graft failure in femoral distal reconstruction. *Surgery* 1981;90:698-706.
37. Haimovici H: Arterial embolism, myoglobinuria and renal tubular necrosis. *Arch Surg* 1970;100:639-645.
38. Ammann J, Seiler H, Vogt B: Delayed arterial embolectomy: a plea for a more active approach. *Br J Surg* 1976;63:73-76.
39. Oblath RW, Buckley FO, Green RM, et al: Prevention of platelet aggregation and adherence to prosthetic vascular grafts by aspirin and dipyridamole. *Surgery* 1978;84:37-44.
40. Green RM, Roedersheimer LR, DeWeese JA: Effects of aspirin and dipyridamole on expanded polytetrafluoroethylene graft patency. *Surgery* 1982;92: 1016-1026.
41. Sharefkin JB, Latker C, Smith M, et al: Early normalization of platelet survival by endothelial seeding of Dacron arterial prostheses in dogs. *Surgery* 1982;92:385-393.
42. Grode GA, Anderson SJ, Grotta HM, et al: Nonthrombogenic materials via a simple coating process. *Trans Am Soc Artif Intern Organs* 1969;15:1-6.

43. Tyler HM, Saxton CAPD, Parry MJ: Administration to man of UK-37,248-01, a selective inhibitor of thromboxane synthetase. *Lancet* 1981; 1:629–632.
44. Blaisdell FW, Steele M, Allen RE: Management of acute lower extremity arterial ischemia due to embolism and thrombosis. *Surgery* 1978;84:822–834.

8 · Arterial Occlusive Disorders in the Coronary Arterial System

Paul D. Hirsh
James T. Willerson

Recently published statistics indicate that over 5 million physician-patient contacts occur monthly in the United States due to heart disease.[1] The majority of these contacts are a result of ischemic heart disease, with over 1.3 million patients suffering a myocardial infarction in the United States each year.[2] The in-hospital mortality rate for acute infarction is approximately 15%, with an additional 10% mortality in the first year postinfarction.[3] These statistics emphasize the magnitude of the public health issue of ischemic heart disease. This chapter will (a) review the factors associated with increased risk of coronary artery disease, and (b) discuss the pathogenesis, clinical manifestations, treatment, and prognosis of the acute and chronic ischemic heart disease syndromes.

RISK FACTORS

Epidemiologic studies have shown that coronary artery disease does not occur randomly in the population. Various demographic, biologic, biochemical, environmental, social, psychological, and genetic factors have been associated with an increased occurrence of ischemic heart disease. The currently identified risk factors do not explain all of the differences in disease incidence among various groups. Thus, further investigation is required to find new risk factors or identify new relationships among the known factors. Nevertheless, the following discussion will point out what has been discovered in this regard during the past 30 to 40 years of epidemiologic research, with some speculative remarks concerning mechanisms and some guidelines for the primary prevention of coronary disease through risk-factor modification.

Age and Sex Hormones

Increasing age and male sex are both associated with significantly increased mortality rates from coronary artery disease.[4] Specifically, the mortality rate due to ischemic heart disease for women lags behind that for men by approximately seven to ten years. The mechanism by which these age- and sex-related differences occurs remains undefined. However, sex hormones are known to influence many metabolic pathways and vascular adrenergic receptor density.[5,6] It is likely that various

166

hormonal patterns and the changes that occur in these patterns with aging have an impact on atherogenesis and subsequent myocardial ischemia. The inability to identify a specific mechanism responsible for the effects of age and sex hormones on the incidence of coronary artery disease may be a reflection of the multifactorial nature of the metabolic effects of these processes.

Genetics

Racial differences in mortality rates due to coronary artery disease in the United States have been inconsistent over the past 30 years, suggesting that any apparent racial differences are secondary to other, nongenetic factors. However, there are ethnic groups within the United States with different incidence rates of coronary artery disease. In particular, Japanese men in Hawaii and California have approximately one-half the incidence of coronary disease as white males in the same regions.[7] The mechanism for these genetic differences remains unknown. Additionally, there is a strong intrafamily risk for acquiring coronary artery disease prematurely in families with members who have had myocardial infarction prior to age 45.

It has recently been pointed out that Greenland Eskimos have a markedly reduced incidence of ischemic heart disease. In addition, a hemostatic abnormality has been described in this group with a resultant prolongation of the bleeding time.[8] This, in turn, has been attributed to their intake of large quantities of saltwater fish (such as cod and mackerel). In fact, this same hemostatic abnormality has been reproduced in individuals on a Western diet by supplementation with cod liver oil or increased fish intake.[9] The platelet function abnormality and alteration in prostaglandin and thromboxane production which occur as a result of these dietary differences may play a role in the reduced incidence of ischemic heart disease and atherosclerosis in the Eskimos. Whether this is, in fact, the mechanism involved and whether long-term dietary changes can result in a similar benefit to other groups remain unproven and intriguing hypotheses.

Environment

There are striking differences in the mortality rates from coronary artery disease within countries and between countries. For example, within the United States, there are high mortality rates in the southern Atlantic seaboard states and in the Northeast, and low rates in the Great Plains and Rocky Mountain states. The weather (and temperature) conditions, the hardness of the drinking water, and a variety of other ecological factors have been implicated,[10,11] although none has been clearly proved.

The strongest available evidence for the importance of environmental factors in the incidence of coronary events comes from the study of Japanese men living in different areas of the world.[12] The low rate of atherosclerotic coronary artery disease in Japanese men living Japan is increased toward that of Western whites after they move to and live in the United States.

Hyperlipidemia

Hypercholesterolemia has been clearly associated with the development of atherosclerosis. In fact, the incidence of coronary artery disease correlates well with the plasma cholesterol concentration, particularly in individuals less than 65 years old.[13] By contrast, plasma triglyceride elevations have been associated with an increased risk of atherosclerosis in some studies, but the association appears weak and is unsupported in other large-scale epidemiologic studies.[14]

Cholesterol is transported within the body in various lipoprotein complexes. Quantifying these lipoproteins provides much more information regarding cardiovascular risk than simply utilizing the absolute plasma cholesterol level. The major cholesterol lipoprotein groups are chylomicrons, very-low-density lipoproteins (VLDL), low-density lipoproteins (LDL), and high-density lipoproteins (HDL), as defined by various physiochemical properties. Since generally two thirds of plasma cholesterol is in the LDL fraction, plasma LDL concentrations correlate well with the incidence of atherosclerotic coronary artery disease. High-density lipoproteins generally constitute approximately one fourth of plasma cholesterol. There is an inverse relationship between HDL levels and the incidence of coronary artery disease. In fact, in individuals over 50 years old, this relationship of HDL cholesterol is the most predictive factor regarding plasma cholesterol and coronary risk.[15]

The mechanism(s) by which blood lipids influence atherogenesis and the clinical expression of coronary disease is unknown. The predominant cellular component of the human atherosclerotic plaque is smooth muscle cells that have migrated and proliferated from the inner media. Cholesterol and cholesterol esters in these plaques are derived principally from LDL. Current research is focused on the causes of smooth muscle cell proliferation and the mechanisms of LDL-derived cholesterol localization in and around smooth muscle cells. A platelet-derived peptide has been described which stimulates arterial smooth muscle cell growth.[16] In some situations, repeated, sustained, and/or severe vascular endothelial injury may result in a pathologic repair process involving platelet deposition, smooth muscle cell stimulation, and ultimately, plaque formation.

It has been postulated on theoretical grounds that thromboxane A_2, a potent vasoconstrictor and platelet aggregator, which is synthesized and released by circulating platelets, might contribute to atherogenesis and to ischemic coronary events.[17] In this regard, cholesterol-rich platelets have been observed to have increased thromboxane formation in comparison to cholesterol-poor platelets. Furthermore, vascular endothelial cells and smooth muscle cells synthesize prostacyclin, a powerful vasodilator and inhibitor of platelet aggregation. It has been suggested that prostacyclin may serve to prevent platelet clumping on endothelial surfaces and thereby protect against thrombus formation and atherosclerosis. In light of this hypothesis, it is interesting that HDL has been shown to stimulate arterial endothelial prostacyclin synthesis.[18] Whether this represents even part of the mechanism by which HDL exerts its beneficial effect remains speculative.

Hypertension

Elevations of systolic and diastolic blood pressure are both risk factors for the development of atherosclerotic coronary artery disease.[19] In fact, there is a direct relationship between the levels of systolic and diastolic pressures and the risk of atherosclerotic disease over the entire range of blood pressures. This relationship applies equally to men and women and is based on the casual measurement of blood pressure in a routine office setting.

Cigarette Smoking

Cigarette smoking may contribute to the development of atherosclerosis.[20] Furthermore, cardiovascular morbidity and mortality are markedly increased among cigarette smokers,[21] even in the absence of atherosclerotic coronary artery disease.[22] The risk increases linearly according to the number of cigarettes smoked per day[23,24] and diminishes with discontinuation of smoking.[25] Pipe and cigar smokers have only a slightly increased risk.[21]

The mechanism by which cigarette smoking affects atherogenesis and ischemic heart disease remains undefined, although there have been several intriguing suggestions. Catecholamine release associated with smoking may play a role in the etiology of acute ischemic coronary events.[26] In addition, smoking and nicotine adversely alter the thromboxane/prostacyclin ratio[27] and increase platelet reactivity.[28] Whether these deleterious physiologic phenomena are pathogenetically important in cardiovascular disease remains to be proved.

Diabetes Mellitus

Diabetes mellitus is a precursor of atherosclerotic vascular disease.[29] Glucose intolerance, an elevated fasting blood sugar, and even random hyperglycemia have all been associated with an increased risk of coronary artery disease.[30,31]

There is evidence of altered platelet function and abnormal prostaglandin synthesis in diabetes. In particular, increased platelet adhesiveness,[32] increased platelet sensitivity to adenosine diphosphate (ADP)[33] and arachidonic acid,[34] and increased thromboxane generation rates[35] have all been observed in platelets from diabetics. Furthermore, prostacyclin production appears to be diminished in vascular tissue from diabetic rats[36] and humans.[37] It is of concern that most of these abnormalities have been determined by in vitro technics and may not reflect the in vivo situation. Therefore, it is encouraging that altered platelet turnover[38] and increased plasma beta thromboglobulin concentrations[39] have been reported in diabetics, presumably reflecting in vivo abnormalities. These results support the extensive in vitro studies suggesting a potential role for platelets and prostaglandins in the pathophysiology of diabetic vascular disease.

Stress

A "coronary-prone" personality has been described by Friedman and Rosenman and is defined as "an individual who is engaged in a relatively chronic and excessive struggle to obtain an unlimited number of things from the environment in the shortest period of time and/or against the opposing efforts of other persons or things in the same environment."[40] The Western Collaborative Group Study has confirmed the increased incidence of coronary events among these so-called type A individuals.[41] The observation that stress is a risk factor for the development of atherosclerotic coronary artery disease has been supported by other studies as well.[42]

Studies in healthy volunteers have shown that stress causes increased platelet aggregability.[43] The basis for this may be through catecholamine release, which is a potent stimulus for platelet activity.[44] However, this is speculative and further research is needed to elucidate the mechanisms by which stress influences atherogenicity and cardiovascular events.

Diet

There are several intriguing aspects of the relation between diet and coronary risk. First, plasma concentrations of LDL are directly proportional to the ingestion of saturated fats and cholesterol, while the ingestion of polyunsaturated fats depresses LDL levels. Vegetarians (with low levels of saturated fats and cholesterol) have one-third the mortality rate from coronary disease of nonvegeterians.[45] The role of LDL in coronary heart disesase has been reviewed above.

Second, there appears to be an inverse relationship between the hardness of drinking water and local cardiovascular mortality rates.[46] The specific trace elements in water that are responsible for altering cardiovascular risk have not yet been identified. Third, daily alcohol intake may help to prevent atherosclerotic coronary disease,[47] although not all studies have confirmed this finding. Alcohol intake has been correlated with HDL cholesterol levels and this may explain its beneficial effect.[48]

Fourth, Greenland Eskimos have a reduced incidence of coronary vascular disease. In addition, they have a hemostatic abnormality, which has been attributed to their high intake of saltwater fish. Their diet of predominantly mackerel and cod provides increased amounts of eicosapentaenoic acid (EPA, C-20:5) rather than eicosatetraenoic acid (arachidonic acid, C-20:4) substrate. The resultant prostaglandin products of the 3-series (rather than the 2-series) are relatively antiaggregatory. The hypothesis is that, by substituting for arachidonic acid in tissue phospholipid stores, EPA is released and metabolized to vasodilatory and antiaggregatory prostaglandin end-products and this may play a role in reducing cardiovascular risk.[59] The contribution of plasma lipid alterations associated with these dietary differences remains unknown. Validation of the EPA hypothesis will require a long-term dietary crossover trial.

ISCHEMIC HEART DISEASE SYNDROME

Stable (Exertional) Angina Pectoris

Pathogenesis Chronic stable angina connotes a symptom complex of chest pain which occurs predictably at a specific stress level or under a specific set of circumstances, with stability in the daily frequency of anginal episodes. Symptoms occur due to myocardial ischemia which develops as a result of an increase in myocardial oxygen demand in the presence of limited coronary arterial oxygen supply. The most important determinants of myocardial oxygen demand are (a) The intramyocardial systolic tension, (which is proportional to the blood pressure and ventricular size); (b) the heart rate; and (c) the contractile state of myocardium.

"Normal" persons do not develop angina because they are protected by limitations in physical capacity (skeletal muscle fatigue and dyspnea). Therefore, the predisposing factor is a limitation in coronary arterial flow due to atherosclerotic coronary artery disease. Other causes of angina, such as mechanical factors that increase left ventricular systolic pressure (eg, aortic stenosis), will not be discussed here.

Clinical manifestations The quality of chest discomfort which patients experience due to myocardial ischemia is variable. Frequently used adjectives include "viselike," "constricting," "pressure," "crushing," "squeezing," and "suffocating." There are many others, some of which are relatively vague. The major pain is generally retrosternal, although radiation is common to the left arm and less commonly to the right arm, neck, jaw, and teeth. Angina is occasionally felt only as breathlessness.

The typical anginal episode occurs in response to an increase in cardiac work brought on by effort, emotion, eating, excessive metabolic demands (chills, fever), thyrotoxicosis, tachycardia from any cause, anemia, exposure to cold air or a cold drink, and cigarette smoking. The discomfort increases steadily over several minutes and then dissipates, generally after the stimulus has been removed.

Physical examination is of limited value for the diagnosis of chronic stable coronary artery disease. Signs suggesting the presence of risk factors for coronary atherosclerosis may be observed, eg, hypertension or xanthomas (resulting from hypercholesterolemia). Abnormal findings may also suggest ischemic left ventricular dysfunction, particularly if they occur only during an anginal attack or in response to an applied stress. Such findings include a third or fourth heart sound (diastolic filling sounds), a dyskinetic apical bulge, a systolic murmur of papillary muscle dysfunction, and paradoxical splitting of the second heart sound.

Laboratory findings   The electrocardiogram obtained at rest is normal in up to 50% of patients with stable angina pectoris. The most common abnormality is a nonspecific ST-T change. A variety of conduction disturbances, particularly left bundle branch block and left anterior hemiblock, are also seen in association with ischemic heart disease. Arrhythmias, especially premature ventricular beats, are a nonspecific finding in some patients.

Routine laboratory tests are generally within normal limits in patients with chronic stable coronary disease. Chest films occasionally reveal cardiomegaly. Coronary artery calcification detected fluoroscopically is somewhat more specific, particularly in younger people, and in combination with a positive stress test, greatly raises the likelihood of the presence of coronary artery disease.[50]

There are several newer methods for evaluating left ventricular function noninvasively. Evidence of left ventricular damage or ischemia may be reflected in abnormal regional wall motion detected by echocardiography (M-mode or cross-sectional) or technetium 99m radionuclide angiography (first-pass or gated blood pool).

The sensitivity and specificity of these noninvasive procedures is increased markedly when they are combined with an applied stress. A nonspecific finding on physical examination, the ECG, an echocardiogram, or radionuclide scintigraphy becomes much more significant for the diagnosis of coronary artery disease if it occurs at peak stress and resolves with rest. In this regard, the most accurate noninvasive procedure for the diagnosis of physiologically significant coronary artery disease at the present time involves symptom-limited exercise testing coupled with repeated physical examinations, continuous ECG monitoring, and serial radionuclide scintigraphy (technetium 99m-gated blood pool angiography or thallium 201 myocardial perfusion scanning).[51]

The definitive assessment of the presence and anatomic severity of atherosclerotic artery disease requires cardiac catheterization. This includes left heart catheterization with intraventricular pressure measurement, left ventricular angiography, and coronary arteriography.

Treatment and prognosis   There are five aspects to the treatment of patients with chronic stable angina pectoris. First, risk factor modification should be undertaken. Second, general life-style adjustment may be beneficial. Third, medical therapy can be extremely rewarding because of the constantly increasing pharmacologic armamentarium available. Fourth, percutaneous transluminal angioplasty is a nonsurgical intervention which can dilate coronary stenoses and offers promise in the treatment of some patients with angina pectoris. Fifth, surgical intervention can provide symptomatic improvement for many patients through coronary revascularization.

Risk factor modification is an appropriate goal in the prophylaxis of atherosclerotic heart disease. However, proof that these efforts are justified is only now slowly becoming available. To date, evidence for regression of the atherosclerotic process in humans is even more uncertain. Therefore, risk factor reduction in patients with established coronary disease requires some reliance upon a belief in the soundness of the hypothesis. Reduction in elevated cholesterol levels may be achieved usually through diet modification and appropriate weight reduction. Pharmacologic agents to reduce serum cholesterol concentrations should generally be reserved for those with severe hypercholesterolemia, especially those with familial hypercholesterolemia characterized by extremely high values. Pharmacologic intervention may also be warranted in individuals with multiple risk factors and a strongly positive family history of early-onset ischemic heart disease, despite a lack of clear-cut evidence to prove the efficacy of this approach. Control of hypertension, discontinuation of cigarette smoking, and normalization of blood glucose concentrations may help to prevent atherogenesis and retard its progression.

Under the category of general life-style adjustments, avoidance or modification of strenuous activities may be necessary, eg, use of an elevator instead of stairs. Eliminating or reducing the factors that precipitate angina is an individual trial-and-error process which has obvious benefits. Decisions regarding changes in work and retirement need careful consideration. Avoidance of extremely cold weather and ice-cold drinks, as well as hot, humid environments, may be important. Large meals and emotional outbursts may also precipitate anginal attacks and should be avoided.

Specific antianginal drugs currently include various nitrate preparations, beta-adrenergic blocking agents, and calcium antagonists. Nitrates appear to work primarily by reducing cardiac work through a decrease in systemic venous tone with a subsequent reduction in preload. Some of their beneficial effect may also be through afterload reduction as well as direct coronary arterial dilation. However, these latter effects are clearly not the principal basis for their antianginal utility. Beta-adrenergic blocking agents reduce myocardial oxygen requirements for any given level of activity by reducing heart rate, arterial pressure, and myocardial contractility. Calcium antagonists demonstrate some individual variability in their relative effects on different organ systems in vivo. Nevertheless, as a group they cause coronary artery dilation, afterload reduction, and a decrease in cardiac contractility. As a result, they are all effective antianginal agents.

Percutaneous balloon angioplasty can, in carefully selected patients, effectively dilate stenotic coronary arteries and provide immediate improvement in myocardial perfusion with subjective and objective improvement. Insofar as the long-term effects, risks, indications, and contraindications are still not fully recognized, this procedure must still be considered experimental. Nevertheless, for patients considering coronary bypass surgery for relief of angina pectoris, balloon angioplasty has offered a nonsurgical alternative since its introduction in 1977 by Gruntzig et al.[52]

Modern surgical management of ischemic heart disease was introduced by Garrett et al[53] in 1964, Favaloro et al,[54] and by Johnson et al[55] with the saphenous vein bypass procedure. This procedure is now performed on more than 10,000 patient each year in the United States alone. Criteria for the procedure vary among institutions, but there is general agreement that it is indicated for patients with chronic stable angina with significant disability due to angina despite optimal medical therapy. There is a growing trend to operate on patients with significant left main coronary artery disease regardless of symptoms, in order to prolong life. Patients with critical proximal disease in the three major epicardial vessels, with severe angina persisting despite therapy, are also considered candidates for surgery by some cardiologists.

The natural history of coronary artery disease has been well defined. The annual mortality of patients with angina is about 4%.[56] Mortality rates correlate well with the number of epicardial vessels showing angiographic disease: the annual mortality rate for single-vessel disease is 2%; two-vessel disease, 7%; and three-vessel disease, 11%.[57] The major exception to this is high-grade stenosis of the left main coronary artery, which has a two-year mortality of 44%.[58] Since the widespread, adoption of beta-adrenergic blocking agents, it appears that the annual mortality rate in patients with angina has decreased from 6 or 7% to 4%, but other factors may be involved. Evidence from several European studies suggests that these agents improve survival following myocardial infarction.[59]

Coronary Arterial Spasm

Pathogenesis Variant angina pectoris (Prinzmetal's angina) is caused by focal coronary arterial spasm. Maseri and coworkers have argued that coronary vasospasm is ubiquitous in ischemic heart disease, occurring not just in variant angina but also in many cases of rest angina, unstable angina, and acute myocardial infarction.[60] This hypothesis also has been suggested by Oliva and Breckinridge, who observed coronary obstruction reversed with intracoronary nitroglycerin in six of 15 patients (40%) with acute infarction.[61] However, more recently most other investigators have been unable to demonstrate evidence for coronary spasm at the time of streptokinase infusion for thrombolytic therapy in patients with acute myocardial infarction.

The pathogenesis of coronary spasm is unknown. What initiates the spasm, what causes it to terminate spontaneously, what determines the location of the spasm—all of these questions remain unanswered. Various neurogenic and humoral mechanisms have been postulated, but none has been proved. Because it is a potent arterial constrictor, there has been great interest recently in the role of thromboxane A_2 (TxA_2) in this syndrome. In sampling from coronary sinus in five patients during eight anginal attacks within the first two minutes after onset of ischemic ECG changes, coronary sinus thromboxane B_2 (TxB_2, the stable TxA_2 hydration product) increased in seven, dramatically so in five.[62] However, low-dose aspirin and indomethacin (cyclooxygenase inhibitors), which effectively block TxA_2 synthesis, have no effect on Prinzmetal's syndrome.[62,63] These studies suggest that although TxA_2 may be involved in the pathophysiology of Prinzmetal's angina, it is probably not the principal mediator. High doses of aspirin (4 g/day) have been reported to worsen variant angina,[64] suggesting that prostacyclin (PGI_2) may be protective in vivo and that a TxA_2:PGI_2 balance may play a role in the pathophysiology of coronary spasm. Chierchia et al recently reported complete and repeated abolition of Prinzmetal's angina attacks in one of five patients treated with intravenous prostacyclin,[65] suggesting that the etiology and pathophysiology of coronary spasm may be multifactorial.

Clinical manifestations Variant angina is a syndrome characterized by chest pains at rest associated with ST segment elevation on the ECG. Pain is not precipitated by physical exertion or emotional stress, although some patients do experience symptoms during or after exertion as well as at rest. Physical examination is often notable for the absence of coronary risk factors. Cardiac examination is generally normal in the absence of pain but reveals the signs of left ventricular dysfunction during ischemia, just as described in patients with exertional angina pectoris. Coronary spasm may result in angina, arrhythmias, and acute myocardial infarction. Furthermore, there is a clinical association between coronary spasm and peripheral vasospasm (Raynaud's phenomenon) and migraine headache. The basis for this association is unknown.

Laboratory findings The electrocardiogram during an attack of variant angina is pathognomonic. The ST segment, normal at rest, becomes characteristically elevated during pain. This can and does often occur in the absence of pain (subclinical myocardial ischemia).

Cardiac catheterization with coronary angiography is used to confirm the diagnosis when the clinical picture is unclear. Provocative agents, such as ergonovine maleate, can be administered intravenously during clinical, hemodynamic, and ECG monitoring. Ergonovine will induce spasm in patients with Prinzmetal's angina and these episodes can be documented with coronary arteriography. This is a relatively safe procedure, but because of the hazard of prolonged spasm and myocardial infarction, ergonovine should be administered in low, gradually increasing doses. This provocative test is relatively sensitive and specific for Prinzmetal's angina.[66]

Treatment and prognosis The treatment of variant angina has improved dramatically over the past decade. Nitrates, both short- and long-acting, and calcium antagonists are effective in aborting and preventing attacks of Prinzmetal's angina. Beta-adrenergic antagonists result in improvement in some patients, but no change or worsening in others. As a result, these agents are generally avoided in patients with this syndrome.

Patients with variant angina and no atherosclerotic coronary disease generally have a good prognosis.[67] Although myocardial infarction can occur, there is a tendency for its symptoms to stabilize and diminish.[68] Sudden death is the major risk of coronary spasm and has been reported in up to 15% of patients, many within the first three months after onset of symptoms.[69] The effect of medical therapy on these statistics is currently being evaluated.

Unstable Angina Pectoris

Pathogenesis This syndrome has been called preinfarction angina, crescendo angina, the intermediate coronary syndrome, and acute coronary insufficiency. It is characterized by primary reductions in coronary arterial flow,[60] which in turn may be caused by an increase in coronary arterial tone (ie, spasm) or transient platelet "plugging." The mechanism responsible for these events remains unknown. Various mechanical (spontaneous rupture of, and hemorrhage into an atherosclerotic plaque), neurogenic (an increase in alpha-adrenergic tone), and humoral (ADP, serotonin, and prostaglandin) mechanisms have been proposed. All have received some support from cardiovascular research efforts. For example, regarding the prostaglandin hypothesis, it has been postulated that an increase in TxA_2 relative to PGI_2 (ie, an increased $TxA_2:PGI_2$

ratio), with its resultant vasoconstrictive and proaggregatory humoral imbalance, might initiate or sustain an attack of unstable angina.[17,70] This hypothesis has received support from the observation that patients with unstable angina have increased transcardiac levels of TxA_2[70] which do not appear to be simply a metabolic response to myocardial ischemia.[71] It is likely that unstable angina is a heterogeneous syndrome of multiple etiology.

Clinical manifestations The unstable angina syndrome is intermediate between stable angina and acute myocardial infarction. It is characterized by: (a) angina pectoris that is progressive (accelerated) in nature or that occurs at rest; (b) the deterioration of chronic, stable angina pectoris to a more frequent, more easily provoked, and more severe angina; and/or (c) one or more episodes of angina pectoris that last in excess of 15 minutes, with poor or no relief with rest and nitroglycerin.[72]

Physical examination in patients with unstable angina pectoris may reveal any of the signs associated with myocardial dysfunction, notably a diastolic (third or fourth) heart sound, a dyskinetic apical impulse, a transient mitral regurgitation murmur, and/or a paradoxically split second heart sound.

Laboratory findings The diagnosis of unstable angina pectoris depends solely on the clinical history. Nevertheless, the ECG is frequently helpful in that most patients will have transient deviations of the ST segment, often with T-wave inversions. It should be emphasized, however, that a normal ECG does not exclude the diagnosis.

Cardiac enzymes are not usually elevated, although they may frequently approach the upper limits of normal. Indeed, serum creatine kinase (CK) may be slightly elevated, probably indicating a small amount of myocardial necrosis. Microinfarcts do occur during unstable angina, suggesting that there is a continuum between chest pain and infarction with unstable angina covering a spectrum in between the two. Technetium 99m stannous pyrophosphate myocardial scintigrams are positive in up to one third of these patients, suggesting diffuse subendocardial necrosis.[73]

Exercise stress testing is contraindicated in patients with unstable angina because of the hazard of provoking a myocardial infarction. Coronary angiography in patients with unstable angina reveals the same distribution of epicardial vascular involvement as in patients with stable angina, except for a higher incidence of left main coronary artery stenosis.[73]

Treatment and prognosis Treatment of unstable angina should be aggressive to prevent infarction: bed rest (with cardiac monitoring), sedation, narcotic analgesia, oxygen, nitrates, beta-adrenergic blocking agents, and intra-aorta balloon counterpulsation if necessary to control anginal pain. Calcium antagonist drugs are currently being tested in this syndrome. In light of the recent experience with thrombolytic therapy in dissolving acute coronary thrombi in acute myocardial infarction, anticoagulation (with heparin) may be considered for prevention of infarction.[75] If a subset of patients with unstable angina can be shown to have thromboxane-mediated events (recurrent chest pain, infarction, arrhythmias, or sudden death), then cyclooxygenase inhibition with aspirin or similar agents may be efficacious. Even more helpful would be the availability of a specific thromboxane synthetase inhibitor; such inhibitors have become available recently and are being tested clinically and experimentally.

The early mortality rate for unstable angina (within the first month) is generally 1% to 2%, with a myocardial infarction rate as high as 15%.[76] The recurrence rate within a 24-month period is substantial, even with medical intervention, but is lower with surgical therapy.[73] Emergency coronary revascularization is reserved for those with refractory unstable angina.

Acute Myocardial Infarction

Pathogenesis Most myocardial infarcts are associated with atherosclerotic coronary artery disease. Recent results with coronary thrombolysis therapy suggest that thrombi are present at the site of occlusion in most patients with acute transmural myocardial infarction.[77,78] However, many nontransmural myocardial infarcts occur without thrombotic occlusion of the infarct-related artery. Thrombosis may be a secondary event resulting from hemorrhage into a plaque, with plaque enlargement, plaque rupture with intimal disruption and collagen exposure, or plaque ulceration.[78,79] The role of other thrombogenic humoral substances, such as thromboxane A_2, in the pathogenesis of acute infarction is speculative at this writing.

Clinical manifestations A history of unstable angina is present in many patients with acute myocardial infarction. The pain of infarction is generally severe and prolonged, lasting for several hours in most cases. It is generally similar in quality to angina pectoris but far more intense. Nausea and vomiting occur frequently. Weakness and a sense of impending doom are common. In spite of this, perhaps 10% to 20% of infarcts are unrecognized clinically, either because they are truly "silent" (as in some patients with diabetes mellitus) or more likely because the patient ignores what he might consider as relatively mild discomfort.

Physical examination reveals an individual in severe distress occasionally with the signs of myocardial dysfunction mentioned above. Complications of acute infarction may also be present, including hypertension, hypotension, arrhythmias, congestive heart failure, and/or cardiogenic shock.[79]

Laboratory findings Myocardial cellular release of enzymes into the circulation is the hallmark of myocardial necrosis. A pattern of appearance is characteristic, such that the serum CK rises early (within two to three hours) and peaks at ten to 12 hours after the onset of infarction, SGOT peaks at 18 to 36 hours, and lactic dehydrogenase (LDH) peaks at three to six days after the onset of pain.[79] Each of the enzymes has isoenzymes that are somewhat more specific for cardiac muscle, although none is contained exclusively within heart muscle. Therefore, these isoenzymes, particularly the CK-MB or CK-B fraction, are helpful in differentiating cardiac from noncardiac cellular damage.[79]

The ECG is abnormal in the majority of patients with acute myocardial infarction, particularly when obtained serially over several days. In transmural infarction, the ECG is useful for the detection and localization of the damage. In nontransmural infarction, the ECG is considerably less sensitive and specific.

Radionuclide technics are also helpful in diagnosing acute infarction. Technetium 99m stannous pyrophosphate scanning, thallium 201 imaging, and gated blood pool scintigraphy can all contribute valuable information.[79]

Coronary angiography is not indicated acutely to confirm the diagnosis. However, new approaches to limit infarct size have employed acute infarct angiography safely. As mentioned earlier, acute transmural infarction is generally associated with complete occlusion of the infarct-related coronary artery.[78,79]

Treatment and prognosis Most deaths associated with acute myocardial infarction occur as a result of ventricular fibrillation within the first hour after its onset. Since this is generally reversible if treated with immediate electrical defibrillation, rapid transportation to the hospital by a well-equipped ambulance staff is of primary importance. Cardiac monitoring and aggressive therapy in the coronary care unit has reduced the mortality due to this disease from 30% to 15%.[79,80] Prevention and treatment of life-threatening arrhythmias is the principal cause of this improved prognosis.

Acute infarction is treated with bed rest, oxygen and analgesia. Anticoagulant therapy is generally employed only to prevent deep venous thrombophlebitis (heparin 5000 IU subcutaneously every 8 to 12 hours). Fibrinolytic therapy is currently under intense investigation as are many other forms of therapy designed to attempt to limit infarct size (beta-adrenergic blocking agents, calcium antagonist drugs, glucose-insulin-potassium, and urgent coronary revascularization.[79] Because ventricular fibrillation is common in this setting, prophylactic pharmacologic therapy (eg, lidocaine) is often administered for the first 12 to 24 hours. Other arrhythmias, and all other complications of infarction, are treated as necessary.

REFERENCES

1. IMA America: National Disease and Therapeutic Index (NDTI), Oct 1981, section 3.
2. Stamler J: The primary prevention of coronary heart disease, in Braunwald E (ed): *The Myocardium: Failure and Prevention*. New York, HP Publishing Co, 1974, p. 219.
3. Blackburn H: Progress in the epidemiology and prevention of coronary heart disease, in Yu PN, Goodwin JF (eds): *Progress in Cardiology*. Philadelphia, Lea & Febiger, 1974, p. 1.
4. Kuller LH: Epidemiology of cardiovascular diseases: current perspectives. *Am J Epidemiol* 1976;104:425–456.
5. Wallace RB, Hoover J, Barrett-Conner E, et al: Altered plasma lipid and lipoprotein levels associated with oral contraceptive and estrogen use. *Lancet* 1979;2:111–114.
6. Nordoy A, Svensson B, Haycraft D, et al: The influence of age, sex, and the use of oral contraceptives on the inhibitory effects of endothelial cells and PGI_2 (prostacyclin) on platelet function. *Scand J Haematol* 1978;21:177–187.
7. Gordon T, Garcia-Palmieri MR, Kagan A, et al: Differences in coronary heart disease in Framingham, Honolulu and Puerto Rico. *J Chronic Dis* 1974;27:329–344.
8. Dyerberg J, Bang HO: Hemostatic function and platelet polyunsaturated fatty acids in eskimos. *Lancet* 1979;2:433–435.
9. Seiss W, Scherer B, Bohlig B, et al: Platelet-membrane fatty acids, platelet aggregation, and thromboxane formation during a mackerel diet. *Lancet* 1980;1:441–444.
10. Rogot E, Padgett SJ: Associations of coronary and stroke mortality with temperature and snowfall in selected areas of the United States, 1962–1966. *Am J Epidemiol* 1976;103:565–575.
11. Sharrett AR, Feinleib M: Water constituents and trace elements in relation to cardiovascular disease. *Prev Med* 1975;4:20–36.
12. Marmot MG, Syme SL, Kagan A, et al: Epidemiologic studies of coronary heart disease and stroke in Japanese men living in Japan, Hawaii and California: prevalence of coronary and hypertensive heart disease and associated risk factors. *Am J Epidemiol* 1975;102:514–525.
13. Kannel WB, Castelli WP, Gordon T, et al: Serum cholesterol, lipoproteins and the risk of coronary heart disease: the Framingham study. *Ann Intern Med* 1971;74:1–12.
14. Rifkind BM, Lawson D, Gale M: Diagnostic value of serum lipids and frequency of lipoprotein patterns in myocardial infarction. *J Atheroscler Res* 1968;8:167–176.
15. Gordon T, Castelli W, Hjortland M, et al: High density lipoprotein as a protective factor against coronary artery disease: the Framingham study. *Am J Med* 1977;62:707–714.
16. Ross R, Glomset J, Kariya B, et al: A platelet-dependent serum factor that stimulates the proliferation of arterial smooth muscle cells in vitro. *Proc Natl Acad Sci USA* 1974;71:1207–1210.
17. Hirsch PD, Campbell WB, Willerson JT, et al: Prostaglandins and ischemic heart disease. *Am J Med* 1981;71:1009–1026.
18. Fleisher LN, Tall AR, Witte LD, et al: Stimulation of arterial endothelial cell prostacyclin synthesis by high density lipoproteins. *J Biol Chem* 1982;257:6653–6655.

19. Kannel WB: Role of blood pressure in cardiovascular disease: the Framingham study. *Angiology* 1975;26:1–14.
20. Auerbach O, Hammond EC, Garfinkel: Smoking in relation to atherosclerosis of the coronary arteries. *N Engl J Med* 1965;273:775–779.
21. Feinleib M, Williams RR: Relative risks of myocardial infarction, cardiovascular disease and peripheral vascular disease by type of smoking. *Proc 3rd World Conf Smoking Health* 1976;1:243.
22. McKenna WJ, Chew CYC, Oakley CM: Myocardial infarction with normal coronary angiogram—possible mechanism of smoking risk in coronary artery disease. *Br Heart J* 1980;43:493–498.
23. Kannel WB, McGee D, Gordon T: A general cardiovascular risk profile: the Framingham study. *Am J Cardiol* 1976;38:46–51.
24. Rosenman RH, Brand RJ, Sholtz RI, et al: Multivariate prediction of coronary heart disease during 8.5 year follow-up in the Western Collaborative Group Study. *Am J Cardiol* 1976;37:903–910.
25. Gordon T, Kannel WB, McGee D, et al: Death and coronary attacks in men after giving up cigarette smoking. A report from the Framingham study. *Lancet* 1974;2:1345–1348.
26. Cryer PE, Haymond MW, Santiago JV, et al: Norepinephrine and epinephrine release and adrenergic mediation of smoking-associated hemodynamic and metabolic events. *N Engl J Med* 1976;295:573–577.
27. Wennmalm A: Interaction of nicotine and prostaglandins in the cardiovascular systems. *Prostaglandins* 1982;23:139–144.
28. Levine PH: An acute effect of cigarette smoking on platelet function. *Circulation* 1973;48:619–623.
29. Garcia MJ, McNamara PM, Gordon T, et al: Morbidity and mortality of diabetes in the Framingham population. Sixteen year follow-up study. *Diabetes* 1976;23:105–111.
30. Coronary Drug Project Research Group, Baltimore: The prognostic importance of plasma glucose levels and the use of oral hypoglycemic drugs after myocardial infarction in men. *Diabetes* 1977;26:453–465.
31. Ostrander LD Jr, Block WD, Lamphiear DE, et al: Altered carbodydrate and lipid metabolism and coronary heart disease among men in Tecumseh, Michigan, in Camerini-Davalos R, Cole HS (eds): *Vascular and Neurological Changes in Early Diabetes*. New York, Academic Press, 1973, p 73.
32. Shaw S, Pegrum GD, Wolff S, et al: Platelet adhesiveness in diabetes mellitus. *J Clin Path* 1967;20:845–847.
33. Breddin K: Experimental and clinical investigations on the adhesion and aggregation of human platelets. *Exp Biol Med* 1968;3:14–23.
34. Halushka PV, Lurie D, Colwell JA: Increased synthesis of prostaglandin-E-like material by platelets from patients with diabetes mellitus. *N Engl J Med* 1977;297:1306–1310.
35. Halushka PV, Rogers BC, Loadholt CB, et al: Increased platelet thromboxane synthesis in diabetes mellitus. *J Lab Clin Med* 1981;97:87–96.
36. Harrison HE, Reece AH, Johnson M: Decreased vascular prostacyclin in experimental diabetes. *Life Sci* 1978;23:351–355.
37. Silberbauer K, Schernthaner G, Sinzinger H, et al: Decreased vascular prostacyclin in juvenile-onset diabetes. *N Engl J Med* 1979;300:366–367.
38. Garg SK, Lackner H, Karpatkin S: The increased percentage of megathrombocytes in various clinical disorders. *Ann Int Med* 1972;77:361–369.
39. Burrows AW, Chavin SI, Hockaday TDR: Plasma-thromboglobulin concentrations in diabetes mellitus. *Lancet* 1978;1:235–237.
40. Rosenman RH: History and definition of the Type A coronary-prone

behavior pattern, in Dembroski TM, Feinleib M, Haynes SG, et al (eds): *Proceedings of the Forum on Coronary-Prone Behavior*. Washington, 1978, DHEW Publ. No. (NIH) 78-1451, p 13.

41. Rosenman RH, Brand RJ, Sholtz RI, et al: Multivariate prediction of coronary heart disease during 8.5 year follow-up in the Western Collaborative Group Study. *Am J Cardiol* 1976;37:903–910.

42. Blumenthal JA, Williams RB, Kong Y, et al: Type A behavior pattern and coronary atherosclerosis. *Circulation* 1978;58:634–639.

43. Arkel YS, Haft JI, Kreutner W, et al: Alteration in second phase platelet aggregation associated with an emotionally stressful activity. *Thromb Haemost* 1977;38:552–561.

44. Vlachakis ND, Aledort L: Hypertension and propranolol therapy: effect on blood pressure, plasma catecholamines and platelet aggregation. *Am J Cardiol* 1980;45:321–325.

45. Phillips RL, Lemon FR, Beeson L, et al: Coronary heart disease mortality among Seventh-Day Adventists with differing dietary habits: a preliminary report. *Am J Clin Nutr* 1978;31:S191–198.

46. Sharrett AR, Feinleib M: Water constituents and trace elements in relation to cardiovascular disease. *Prev Med* 1975;4:20–36.

47. Yano K, Rhoads GG, Kagan A: Coffee, alcohol and risk of coronary heart disease among Japanese men living in Hawaii. *N Engl J Med* 1977;297:405–409.

48. Castelli WP, Gordon T, Hjortland MC, et al: Alcohol and blood lipids. The Cooperative Lipoprotein Phenotyping Study. *Lancet* 1977;2:153–155.

49. Dyerberg J, Bang HO: Hemostatic function and platelet polyunsaturated fatty acids in eskimos. *Lancet* 1979;2:433–435.

50. Diamond GA, Forrester JS: Analysis of probability as an aid in the clinical diagnosis of coronary artery disease. *N Engl J Med* 1979;300:1350–1358.

51. Bonte FJ, Parkey RW, Willerson JT: Past, present and future of nuclear cardiology, in Willerson JT (ed): *Nuclear Cardiology*. Philadelphia, FA Davis Co., 1979, pp. 1–7.

52. Gruntzig AR, Senning A, Siegenthaler WE: Nonoperative dilation of coronary-artery stenosis. Percutaneous transluminal coronary angioplasty. *N Engl J Med* 1979;301:61–68.

53. Garrett HE, Dennis EW, DeBakey M: Aorto-coronary bypass with saphenous vein graft. Seven-year follow-up. *JAMA* 1973;233:792–794.

54. Favoloro RG: Saphenous vein graft in the surgical treatment of coronary artery disease: operative technique. *J Thor Cardiovasc Surg* 1969;58:178–185.

55. Johnson WD, Flemma RJ, Leppley Jr D: Direct coronary surgery utilizing multiple-vein bypass grafts. *Ann Thorac Surg* 1970;9:436–444.

56. Kannel WB, Feinleib: Natural history of angina pectoris in the Framingham study: progress and survival. *Am J Cardiol* 1972;29:154–163.

57. Reeves RJ, Oberman A, Jones WB, et al: Natural history of angina pectoris. *Am J Cardiol* 1974;33:423–430.

58. Cohen MV, Gorlin R: Main left coronary artery disease. *Circulation* 1975;52:275–285.

59. Wilhelmsen L, Vedin A, Wilhelmsson C: Beta blockade and sudden death following myocardial infarction. *Cardiovasc Med* 1978;3:557–563.

60. Chierchia S, Brunelli C, Simonetti I, et al: Sequence of events in angina at rest: primary reduction in coronary flow. *Circulation* 1980;61:759–768.

61. Oliva PB, Breckinridge JC: Arteriographic evidence of coronary arterial spasm in acute myocardial infarction. *Circulation* 1977;56:366–374.

62. Robertson RM, Robertson D, Roberts LJ, et al: Thromboxane A_2 in vasotonic angina pectoris: evidence from direct measurements and inhibitor trials. *N Engl J Med* 1981;304:998–1003.
63. Chierchia S, deCaterina R, Crea F, et al: Failure of thromboxane A_2 blockade to prevent attacks of vasospastic angina. *Circulation* 1982;66:702–705.
64. Miwa K, Kambara H, Kawai C: Exercise-induced angina provoked by aspirin administration in patients with variant angina. *Am J Cardiol* 1981;47:1210–1214.
65. Chierchia S, Patrono C, Crea F, et al: Effects of intravenous prostacyclin in variant angina. *Circulation* 1982;65:470–477.
66. Curry RC, Pepine CJ, Sabom MB, et al: Hemodynamic and myocardial metabolic effects of ergonovine in patients with chest pain. *Circulation* 1978;58:648–654.
67. Selzer A, Langston M, Ruggeroli C, et al: Clinical syndrome of variant angina with normal coronary arteriogram. *N Engl J Med* 1976;295:1343–1347.
68. Kerin NZ, Rubenfire M, Naini M, et al: Arrhythmias in variant angina pectoris: relationship of arrhythmias to ST-segment elevation and R-wave changes. *Circulation* 1979;60:1343–1350.
69. Silverman ME, Flamm MD: Variant angina pectoris: anatomic findings and prognostic implications. *Ann Intern Med* 1971;75:339–343.
70. Hirsh PD, Hillis LD, Campbell WB, et al: Release of transcardiac prostaglandins and thromboxane into the coronary circulation in patients with ischemic heart disease. *N Engl J Med* 1981;304:685–691.
71. Hirsh PD, Firth BG, Campbell WB, et al: Effects of provocation on transcardiac thromboxane in patients with coronary artery disease. *Am J Cardiol* 1983;51:727–733.
72. Fowler NO: "Preinfarctional" angina. A need for an objective definition and for a controlled clinical trial of its management. *Circulation* 1971;44:755–758.
73. Pugh B, Platt MR, Mills LJ, et al: Unstable angina pectoris: A randomized study of patients treated medically and surgically. *Am J Cardiol* 1978;41:1291–1298.
74. Donsky MS, Curry GC, Parkey RW, et al: Unstable angina pectoris. Clinical, angiographic and myocardial scintigraphic observations. *Br Heart J* 1976;38:257–263.
75. Telford AM, Wilson C: Trial of heparin versus atenolol in prevention of myocardial infarction in intermediate coronary syndrome. *Lancet* 1981;1:1225–1228.
76. Cairns JA, Fantus IG, Klassen GA: Unstable angina pectoris. *Am Heart J* 1976;92:373–386.
77. Rentrop P, Blanke H, Karsch KR, et al: Selective intracoronary thrombolysis in acute myocardial infarction and unstable angina pectoris. *Circulation* 1981;63:307–317.
78. Buja LM, Willerson, JT: Clinicopathologic findings in 100 episodes of acute ischemic heart disease (acute myocardial infarction or coronary insufficiency) in 83 patients. *Am J Cardiol* 1981;47:343–356.
79. Willerson JT, Hillis LD, Buja LM: *Ischemic Heart Disease: Clinical and Pathophysiological Considerations*. Raven Press, New York, 1982.

9 *Cerebrovascular Disease*

Robert W. Stein
William J. Weiner

Stroke comprises a heterogeneous group of disorders with different mechanisms. Despite a decreased incidence of stroke in recent years,[1] as the population ages stroke remains prevalent. In 1977, it was the third most common cause of death in the United States with 83,000 deaths attributed to stroke, and with more than 1 million disabled survivors.[2]

Categorization of cerebrovascular disease has changed over the years as the technologies available to investigate mechanisms have improved, and concepts changed. Aring and Merritt in a retrospective postmortem study estimated that 82% of strokes were secondary to large vessel thrombosis, 3% to embolism and 15% to all types of hemorrhages.[3] Whisnant et al[4] and Matsumoto et al[5] later reported similar frequencies with 75% thrombotic, 3-8% emboli, and 10% hemorrhage. In contrast, the most recently published registry data by Caplan, Mohr and coworkers done in the era of the newer imaging technics are quite different.[6] The incidence of embolism increased to 31%, and large vessel thrombosis decreased to 32%. This change in frequency was probably due to both the improved criteria for the diagnosis of embolism, and the recognition of lacunar stroke syndromes. Lacunes accounted for approximately 20% of all strokes in that registry with the remainder consisting of approximately 10% hypertensive hemorrhages and 10% hemorrhages secondary to arteriovenous malformations or aneurysms.

Despite the recent diagnostic advances, often the mechanism of stroke in a particular patient remains speculative. This chapter will address those stroke syndromes of definite or possible thromboembolic etiology, large vessel thrombosis, embolism, and lacunes. No discussion of hemorrhage will be undertaken.

VASCULAR ANATOMY

An understanding of cerebrovascular disease requires knowledge of the vascular anatomy. The cerebral blood supply is provided by an anterior and a posterior circulation joined together by the circle of Willis. The anterior circulation is formed primarily by the paired carotid arteries which divide to form the external and internal carotid arteries. Intracranially, the first major branches of the supraclinoid carotid artery are the ophthalmic, posterior communicating, and anterior choroidal arteries. The internal carotid then divides to form the anterior cerebral and the main stem of the middle cerebral artery.

The middle cerebral artery after giving off deep penetrating branches (the lenticulostriate arteries) soon divides into an upper trunk and lower trunk. The upper trunk supplies the lateral and inferior aspects of the frontal lobe while the lower trunk supplies the lateral portions of the parietal lobe and superior portions of the temporal lobe and insula. The lenticulostriate arteries supply the basal ganglia, internal capsule, and corona radiata.

The anterior cerebral arteries are joined by the anterior communicating arteries. The anterior cerebral artery supplies the anterior three fourths of the medial surface of the cerebral hemispheres. Deep penetrating branches from the anterior cerebral artery supply the head of the caudate and anterior limb of the internal capsuli.

The posterior circulation supplies the brain stem, cerebellum, and the hemispheral areas not supplied by the anterior circulation. The posterior circulation originates from the paired vertebral arteries. After giving off branches which form the anterior spinal artery and the posterior inferior cerebellar artery (PICA), the vertebrals terminate by forming the large, single basilar artery. The basilar artery runs the course of the pons and midbrain before it terminates by forming the biolateral superior cerebellar and the posterior cerebral arteries. En route, the basilar artery has numerous branches including the anterior inferior cerebellar artery (AICA) and innumerable paramedian short and long perforators.

In general, the blood supply of the brain stem can be divided into a medial and lateral supply. The medial medulla, pons, and midbrain are supplied by penetrators from the anterior spinal, basilar, and posterior cerebral arteries, respectively. The lateral portions of the brain stem are supplied by circumferential vessels. The PICA supplies the lateral medulla, the AICA the inferior lateral pons, the superior cerebellar artery the superior pons, and the posterior cerebral artery the lateral midbrain.

The thalamus receives blood from the deep penetrators from the basilar and posterior cerebral arteries. The terminal branches of the posterior cerebral artery supply the medial occipital cortex and the inferomedial part of the temporal lobe.

CLASSIFICATION AND PATHOGENESIS

The diagnosis of a stroke syndrome is rarely in doubt. Its hallmark is the sudden onset of a focal, nonconvulsive neurologic deficit.[2] The deficit can range from a severe hemiplegia, aphasia, or coma to a mild transient sensory deficit. It is the time course of the onset of deficit, developing over seconds to minutes to hours that give stroke its characteristic picture. Transient ischemic attack (TIA), reversible ischemic neurologic deficit (RIND), and completed stoke are artificial categorizations of stroke which represent a spectrum of ischemia and recovery of function. A TIA is defined as a focal deficit of vascular origin which resolves over 24 hours. However, it is speculated that the duration of a TIA may vary according to its mechanism. The TIA preceding large vessel occlusion may be stereotyped, frequent, and of short duration (30 minutes or less) while the one-time focal deficit which has abrupt onset but resolves in less than 24 hours may be embolic in origin. A RIND is defined as a deficit which almost entirely resolves within three weeks. In a completed stroke the deficit persists.

A more useful classification of stroke is the mechanistic one intimated previously. In this classification ischemic stroke is divided into embolic (cardiac, arterial, or venous source) lacune, large vessel arthero-thrombosis, or some combination.

EMBOLIC STROKE

It has long been suspected that emboli may cause stroke. Chiari at the turn of the century is said to have discussed eight patients who at postmortem had thrombosis of the bifurcation of the common carotid artery.[7] Chiari suggested that portions of this thrombus might embolize to the cerebral arteries. Emboli arise from two major sources, the heart and large vessels with less common sources being tumor, marrow of long bones (fat), or air. Regardless of its source the embolus travels distally until it becomes lodged in a vessel of smaller diameter than the embolus. Emboli have a predilection for points of arterial bifurcation, particularly the middle cerebral stem, upper or lower trunk of the middle cerebral artery, top of the basilar artery, or posterior cerebral artery.

Emboli can reach any of the intracerebral arteries.[8] Gacs et al have shown that emboli of cardiac origin that enter the carotid circulation most repeatedly lodge in the middle cerebral artery or one of its branches (93%). The anterior cerebral artery is a rare destination (7%).[9] Emboli to the posterior cerebral artery arc not uncommon. The embolus may directly traverse the vertebral basilar system or reach that circulation via a posterior cerebral artery which is derived from the internal carotid artery. Emboli may also lodge within large vessels around which a thrombus develops. Such a mechanism is well described in Kubik and Adams's description of basilar artery occlusion.[10]

Embolic infarction, in addition to being composed of areas of ischemic necrosis (pale infarction), may have frankly hemorrhagic features consisting of petechial zones. Either the embolus fragments or anastomotic reperfusion occurs, allowing the reirrigation by damaged

186

capillaries of infarcted tissue. These hemorrhagic areas may cover the entire zone of infarction but tend to predominate along boundary zones between anastomatic circulation, both cerebral-to-cerebral and meningeal-to-cerebral.[11] Unfortunately, to date there is no method to predict if and when embolic strokes will bleed, confusing the issue of therapy.

Cardiac Sources of Embolic Stroke

Emboli from the heart can arise from multiple disease processes. Embolic strokes are well recognized as a complication of dysfunction of heart muscle including idiopathic, ischemic, and other secondary cardiomyopathies. In the Framingham study, congestive heart failure alone increased the risk of brain infarction ninefold.[12] The embolic material in this setting is usually composed of platelet fibrin material. The pathologic study of congestive heart failure has demonstrated platelet fibrin thrombi in 50% of cases, with a predilection for the thrombi to be multiple, at the apex, and entrapped within the trabeculae carnae.[13]

The incidence of stroke in recent myocardial infarction has been estimated to be 2% maximal between the first and second week. A greater risk (24-fold) is associated with large myocardial infarctions as demonstrated by creatinine phosphokinase values greater than 1160 IU/I.[14] The endocardial lesion will heal and will no longer be a source of embolic material. Beam demonstrated a crescendo-decrescendo frequency of emboli after myocardial infarction, again with maximal incidence in the second week and with less than 14% of such emboli occurring after the first month.[15] In contrast to the endothelium, which can heal, the heart muscle may be severely damaged with production of akinetic segments and ventricular aneurysms. In these areas of abnormal nonfunctioning, stagnant heart muscle clots may form and be the source of emboli.

Atrial fibrillation in the setting of rheumatic heart disease has long been known to be a source of systemic emboli.[16] Wolf et al reaffirmed this finding and in addition showed a fivefold increased risk of stroke in atrial fibrillation in the absence of rheumatic heart disease.[17] Hinton et al reported similar findings in a pathologic study of 333 patients with atrial fibrillation. Embolism occurred in 35% of those with atrial fibrillation and ischemic heart disease, compared to only 7% of a control group of autopsy patients with ischemic heart disease without atrial fibrillation.[18] Stroke occurrence increases as the duration of atrial fibrillation increases without evidence of a particularly vulnerable period.[17] The origin of this clot is probably the left atrium of left auricular appendage as a clot in these areas was far more common in those individuals with cerebral emboli than in those without emboli.[18]

Disease of the heart valves is another source of emboli. Noninfective calcific stenotic values, particularly the mitral but also the aortic, may serve as a template for deposition of platelet and fibrin clots which can embolize.[19] In mitral stenosis the frequency of cerebral embolus is approximately 20%[20] with most occurring after the age of 35.[21] It has been suggested that the risk of embolization is as great for mitral insufficiency as mitral stenosis with the coexistence of atrial fibrillation an additional risk.[22]

Two other mitral valve abnormalities may be the cause of embolic stroke; mitral valve prolapse and mitral annulus calcification. Barnett et al[23] and Scharf et al[24] have clearly demonstrated the association of mitral valve prolapse and cerebral infarction. However, the risk associated with mitral valve prolapse appears greatest before the age of 45 with few strokes credited to this valvular abnormality after that age. The mechanism remains undefined. Speculations include thrombus formation on the atrial side of the prolapsing valve in an area of stagnant flow, clot formation secondary to a hypercoagulable state,[24] or myxomatous change in the valve allowing endothelial tears, platelet adhesion, and agglutination followed by fibrin deposition and embolization.[25]

Calcification of the mitral valve annulus has also been reported to be more common in embolic stroke than in aged-matched controls.[26] In an early clinicopathologic review of this entity four of the 14 patients described suffered cerebral infarctions, one of whom was not in atrial fibrillation.[27] Possible mechanisms include extrusion of calcified material or platelet fibrin emboli.

Infected heart valves are also a source of embolic material. In one large series of patients with infective endocarditis, 33% with natural valve infection and 50% of those with infected prosthetic valves suffered cerebral emboli. In natural valve infections the aortic valve was most commonly infected with *Staphylococcus aureus*. In prosthetic valve endocarditis, *Aspergillus* was the most common early organism while *Streptococcus viridans* became the most common late cause.[28] Occasionally emboli from infected valves are infected themselves producing brain abscesses or mycotic aneurysms. These aneurysms are typically located in unusual sites far beyond the circle of Willis.

Nonbacterial thrombotic endocarditis may be another cause of embolic stroke. This syndrome is usually associated with cancer (pancreas, stomach, prostate, ovary and lung),[29] congestive heart failure, and pneumonia.[30] The mitral is the most commonly involved valve. On the valve surface are located granular friable hemorrhagic platelet fibrin vegetations that may embolize.

Noninfective prosthetic valves may also be a source of embolic material. The incidence of emboli is probably related to valve type with the degree of thombogenicity declining from the noncloth-covered prosthetic valves to cloth-covered prosthetic valves to tissue valves.

Atrial myxomas have been identified as a rare but recognizable and treatable cause of embolic infarction. In one series, 27% of the atrial myxomas presented with cerebral ischemia but in most cases cardiac and constitutional symptoms predominate in particular heart murmur, congestive heart failure, polymyalgias, fever, weight loss, and anemia.[31] Emboli take the form of thrombi or tumor fragments. Cerebral aneurysms and tumors have been reported as late sequelae of myxoma[32] but their occurrence appears unusual.[31]

Large Vessel Occlusion as Embolic Source

Although the heart is overwhelmingly the largest contributor of emboli, embolism can also arise from the arterial circulation. As previously mentioned Chiari observed that a large vessel occlusion could be the source of an embolic stroke.[7] It is now apparent that there are presumably three different time periods (immediate, early, and late) for embolic stroke to occur after large vessel occlusion. Pessin et al observed a group of patients who clinically appeared to have an embolic occlusion of a distal vessel but at angiography had occlusion of the more proximal carotid artery.[33] Two other groups have reported the occurrence of stroke in the early time period (less than one week) after vessel occlusion.[34,35] In this early group Finklestein et al[34] documented pathologically that the embolus originated from the distal "tail" of the carotid thrombus. Barnett reported stroke occurring (weeks to years) after vessel occlusion.[35] In the acute and early groups it could be speculated that the embolus is composed of material from the thrombotic occlusion, as demonstrated by Finklestein et al.[34] In the late group Barnett has suggested that turbulence in the arterial stump would predispose to atheroma and platelet-fibrin aggregation. This material could then embolize through collateral circulation.[35] Thrombosis of the subclavian artery with retrograde propagation of the thrombus and subsequent embolization to the cerebral circulation has also been documented.[36]

Large Vessel Stenosis as Embolic Source

Emboli also arise from the stenotic atherosclerotic areas both intra- and extracranially. The frequency and severity of atherosclerotic lesions in the cervicocerebral tree is shown in Figure 9-1, which is redrawn from Escourelle and Poirier.[11] The existence of emboli from these sources has been well documented. For example, Pessin et al,[33] in their series on acute carotid stroke, reported a group of patients with embolic stroke who had internal carotid artery lumens less than 2 mm. The emboli are probably composed of two types of materials, platelet-fibrin clots and atheromatous cholesterol debris. Fisher[37] in 1959 first suggested the existence of platelet-fibrin emboli when he noted white bodies passing through the retinal arterioles during an episode of transient monocular blindness. In 1964, Gunning et al reported 16 patients with atheromatous carotid disease and episodes of TIAs, cerebral infarction, transient monocular blindness, and retinal infarction.[7] In a subgroup of these patients platelet fibrin emboli were demonstrated in the retinal and cerebral

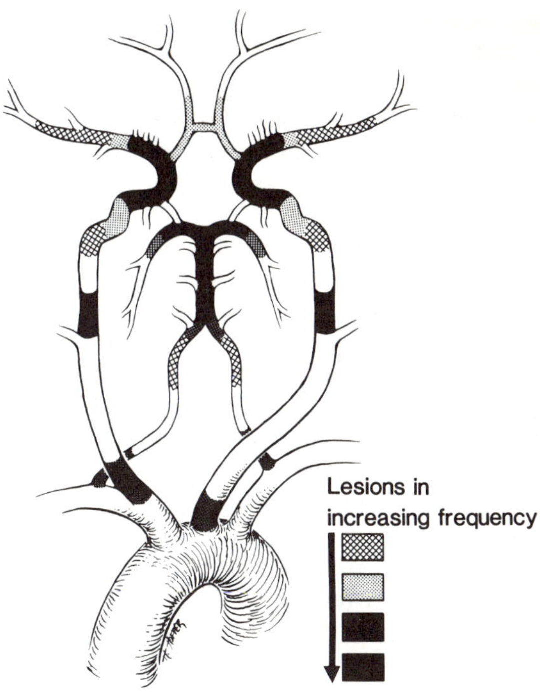

Figure 9-1 Frequency and severity of atherosclerotic lesions in the cervicocerebral vessels. (Redrawn with permission from Escourolle R, Poirier J: *Manual of Basic Neuropathology*. Paris, Masson, S.A., 1978.)

vessels. Adams and Gross[38] reported a remarkable case in which a platelet-fibrin embolus was observed to move to a middle cerebral artery stenosis during superficial temporal-middle cerebral artery bypass surgery.

In addition to platelet-fibrin emboli, atheromatous debris emboli are a cause of stroke. Hollenhorst in 1961 described bright plaques in the retinal circulation in patients with carotid disease and stroke.[39] Beal et al[40] reported a case of cholesterol emboli originating from a severely ulcerative atheromatous area of thoracic aorta. These emboli caused multiple episodes of numbness or weakness. At postmortem many small cerebral arteries were found to be occluded by these cholesterol emboli.

Despite their characterization, a complete understanding of how these emboli are formed and what conditions are essential for their formation is still lacking. The following scheme can be proposed based upon the work of Imparato et al who reviewed the clinical and pathologic findings from 50 patients who underwent 69 carotid endarterectomies.[41] The plaque represents an area of fibrointimal thickening. It evolves to a symptomatic stage by the occurrence of one of the following processes:

(1) intraplaque hemorrhage with severe stenosis of the lumen, with extension of the hemorrhage through the vessel wall with a thrombus forming in the area; (2) intraplaque accumulation of atheromatous debris (often following plaque hemorrhage) with subsequent ulceration and release of the material into the circulation; (3) formation of a laminated thrombus on either a smooth or ulcerative area of stenotic fibrous thickening.

Whether the ulcerative nonstenotic plaque is a nidus for embolus formation is uncertain. A review of the pathology of 44 carotid plaques from the side appropriate to focal cerebral symptoms revealed no cases of isolated plaque.[41] Rather, all symptomatic plaques were associated with either intramural plaque hemorrhage, greater than 70% stenosis of the vessel lumen, or both.[41] Furthermore, Durward et al reported that when previously asymptomatic plaques became symptomatic, it was always in the presence of progression of the plaque.[42]

Experimental models have provided support for the concept that the endothelium must be damaged to be thrombogenic. Denny-Brown reported that after the production of traumatic lesions in the proximal middle cerebral artery of rats, he was able to observe and photograph a platelet-fibrin embolus lodged in a small peripheral branch artery.[43]

The prostaglandin system and its metabolic products have been implicated to play a role in the formation of platelet-fibrin emboli. The potential role of prostaglandins in vascular patency and platelet reactivity was suggested by Piper and Vane in 1969.[44] They observed that an unidentified unstable substance released from guinea pig lung during anaphylaxis caused transient contraction of rabbit aorta. This action was blocked by aspirin or indomethacin. This substance was eventually identified by Hamberg et al in 1975 to be composed to three prostaglandins with the most potent effect produced by thromboxane A_2.[45] In addition it was found that thromboxane also caused irreversible platelet aggregation.[45] In 1976 Moncada et al[46] isolated prostacyclin which inhibited platelet aggregation and relaxed smooth muscle. It is these two substances, thromboxane A_2 and prostacyclin, which have been identified as the two most likely candidates for playing a significant role in platelet aggregation and vascular reactivity.

Most cells are able to produce prostaglandins but in general one particular prostaglandin is made in relative abundance by a particular cell type. All cells oxidize arachnidonic acid via a cyclooxygenase to an intermediate cyclic endoperoxide. In a particular cell type the cyclic endoperoxides are then metabolized in a unique direction. In platelets thromboxane A_2 is produced by thromboxane synthetase. Thromboxane A_2 is the most potent naturally occurring vasoconstrictor and platelet aggregator known. It has a half-life of approximately 32 seconds at 37°C. Thromboxane A_2 is rapidly converted to thromboxane B_2, an inactive metabolite.

In the endothelial cell of the vessel wall the cyclic endoperoxides are converted to prostacyclin. Prostacyclin is the most potent vasodilator and inhibitor of platelet aggregation known. Prostacyclin is unstable in aqueous solution with a half-life of two minutes. It is rapidly metabolized to 6-keto-$PGF_{1\alpha}$.

As originally suggested by Moncada et al[46] vascular patency may in part be maintained by a balance between the proaggregatory and vasconstrictor forces of thromboxane and the antiaggregatory and vasdilatory action of prostacyclin. A disruption of this balance in favor of thromboxane could lead to an increased thrombotic tendency. Such a disturbed balance has been reported by Wu et al in a patient with thrombotic thrombocytopenic purpura with multiple strokes and an accelerated rate of prostacyclin degradation.[47] It is possible that at a site of stenosis, plaque hemorrhage, and ulceration with disruption of endothelial cells, a local decrease in production of prostacyclin could lead to platelet aggregation and fibrin clot.

Venous Sources of Embolic Stroke

In addition to the heart and arterial vessels, a third source of emboli may be the venous circulation. It is estimated that up to 35% of a general autopsy series will have a probe-patent foramen ovale. An increase in right atrial pressure, particularly during a Valsalva maneuver, might allow an embolus that originated in the venous circulation to pass from the right to left heart and then into the systemic circulation.[48] Jones et al[48] have recently reported five such cases of cerebral emboli of paradoxical origin.

LARGE VESSEL OCCLUSIVE DISEASE

Large vessel atherosclerosis, in addition to being a source of emboli, can lead to severe stenosis and occlusion, making adequate cerebral blood flow unlikely. If other vessels do not allow for collateral circulation stroke will ensue. Such a mechanism might be called low distal perfusion. In the study of acute carotid stroke by Pessin et al a group of patients were identified who were without evidence of emboli and who only showed a widespread delay in cerebral arterial perfusion.[33] In this group of patients stroke is more frequently preceded by TIAs, and less severe deficit results than in the embolic stroke group.[33]

Occlusion of the basilar and vertebral arteries is well described. Kubik and Adams[10] reported the clinical and pathologic findings of basilar artery occlusion in 18 cases. In 11 of their patients thrombotic occlusions occurred in the setting of atherosclerosis. The remainder of cases were of an embolic mechanism. Fisher et al[49] described a group of patients with a lateral medullary syndrome following vertebral artery thrombosis, also in the setting of severe atherosclerosis.

While severe atherosclerosis with stenosis or occlusion is common in the carotid, basilar, and vertebral arteries, such vascular lesions at the origin of the anterior, middle, or posterior cerebral arteries are less common, with more distal involvement even rarer. Middle cerebral artery stenosis was present in only 4.1% of the angiograms done in the joint study of extracranial arterial occlusion.[50] Hinton et al in their report of 16 cases of middle cerebral artery stenosis cited only three cases that had stenosis beyond the stem, and all three were located in the proximal portion of the upper trunk.[51] Similarly Fisher et al[52] in a study of atherosclerosis of the carotid and vertebral arterial distribution failed to find significant atherosclerosis at any site distal to the proximal portion of the superior or inferior division of the middle cerebral artery. Similar to the larger vessels, the anterior, middle, and posterior cerebral arteries can develop symptomatic infarction by thrombosis in an area of atherosclerosis or impact of an embolus in an area of atherosclerotic narrowing.

LACUNES

Lacunar stroke results from infarction deep within the brain in the distribution of small penetrating nonanastomosing end-arteries 150 to 300μ in diameter. These arteries arise as branches of the proximal basilar, vertebral, anterior, middle, and posterior arteries. These penetrating arteries supply the internal capsule, basal ganglia, deep white matter, thalamus, and pons. Lacunes usually occur in the setting of hypertension and diabetes.

The most likely mechanism in this stroke type involves a lipohylanotic thickening of the artery along its course. This process resembles atherosclerosis but features excessive subendothelial accumulation of material that stains like hyaline and fat. There is severe damage to the vessel wall with segmental enlargement of the external diameter, obliteration of the lumen by thrombus with leakage of red blood cells, and edema of surrounding tissue.[53] The size of the infarct will vary according to where along the path of the vessel the occlusion occurs. The more distal occlusion will cause the smaller lacune while proximal occlusions will cause larger infarctions.

Another potential mechanism for lacunar stroke is atheromatous narrowing and occlusion of the origin of the penetrating vessel by large vessel atherosclerosis. This process has been suggested as the possible mechanism for giant lacunes although embolic branch occlusions have also been proposed.

Multiple lacunar syndromes have been described with the clinical features dependent upon the distribution of the infarction. Pure motor hemiplegia with sparing of language, vision, behavior, and sensory abilities occurs most commonly after infarction of the internal capsule or pons[54] although the syndrome might be expected to occur from a lesion anywhere along the corticospinal tract as demonstrated in the report of pure motor hemiplegia due to infarction of the cerebral peduncle.[55] Pure sensory stroke has been shown to result from a thalamic lacune.[53,56] Because the thalamus and internal capsule receive blood supply from different circulations, sensorimotor stroke secondary to a lacunar mechanism although reported, is rare.[57] The major blood supply of the internal capsule is from the lenticulostriates off the middle cerebral artery while the thalamus is supplied by the thalamogeniculate branches of the posterior cerebral artery.

In ataxic hemiparesis pure motor hemiplegia is combined with a cerebellar ataxia. The ataxia is out of proportion to the weakness. This syndrome has been localized by Fisher to the basis pontis at the level of the junction of the upper one third and lower two thirds of the pons of the side opposite the neurologic deficit.[58] Two other reports have described a similar clinical picture with computed tomography (CT) localization to the superior portion of the posterior limb of the internal capsule.[59,60] The syndrome of hemichorea-hemiballismus has been shown by CT to be secondary to lacunar stroke in the anterior portions of the putamen, internal capsule, and caudate.[61] Retrospectively, a lacunar mechanism has been suggested for the syndrome occurring in infarction of the subthalamic nucleus or thalamus.[61] Another remarkable lacunar syndrome, clumsy hand-dysarthria is characterized by severe dysarthria, lower facial weakness, clumsiness, slowness of fine manipulations with the affected hand, minimal weakness, and on the affected side enhanced reflexes and the presence of Babinski's sign. Postmortem study has demonstrated a lacune deep in the base of the pons.[62]

The number of possible lacunar syndromes is limited only by the almost infinite number of possible deep penetrating vessel occlusions which can give rise to clinical symptomatology. Up to 20 syndromes including pure dysarthria, mutism, ocular paresis with cerebellar ataxia, and isolated internuclear ophthalmoplegia have been suggested and await confirmation.

TRANSIENT ISCHEMIC ATTACKS

Since TIAs represent a spectrum of ischemia and recovery of function, one mechanism is unlikely. In considering their pathogenesis it is helpful after eliminating seizure and migraine headaches as causes of transient focal neurologic deficit to divide the spells into two groups. The first group consists of those spells that occur as a single episode and last for hours. In this group the mechanism of ischemia could include any of those previously delineated, with embolus being very common. The transient nature of the TIA may be a result of: (1) relief of the ischemia before significant neuronal damage can result, (2) small size of infarction, (3) rapid compensation by other neuronal tissue.

The second group of TIAs is characterized by short duration (less than 30 minutes), and stereotyped and repetitive episodes. Possible mechanisms include emboli from the heart or artery to artery emboli, extracranial mechanical interference with blood flow, or hemodynamic factors. A single episode that rapidly clears could certainly be of embolic origin, but repetitive stereotyped episodes are less likely to be of embolic origin. Each episode would require that embolic material of different size and shape be carried repetitively in the exact same vascular distribution or that the emboli be consistently the same size and shape allowing them to end continually in the same location. Osteophytes can become large enough to impinge on the vertebral artery and with rotation or extension obstruction of the vessel may occur. This mechanism may be operative in the rare case but it is unlikely to be a frequent cause of vertebrobasilar ischemia.[63,64]

It is argued that reduction of flow through an already narrowed artery will produce symptoms of focal ischemia. This reduction of flow could be secondary to changes in position, fluctuations in blood pressure, or alterations in cardiac function. Opponents of this hypothesis claim that ischemia of this type usually produces diffuse symptomatology such as visual blurring or nonspecific dizziness, and not symptoms referable to the territory beyond the stenosis. In one group of patients with TIAs a deliberate reduction in blood pressure to syncope produced symptoms of prior TIAs in only 1 of 37 patients.[65]

A combination of hemodynamic and embolic mechanisms may be operative. As suggested in the work of Imparato et al[41] and Hutchinson and Yates,[63] perhaps it is the acute changes in the plaque and lining endothelium that allow both a thrombogenic medium for small platelet fibrin emboli and a low flow state conducive to thrombus formation. Fragments of this thrombus may then embolize. Since these emboli originate at a distal site (internal carotid as opposed to heart) the probability that they will traverse the same vascular territory is enhanced. Such a mechanism is compatible with the frequent (66%) discovery of thrombus at early carotid endarterectomy (less than four weeks after the last TIA) but not at late endarterectomy (greater than six weeks after the last TIA).[7,66]

RISK FACTORS

Risk factors for stroke, except for emboli cardiac sources such as atrial fibrillation, have characteristically not been evaluated from a mechanistic viewpoint. For example, although hypertension is a risk for stroke, is it a risk factor for artery-to-artery emboli, carotid bifurcation occlusive disease, siphon stenosis, or some other vascular pathology? Presently, what is known relates to thromboembolic stroke in general. Data from the Framingham study show that increasing age is associated with an increased risk for stroke with incidence rates per 10,000 increasing from 20, to 32, to 83 in the age groups of 45 to 54, 55 to 64, and 65 to 74, respectively. When age is eliminated as a factor, hypertension becomes the most significant risk factor. The degree of elevation for both systolic and diastolic pressure is directly correlated with stroke risk without any pressure separating the stroke-prone from the nonstroke-prone individuals.[67,68]

Glucose intolerance also increases stroke risk twofold. In general diabetes and hypertension are concomitants of lacunar stroke. Birth control pills also increase the risk of stroke, particularly when coexistent with hypertension, migraine, age 35 or older, prolonged use in diabetes, and cigarette use.

Pathologically elevated and high normal hematocrits have been associated with increased stroke and TIA risk even when hypertension and cigarettes are controlled.[69,70] This stroke risk may be related to the increased blood viscosity and decreased blood flow which develop with increasing hamatocrit.[71] The presence of a carotid bruit also correlates with stroke risk but the side of the bruit has failed to predict the side of the stroke.[72]

Data are suggestive but inconclusive regarding cigarettes, hypercholesterolemia, alcohol, and family history as independent risk factors. Coffee, obesity, sedentary life-style, and personality have yet to be clearly associated with stroke.

Once a stroke or TIA has occurred the risk for a recurrent episode is substantial. In studies of previous stroke, stroke recurrence rates of 20% to 40% with mortality of 35% to 65% in five years have been reported.[5,73,74] The risk of stroke after TIA has been variously estimated at four to ten times that of control patients. Within four years 35% of patients with TIAs may have a stroke with the highest risk in the first few months.[75] However, the most frequent cause of death in patients with TIAs is not stroke but heart disease, suggesting that TIAs should be considered a warning for cardiac as well as cerebrovascular disease.[76]

CLINICAL EVALUATION AND THERAPY

The key to correct diagnosis rests with a detailed history and physical examination. From this information the pathophysiologic mechanism underlying a particular episode can be hypothesized and the evaluation of the patient directed and interpreted accordingly. Six crucial historical pieces of information are:

196

1. Activity at onset
2. Severity of deficit at onset
3. Subsequent temporal profile of the deficit
4. Accompanying symptoms such as nausea, vomiting, headache, and stiff neck
5. Prior history of TIAs
6. Associated diseases such as hypertension, diabetes, coronary artery disease, valvular heart disease, peripheral vascular disease, and cardiac arrythmia.

Thrombotic strokes may have a rapid onset of disability but frequently evolve in a stepwise fashion over minutes to hours to days. They are often apparent upon awakening in the morning. Headache when present is described as moderate in intensity and has often been prominent for a few days to weeks preceding the stroke. Historical and physical evidence of other vascular disease (angina, claudication, bruits) is frequently present. The most important clue to thrombotic stroke is the history of preceding stereotyped, short-duration TIAs.

Embolic strokes have a sudden onset and tend to reach maximal deficit within minutes. Often a severe deficit is produced initially as the embolus occludes a large vessel. There is then recovery if collateral circulation is adequate. Subsequently the embolus may fragment and occlude a smaller, more distal vessel, again producing a focal deficit.

Lacunes occur in hypertensive or diabetic patients. Twenty-three percent of lacunar infarcts may be preceded by TIAs.[6] The deficit which may be initially severe tends to evolve less than thrombotic strokes but can progress over one to two days. After this time, recovery is the rule. However, the ultimate deficit is dependent upon size and location of the infarction.

The physical examination is probably most successful in delineating mechanisms when the examination is consistent with one of the lacunar stroke syndromes. If the history is corroborative of a lacune, a mechanistic diagnosis can be made with some certainty although exceptions occur. The clinical data may also be able to provide localizations to one vascular territory, such as middle cerebral stem, upper trunk, lower trunk, anterior cerebral, posterior cerebral, or PICA, which may then imply mechanism.

General Care

After the history and physical examination a working diagnosis can be made which will help to direct and interpret subsequent evaluation and therapy. However, all patients with stroke regardless of mechanism should undergo the following evaluation. Blood should be obtained for multiple chemistry blood screen, complete blood cell count (CBC) with differential, platelet count, prothrombin time, partial thromboplastin time, ESR, and syphilis serology. Serum protein electrophoresis, blood viscosity, platelet function tests, hemoglobin electrophoresis, and drug screening should be obtained in the appropriate clinical situation. Acutely a plain CT scan of the brain may help localize the area of infarction and will help exclude tumor, intracerebral hemorrhage, or subdural hematoma presenting as a stroke-like syndrome. If clinical suspicion exists for an aneurysm, arteriovenous malformation, tumor or abscess, an infusion scan should be performed. If after the history, physical examination, and CT scan, the clinical diagnosis of ischemic stroke is in doubt, a lumbar puncture should be performed to help in the differential diagnosis of intracranial infection (meningitis, encephalitis—viral, bacterial, or fungal), hemorrhage, and vasculitis.

Evidence is accumulating that not only is the heart a potential source of brain injury but that injury to the brain may significantly injure the myocardium as well. In acute stroke a fourfold higher incidence of cardiac arrthymias (paroxsymal atrial tachycardia, frequent premature ventricular contractions, second or third degree heart block) and significant elevations of creatine phosphokinase-MB have been noted. Elevated CPK-MB was correlated with a 50% higher level of serum catecholamines. Pathologically this brain-heart relationship has been confirmed by finding multiple areas of myocardial necrosis in some patients dying from stroke.[77] Because of this significant relationship, clinical cardiac evaluation is necessary with frequent cardiac examinations, ECGs, cardiac enzyme determinations and, when appropriate, continuous long-term rhythm monitoring.

To further direct stroke care, it is useful to look at the causes of death in patients with stroke. Of those who die, 60% die in the first week from cerebral edema, cardiac abnormality, or pulmonary embolus. The remaining 40% die in the second and third week from pneumonia, septicemia, pulmonary embolus, or myocardial infarction.[78] Each problem requires anticipation and surveillance. Attention should also be directed toward fluid and electrolyte management. In an effort to reduce the high frequency of deep venous thrombophlebitis and pulmonary embolus,[79] range-of-motion exercises, early ambulation, and low-dose subcutaneous heparin (5000 units subcutaneously, twice a day) should be prescribed.

Because an infarct is a rapidly evolving process, the type of cerebral edema will vary not only over time but also throughout the lesion.[80] The two main components of the edema will be intracellular cytotoxic edema which results from damage to the Na-K adenosine triphosphatase (ATPase) pump with failure of the cell to maintain the normal osmotic gradient across its membrane, and extracellular vasogenic edema with loss of fluid through a disautoregulated vascular bed, particularly at the edge of an infarction.

198

Cerebral edema may have its onset within hours after an ischemic stroke, but will typically become maximal after two to four days. Significantly increased intracranial pressure from cerebral edema should be clinically suspected when there is a decreasing level of consciousness, change in respiratory pattern or rate, altered pupillary and eye movements, and new weakness and reflex asymmetry. However, some neurologists contend that these are crude findings which can come very late, often after prolonged periods of raised pressure and that only drowsiness may be present in the face of high pressure. They conclude that the only accurate method of determining pressure and evaluating therapeutic responses in an individual patient is through an intracranial pressure monitor.

Presently therapy for increased intracranial pressure is twofold: (1) Avoidance of factors that exacerbate increased pressure; these include unusual head and neck position, fever, increased central venous pressure, overhydration, increased mean airway pressure, and agitation. (2) Specific action to decrease pressure. Hyperventilation with reduction of PCO_2 to between 20 and 30 mmHg will reduce intracranial pressure over the short term but the pressure will soon return to pretreatment levels. Alterations in blood osmolality by infusion of mannitol and glycerol to maintain blood osmolality between 300 and 310 will also decrease pressure. This osmotic therapy will only be effective where endothelial and cell membranes are intact. Thus it will not be effective in the area of infarction but rather will help reduce the extracellular edema that surrounds the infarct.[80] Steroids may also be tried. The efficacy and mechanism of action of steriods in decreasing intracranial pressure is obscure. They may also ameliorate the extracellular edema that surrounds the infarct (as in brain tumors) and in areas where cell membranes are not severely damaged they may protect against free radical generation. Although their efficacy is in doubt, increased risks of gastrointestinal bleeding, infection, and exacerbations of diabetes are frequent.[81,82]

Crucial to the general care of the stroke patient is identification of risk factors and their intensive modification. Leonberg and Elliot[83] reported a reduction of mortality and stroke recurrences from 35% to 65% mortality and 20% to 40% stroke recurrence to 17% mortality and 16% stroke recurrence. They attempted to modify and treat hypertension, diabetes, hyperlipidemia, heart disease, elevated hematocrit, personal life stress, cigarette consumption, and obesity.

In addition to the care outlined above, specific evaluation and therapeutic modalities should be consistent with the presumed etiologic mechanism.

Lacunes

The key to diagnosis of lacunar stroke rests in the recognition of the clinical syndrome. Because lacunes usually only destroy small amounts of deep brain tissue, the EEG is usually normal. The demonstration of the lacunar infarction on CT scans varies according to the size of the lesion, the timing of the test, and the resolution of the scanner. Arteriography can usually be avoided unless the lacune is large and/or the probable mechanism is large parent vessel atherosclerosis. In such cases lacunar disease may be a warning of impending large vessel stroke.

The role of aspirin, other antiplatelet aggregatory drugs, and anticoagulation in lacunar stroke is unknown. Their role will depend upon a better understanding of the mechanism of vascular occlusion. Because the correlation between understanding of the mechanism of vascular occlusion. Because the correlation between blood pressure and lacunar stroke is strong,[84] blood pressure must be controlled. However, the acute lowering of blood pressure should be avoided as the deficit can be made substantially worse. Lacunes have an excellent prognosis for recovery, particularly the smaller lesion.

Embolic Stroke

In embolic stroke evaluation should be directed toward the heart and large vessels as these comprise the most likely sources of embolic material. Computed tomography in cardiac embolic stroke may reveal multiple bilateral areas of infarction while in artery-to-artery stroke the infarct is single or, if multiple, is located in the same vascular distribution. To clarify the extent of cardiac disease, screening with ECGs and chest roentgenography should be done. Even if these preliminary tests are normal, if the clinical picture is not incompatible with embolic disease, a more extensive evaluation with echocardiography, 24-hour Holter monitoring, and gated blood pool scanning should be carried out. Echocardiography can define possible emboligenic lesions or at times even clot. Holter monitoring can identify paroxysmal rhythm disturbances associated with stroke. Gated blood pool scanning may be useful in identifying akinetic segments of ventricular wall or a cardiomyopathy on which clot can form and embolize. Although the yield of a cardiac evaluation performed on all patients with stroke will be low, if hemorrhage, lacunes, or large vessel occlusions are excluded and embolic stroke is suspected, a cardiac embolic source may be identified.

While the noninvasive cardiac evaluation is proceeding, a similar noninvasive screen of the extracranial vasculature can be performed. Absent carotid pulse on the symptomatic side, prominent venous pattern over the ipsilateral frontal skull, unilateral arcus senilis, unilateral sparing of vascular retinopathy, or increased superficial temporal, facial, supraorbital, or supratrochlear artery may be indicative of significant carotid stenosis or occlusion. When a battery of noninvasive vascular tests are performed a probability of significant carotid stenosis can be obtained. Periorbital directional Doppler and oculoplethysmography monitor the anatomy and physiology at the bifurcation. A real time echo imaging device can show the anatomy at the bifurcation while bruit Doppler analysis can identify those bruits with characteristics most likely to be linked with stenosis. Digital intravenous subtraction angiography can demonstrate the extracranial and some of the intracranial circulation. It can be performed as a screening test for extracranial disease or as an alternative to cerebral arteriography if medical contraindications are present but suspicion of carotid disease exists. If in a medical center with expert angiographers surgical treatment is contemplated, or delineation of the underlying mechanism is desired in focal deficits where there is a high probablity of embolic stroke with a low probability of cardiac source, carotid arteriography can be performed. In experienced hands the complication rate for cerebral arteriography for transient monocular blindness, hemispheral transient ischemia, and severe carotid stenosis was approximately 1% with none of the complications permanent.[85,86] It is only with angiography that both the extracranial circulation can be evaluated and abnormalities more distal in the siphon, middle cerebral stem, or small vessels can be seen. The arteriogram in cardiac emboli will frequently show single or multiple cerebral surface branch occlusions if performed within 48 hours of the ictus. An arteriogram done later will often be normal in the area of infarction on CT scan. In artery-to-artery embolus, the stenotic ulcerative proximal internal carotid, siphon, or middle cerebral artery may be visualized with embolus distal.

Most neurologists would agree that emboli of cardiac origin require full anticoagulation. However, the time to initiate such therapy is still in doubt with proposed times varying from immediate anticoagulation with heparin, to slow anticoagulation with immediate use of warfarin sodium, to delayed anticoagulation (6 weeks after the embolus). Delayed anticoagulation runs the risk of recurrent embolization while immediate anticoagulation risks hemorrhage into infarction. It has been suggested that in small infarctions with no blood on CT or lumbar puncture, in a nonhypertensive individual, immediate or subacute anticoagulation with heparin or warfarin be undertaken.

Consensus for therapy for emboli of arterial origin is also lacking. Three treatment modes are available: antiplatelet therapy, anticoagulants, and surgery. Two large studies, the American and Canadian cooperative studies, have investigated antiplatelet aggregating agents in TIA and stroke.[87,88] The American study showed a beneficial trend away from stroke in those patients who used aspirin. The Canadian study with longer follow-up than the American study showed significantly decreased TIAs, stroke, and death in male patients using aspirin compared to those on no therapy. No significant trend was observed among women.

Four separate reactions occur in the production of platelet fibrin clots.[89] First there is adhesion. The platelets adhere to foreign nonendothelial surfaces such as exposed basement membrane in an ulcerative plaque. This adhesion is followed by a release reaction in which the platelets discharge ADP, thromboxane A_2, beta-thromboglobulin, and platelet factor 3. The ADP and thromboxane then cause further platelet aggregation and the formation of a platelet plug. Platelet factor 3 simultaneously activates the coagulation system by activation of factors X and XII, produing the final platelet fibrin plug.

Aspirin's antiplatelet activity is felt to be a result of irreversible inhibition of platelet cyclooxygenase. This inhibition results in decreased synthesis of platelet thromboxane A_2. Thromboxane A_2 is the most potent naturally occurring platelet aggregator and vasoconstrictor. Unfortunately aspirin also inhibits production of vessel wall prostacyclin. Prostacyclin is the most potent naturally occurring vasodilator and antiplatelet aggregator. There is some experimental evidence to suggest — but as yet no clinical documentation — that the optimal dose of aspirin such that thromboxane but not prostacyclin is inhibited may be less than the dose given in the prior aspirin studies.

Dipyramidole is another antiplatelet drug which acts as a phosphodiesterase inhibitor. Inhibition of this reaction results in increased platelet cAMP. This increase in cAMP has two effects. First, the amount of ADP released in the release reaction of hemostasis is decreased, and second the increase in cAMP inhibits the activity of platelet phospholipases, thus limiting the amount of thromboxane A_2 produced by the platelets. Dipyramidole as a therapeutic agent in the prevention and the treatment of stroke and TIA remains clinically undefined. Unfortunately to date, all large studies of antiplatelet drugs are troubled by entry criteria which are symptoms. Such entry criteria allow diverse stroke mechanisms to be grouped together. However, significant prostaglandin-platelet-vessel wall interactions may be prominent in all ischemic strokes so that antiplatelet therapy remains crucial.

The role of anticoagulation is poorly defined. Anticoagulants have been shown in a small number of nonrandomized uncontrolled groups of patients to reduce frequency of TIA with resumption of attacks after their discontinuation.[90] However, in an extensive review, Brust[91] concluded that the value of anticoagulants in TIAs is unclear as all studies to that time lacked either randomized controls or statistical significance. In all cases the use of anticoagulants must be weighed against risk of hemorrhage (both systemic and intracranial) which has been variously estimated to be from 0%[92] to 8%.[93] This risk of anticoagulation must be taken in light of work which reported a 5% rate of intracranial hemorrhage among anticoagulated patients but also a 4% rate among controls.[94]

Carotid endarterectomy is probably useful but only in a select group of patients. Qualified angiographers and surgeons are needed whose morbidity and mortality rate for angiography and surgery is less than 3%. Jonas and Haas[95] in a review of the extracranial arterial occlusion joint study have suggested that this rate of 3% is the highest possible complication rate which would allow surgical therapy to be significantly better than medical therapy. Furthermore, the lumen of the internal carotid artery should be reduced to greater than 90% or to a residual lumen of less than 2 mm. In addition, the symptoms and signs should be related to and explained by the observed carotid lesion. Vertebrobasilar symptoms will not benefit from carotid artery surgery. Finally, there should be evidence of stenotic intracranial disease and no medical contraindications.[64] Unfortunately, carotid artery surgery has yet to be studied in a controlled fashion, particularly since the introduction of antiplatelet aggregating agents.

If the role of carotid endarterectomy is unclear, even more obscure is the role of extracranial-intracranial bypass surgery. In this operative procedure microsurgical anastomosis of the superficial temporal to branches of the middle cerebral artery is accomplished. This surgery has been recommended for complete carotid occlusion, siphon stenosis, carotid plus siphon stenosis, and middle cerebral artery stem stenosis. Presently a multicenter controlled study is in progress and until its results are available this procedure lacks clear indications.

Large Vessel Occlusion

Large vessel occlusion is suggested by an appropriate history, physical examination, and noninvasive carotid artery diagnostic evaluation. CT scan may show an infarction in almost any pattern with only definite proof provided by angiography which will show occlusion of the appropriate middle cerebral stem, internal carotid artery, basilar artery, or vertebral artery.

Patients with complete occlusion should be maintained in bed with head recumbent without significant lowering of blood pressure in an effort to maintain blood flow and help promote collateralization. The role of antiplatelet agents in this setting is unknown. Some suggest acute anticoagulation to acutely minimize the risk of embolization from the clot or to prevent clot propagation but this is unproved. Acute thrombectomy has been attempted but in general is not widely used. Bypass surgery, as previously mentioned, is under study.

REFERENCES

1. Garraway WM, Whisnant JP, Furlan AJ, et al: The declining incidence of stroke. *N Engl J Med* 1979;300:449–452.
2. Adams RD, Victor M: *Principles of Neurology.* New York, McGraw-Hill, 1981.
3. Aring CD, Merritt HH: Differential diagnosis between cerebral hemorrhage and cerebral thrombosis. *Arch Intern Med* 1935;56:435–456.
4. Whisnant JP, Fitzgibbons JP, Kurland LT, et al: Natural history of stroke in Rochester, Minnesota, 1945 through 1954. *Stroke* 1971;2:11–22.

5. Matsumoto N, Whisnant JP, Kurland LT, et al: Natural history of stroke in Rochester, Minnesota, 1955 through 1969: An extension of a previous study, 1945 through 1954. *Stroke* 1973;3:20–29.

6. Mohr JP, Caplan LR, Melski JW, et al: The Harvard cooperative stroke registry: A prospective registry. *Neurology* 1978;29:754–762.

7. Gunning AJ, Pickering GW, Robb-Smith AHT, et al: Mural thrombosis of the internal carotid artery and subsequent embolism. *Q J Med* 1964;129:155–195.

8. Kistler JP: Cardiac embolic cerebrovascular disease. *Primary Care* 1979;6:745–756.

9. Gacs G, Merel MD, Bodosi M: Balloon catheter as a model of cerebral emboli in humans. *Stroke* 1982;13:39–42.

10. Kubik CS, Adams, RD: Occlusion of the basilar artery—A clinical and pathological study. *Brain* 1946;69:6–121.

11. Escourolle R, Poirier J: *Manual of Basic Neuropathology*. Philadelphia, WB Saunders Co, 1978.

12. Wolf PA, Dawber TR, Kannel WB: Heart disease as a precursor of stroke, in, Schoenburg BS (ed): *Advances in Neurology*. New York, Raven Press, 1978, Vol 19, pp. 567–577.

13. Roberts WC, Ferrans VJ: Pathlogical aspects of certain cardiomyopathies. *Circ Res* 1974 (suppl. 2);35:128–144.

14. Thompson PL, Robinson JS: Stroke after acute myocardial infarction; relation to infarct size. *Br Med J* 1978;2:457–459.

15. Bean WB: Infarction of the heart. III Clinical course and morphological findings. *Ann Intern Med* 1938;12:71–94.

16. Daley R, Mattingly TW, Holt CL, et al: Systemic arterial embolism in rheumatic heart disease. *Am Heart J* 1951;42:566–581.

17. Wolf PA, Dawber TR, Thomas HE, et al: Epidemiologic assessment of chronic artrial fibrillation and risk of stroke: The Framingham Study. *Neurology* 1978;28:973–977.

18. Hinton RC, Kistler JP, Fallon JT, et al: Influence of etiology of atrial fibrillation on incidence of systemic embolisms. *Am J Cardiol* 1977;40:509–513.

19. Pleet AB, Massey EW, Vengrow ME: TIA, stroke and the bicuspid aortic valve. *Neurology* 1981;31:1540–1542.

20. Keen G, Leveaux VM: Prognosis of cerebral embolism in rheumatic heart disease. *Br Med J* 1958;2:91–92.

21. Adam GF, Merrett JD, Hutchinson WM, et al: Cerebral embolism and mitral stenosis: Survival with and without anticoagulants. *J Neurol Neursurg Psychiatry* 1974;37:378–383.

22. Coulshed N, Epstein EJ, McKendrick CS, et al: Systemic emboli in mitral valve disease. *Brit Heart J* 1970;32:26–34.

23. Barnett HJM, Boughner DR, Taylor DW, et al: Further evidence relating mitral-valve prolapse to cerebral ischemic events. *N Engl J Med* 1980;302: 139–144.

24. Scharf RE, Hennerici M, Bluschke V, et al: Cerebral ischemia in young patients: Is it associated with mitral valve prolapse and abnormal platelet activity in vivo? *Stroke* 1982;13:454–458.

25. Rice GPA, Boughner DR, Stiller C, et al: Familial stroke syndrome associated with mitral valve prolapse. *Ann Neurol* 1980;7:130–134.

26. De Bono DP, Warlow CP: Mitral-annulus calcification and cerebral or retinal ischemia. *Lancet* 1979;2:383–385.

27. Korn D, DeSanctis RW, Sell S: Massive calcification of the mitral annulus. *N Engl J Med* 1962;267:900–909.

28. Garvey GJ, Neu HC: Infective endocarditis—an evolving disease. *Medicine* 1978;57:105–127.

29. Kooiker JC, MacLean JM, Sumi SM: Cerebral embolism, marantic endocarditis, and cancer. *Arch Neurol* 1976;33:260–264.
30. Remillind GM, Carpenter S: Cerebral emboli due to non-bacterial thrombotic endocarditis. *Can Med Assoc J* 1972;30:487–491.
31. Sandok BA, Von Estorff I, Guiliani ER: CNS embolism due to atrial myxoma. *Arch Neurol* 1980;37:485–488.
32. Roeltgren DR, Weimer GR, Patterson LF: Delayed neurologic complications of left atrial myxoma. *Neurology* 1981;31:8–13.
33. Pessin MS, Hinton RC, Davis KR, et al: Mechanisms of acute carotid stroke. *Ann Neurol* 1979;6:245–252.
34. Finklestein S, Kleinman GM, Baringer JR: Delayed stroke following carotid occlusion. *Neurology* 1980;30:84–88.
35. Barnett HJM: Delayed cerebral ischemic episodes distal to occlusion of major cerebral arteries. *Neurology* 1978;28:769–774.
36. Symmonds C: Cervical rib: thrombosis of subclavian artery, contralateral hemiplegia of sudden onset, probably embolic, in Symmonds C (ed): *Studies in Neurology*. New York, Oxford University Press, 1970.
37. Fisher CM: Observations of the fundus oculi in transient monocular blindness. *Neurology* 1959;9:333–347.
38. Adams HP, Gross CE: Embolism distal to stenosis of the middle cerebral artery. *Stroke* 1981;12:228–229.
39. Hollenhorst RW: Significance of bright plaques in the retinal arterioles. *JAMA* 1961;178:123–129.
40. Beal MF, Williams RS, Richardson EP, et al: Cholesterol embolism as a cause of transient ischemic attacks and cerebral infarction. *Neurology* 1981;31:860–865.
41. Imparato AM, Riles TS, Gorstein F: The carotid bifurcation plaque: Pathologic findings associated with cerebral ischemia. *Stroke* 1979;10:238–245.
42. Durward QJ, Ferguson GG, Ban HW: The natural history of the asymptomatic carotid bifurcation plaques. *Stroke* 1982;13:459–464.
43. Denny-Brown D: Recurrent cerebrovascular episodes. *Arch Neurol* 1960;2:194–210.
44. Piper PJ, Vane JR: Release of additional factors in anaphylaxis and its antagonism by anti-inflammatory drugs. *Nature* 1969;223:29–35.
45. Hamberg M, Stanford N, Majerus PW: Thromboxanes: a new group of biologically active compounds derived from prostaglandin endoperoxides. *Proc Natl Acad Sci USA* 1975;72:2994–2998.
46. Moncada S, Gryglewski R, Bunting S, et al: An enzyme isolated from arteries transforms prostaglandin endoperoxides to an unstable substance that inhibits platelet aggregation. *Nature* 1976;261:663–665.
47. Wu KK, Hall ER, Papp A: Prostacyclin stabilizing factor deficiency in thrombotic thrombocytopenic purpura. *Lancet* 1982;1:460–461.
48. Jones HR, Caplan LR, Come PC, et al: Cerebral emboli of paradoxical origin. *Ann Neurol* 1983;13:314–319.
49. Fisher CM, Karnes WE, Kubik CS: Lateral medullary infarction—The pattern of vascular occlusion. *J. Neuropath Exp Neurol* 1961;20:323–379.
50. Hass WK, Fields WS, North RR, et al: Joint study of extracranial artherial occlusions. *JAMA* 1968;203:961–968.
51. Hinton RC, Mohr JP, Ackerman RH, et al: Symptomatic middle cerebral artery stenosis. *Ann Neurol* 1979;5:152–157.
52. Fisher CM, Gore I, Okabe N, et al: Atherosclerosis of the carotid and vertebral arteries—extracranial and intracranial. *J Neuropath Exp Neurol* 1965;24:455–476.

53. Fisher CM: Thalamic pure sensory stroke: A pathologic study. *Neurology* 1978;28:1141–1144.

54. Fisher CM, Curry HD: Pure motor hemiplegia of vascular origin. *Arch Neurol* 1965;13:30–44.

55. Ho KL: Pure motor hemiplegia due to infarction of the cerebral peduncle. *Arch Neurol* 1982;39:524–526.

56. Fisher CM: Pure sensory stroke involving face, arm and leg. *Neurology* 1965;15:76–80.

57. Mohr JP, Kase CS, Meckler RJ, et al: Sensorimotor stroke due to thalamocapsular ischemia. *Arch Neurol* 1977;34:739–741.

58. Fisher CM: Ataxic hemiparesis. *Arch Neurol* 1978;35:126–128.

59. Iragui, VJ, McCuthchin CB: Capsular ataxic hemiparesis. *Arch Neurol* 1982;39:528–529

60. Perman CP, Racy A: Homolateral ataxia and crural paresis: Case report. *Neurology* 1980;30:1013–1015.

61. Kase CP, Maulsby GO, de Juan E, et al: Hemichorea, hemiballism and lacunar infarction in the basal ganglia. *Neurology* 1981;31:452–455.

62. Fisher CM: A lacunar stroke: The dysarthsia-clumsy hand syndrome. *Neurology* 1967;17:614–617.

63. Hutchinson EC, Yates PO: Carotico-vertebral stenosis. *Lancet* 1957;1:2–11.

64. Barnett HJM: Progress toward stroke prevention. *Neurology* 1980;30:1212–1224.

65. Kendell RE, Marshall J: Role of hypotension in genesis of transient focal cerebral ischemia. *Br Med J* 1962;2:344–348.

66. Harrison MJG, Marshall J: The finding of thrombosis at carotid endarterectomy and its relationship to the timing of surgery. *Br J Surg* 1977;64:511–512.

67. Whisnant JP: Epidemiology of stroke: Emphasis on transient cerebral ischemic attacks and hypertension. *Stroke* 1974;5:68–75.

68. Kannel WB: Current status of the epidemiology of brain infarction associated with occlusive arterial disease. *Stroke* 1971;2:295–318.

69. Tohgi H, Yamanouchi H, Murakami M, Kameyama M: Importance of the hematocrit as a risk factor in cerebral infarction. *Stroke* 1978;9:369–374.

70. Harrison MJG, Pollock S, Thomas D, et al: Hematocrit, hypertension, and smoking in patients with transient ischemic attacks and in age and sex matched controls. *J Neurol Neurosurg Psychiatry* 1982;45:550–551.

71. Thomas DJ, Marshall J, Ross Russell RW, et al: Effects of haematocrit on cerebral blood flow in man. *Lancet* 1977;2:940–943.

72. Heyman A, Wilkinson WE, Heyden S, et al: Risk of stroke in asymptomatic persons with cervical arterial bruits. *N Engl J Med* 1980;302:838–841.

73. Baker RN, Schwartz WS, Ramsey JC: Prognosis among survivors of ischemic stroke. *Neurology* 1968;18:933–941.

74. Eisenberg H, Morrison JT, Sullivan P, et al: Cerebrovascular accidents. *JAMA* 1964;189:833–888.

75. Mohr JP: Transient ischemic attacks and the prevention of stroke. *N Engl J Med* 1978;299:93–95.

76. Toole JF, Yusan CP, Janeway R, et al: Transient ischemic attacks: A prospective study of 225 patients. *Neurology* 1978;28:746–753.

77. Myers MG, Norris JW, Hachinski VC, et al: Cardiac sequelae of acute stroke. *Stroke* 1982;13:838–842.

78. Millikan CH: Stroke intensive care units. *Stroke* 1979;10:235–237.

79. Warlow C, Ogston D, Douglas AS: Deep venous thrombosis of the legs after stroke. Part I: Incidence and predisposing factors. *Br Med J* 1976;1:1178–1181.

80. O'Brien MD: Ischemic cerebral edema: A review. *Stroke* 1979;10:623–628.

81. Norris JW: Steroid therapy in acute cerebral infarction. *Arch Neurol* 1976;33:69–71.
82. Ottonello GA, Premavere, A: Gastrointestinal complication of high dose corticosteroid therapy in acute cerebrovascular patients. *Stroke* 1979; 10:208–210.
83. Leonberg SC, Elliot FA: Prevention of recurrent stroke. *Stroke* 1981; 12:731–735.
84. Fisher CM: Lacunes: Small deep cerebral infarcts. *Neurology* 1964;15:775–784.
85. Eisenberg RL, Bank WO, Hedgcock MW: Neurologic complication of angiography in patients with critical stenosis of the carotid artery. *Neurology* 1980; 30:892–895.
86. Eisenberg RL, Bank WO, Hedgcock MW: Neurologic complication of angiography for cerebrovascular disease. *Neurology* 1980;30:895–897.
87. Canadian Cooperative Study Group: A randomized trial of aspirin and sulfinpyrazone in threatened stroke. *N Engl J Med* 1978;299:53–59.
88. Fields WS, Lemak NA, Frankowski RF, et al: Controlled trial of aspirin in cerebral ischemia. *Stroke* 1977;8:301–316.
89. Yatsu FM: Acute medical therapy of strokes. *Stroke* 1982;13:524–526.
90. Fisher CM: The use of anticoagulants in cerebral thrombosis. *Neurology* 1958;8:311–332.
91. Brust JCM: Transient ischemic attacks: Natural history and anticoagulations. *Neurology* 1977;29:701–707.
92. Bradshaw P, Brennan S: Trial of long term anticoagulant therapy in the treatment of small stroke associated with normal arteriogram. *J Neurol Neurosurg Psychiatry* 1978;38:642–647.
93. Siekert RG, Whisnant JP, Millikan CH: Surgical and anticoagulant therapy of occlusive cerebrovascular disease. *Ann Intern Med* 1963;58:637–641.
94. Whisnant JP, Matsumoto N, Elveback LR: The effects of anticoagulant therapy on the prognosis of patients with transient cerebral ischemic attacks in a community. *Mayo Clin Proc* 1973;48:844–848.
95. Jonas J, Haas WK: An approach to the maximal acceptance stroke complication rate surgery for transient cerebral ischemia. *Stroke* 1979;10:104.

10   *Mesenteric Artery Thrombosis*

John A. Payne

Mesenteric arterial occlusion may occur without noticeable effect or may result in a catastrophic syndrome of intestinal infarction. After a brief review of the arterial anatomy and the compensatory mechanisms which protect against bowel infarction, the clinical syndromes associated with mesenteric artery thrombosis or hypoperfusion and the measures to minimize or prevent bowel infarction will be discussed.

ANATOMY

The splanchnic circulation is derived from three major arteries: the celiac axis, the superior mesenteric artery, and the inferior mesenteric artery. The celiac axis supplies the liver, stomach, duodenum, pancreas, and spleen. Collateral circulation under control of local metabolic responses is extremely efficient; infarction of these organs is generally found only in conditions of profound hypotension, hypoxia, or extensive occlusion of regional arterioles. Angiographic studies have shown that constriction or occlusion of the celiac axis by the diaphragmatic crus occurs frequently. Efforts to associate such occlusion with clinical syndromes have been unconvincing.

The blood supply to the small bowel and proximal colon is delivered by the superior mesenteric artery, which also augments the circulation of the pancreas and duodenum. A series of vascular arcades join the intestinal, ileocolic, right colic, and middle colic branches of the superior mesenteric artery and permit extensive collateral flow to develop. The small arteriae rectae, which supply the bowel wall and mucosa, do not permit significant collateral flow within the bowel itself. A large diameter and oblique take-off from the aorta predispose the superior mesenteric artery to embolic occlusion.

The inferior mesenteric artery supplies the distal transverse colon, the descending and sigmoid colon, and proximal rectum. Occasionally, a major anastomosis called the arc of Riolan or meandering mesenteric artery provides collateral supply to the superior mesenteric artery and celiac axis (Figure 10-1). The marginal artery of Drummond is an inconstant collateral vessel composed of the final vascular arcade of vessels that originate from the superior and inferior mesenteric arteries and run parallel to the colon (Figure 10-2).

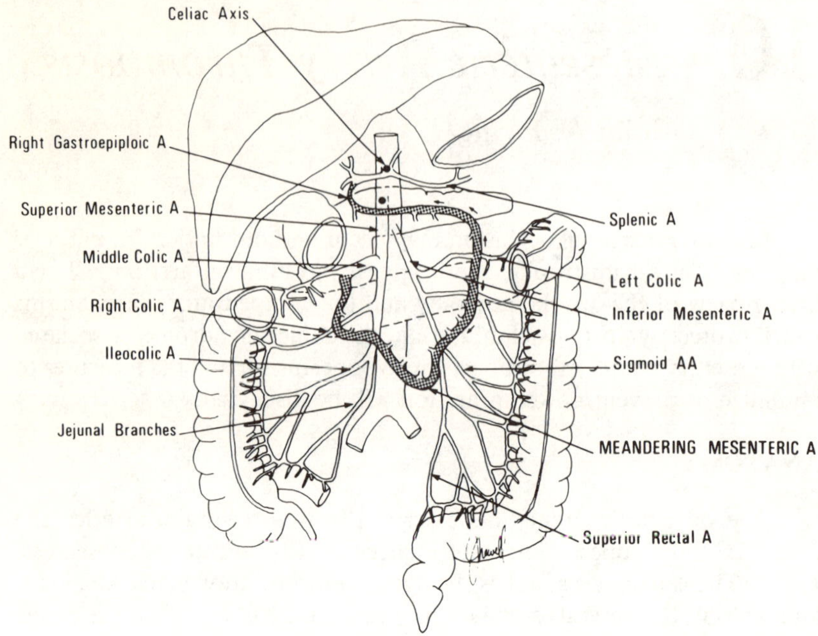

Figure 10-1 Graphic representation of a meandering mesenteric artery (arc of Riolan). This collateral vessel develops in response to occlusion of one or two of the major splanchnic arteries and may prevent any manifestation of ischemic injury. Sites of occlusion are indicated by dots.

Because of these anatomic features, three principles have become accepted. First, with the gradual onset of vascular occlusion limited to major vessels, it is possible to sustain normal bowel function in the face of total occlusion of two of the three major splanchnic arteries. Second, occlusive processes that affect the terminal vessels, penetrating the bowel wall to supply the mucosa, will cause intestinal ischemia without regard to the rate of onset of occlusion. Third, two regions that are relatively susceptible to ischemia because collaterals are poorly developed are the proximal third of the rectum and the junction of the transverse and the splenic flexure of the colon.

PHYSIOLOGY

Given the vital role of nutrient intake and the complexity of the vascular supply to the intestine, it is not surprising that the physiologic control of gut perfusion should be governed by several overlapping "systems" to assure oxygenation and nutrient supply sufficient for basal and active metabolic phases of gut function.

Jacobsen et al have proposed a two-phase model to account for the marked variation of blood flow and oxygen extraction demonstrable under widely diverse situations.[1] The model proposes that the relation between oxygen extraction and blood flow across a segment of bowel is the result of two parallel components, a flow-independent system and a flow-dependent system. Oxygen extraction in the flow-independent system is unaffected by a wide range of blood flow rates because of the small tissue requirement for oxygen relative to the usual amount of flow. In contrast, the flow-dependent system appears to be driven by the metabolic demand for oxygen and to operate in a setting of modest ischemia, analogous to the circulation of the lung apex in the upright position.

The probable anatomic counterpart of the flow-independent system is the mesenteric arteriole and, of the flow-independent system, the precapillary sphincter. The precapillary sphincter regulates the number of capillaries perfused in a segment of gut. Additional factors, such as distention of the gut lumen, oxygen-carrying capacity (eg, hemoglobin content) of the blood, the counter-current exchange mechanism of the villi, and drug effects on parenchymal cell metabolism, increase or decrease metabolic demand considerably (Figure 10-3).

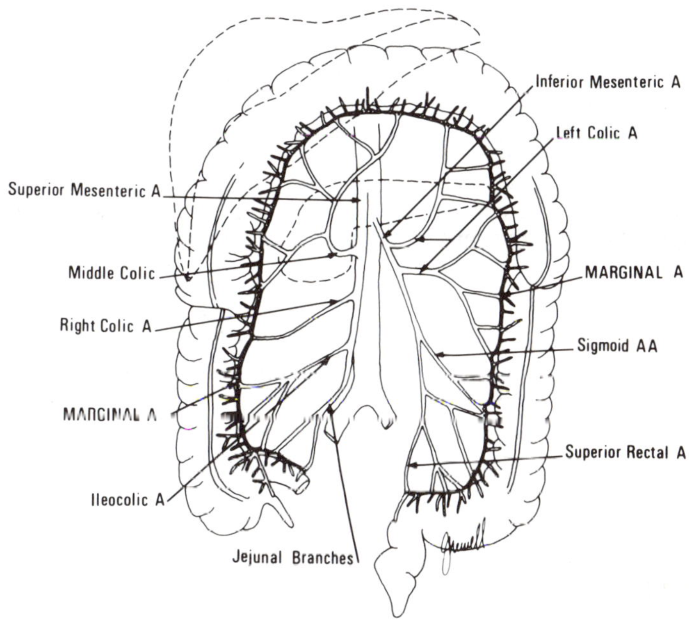

Figure 10-2 Graphic representation of the marginal artery of Drummond, an inconstant vascular arcade that, when present, provides collateral flow to the colon.

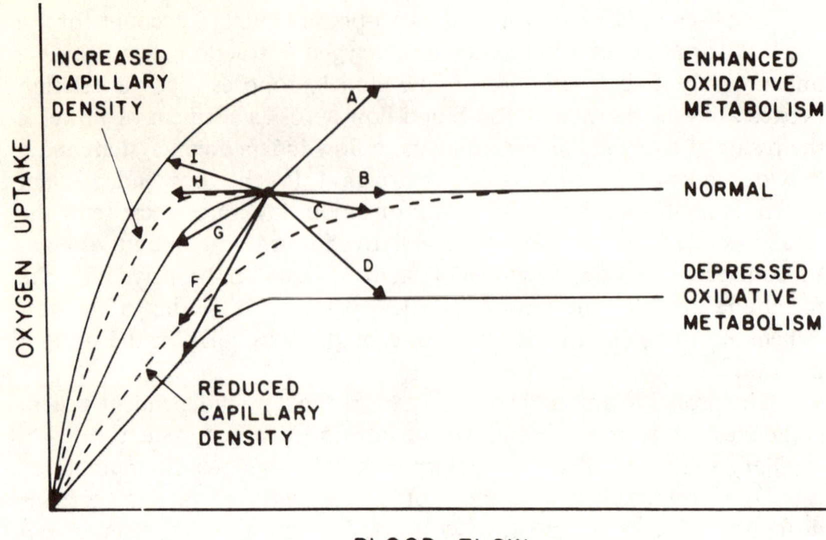

Figure 10-3 Diagrammatic representation of relation between blood flow and oxygen uptake and factors that alter this relationship. Note that alterations in tissue oxidative metabolism shift curves vertically, whereas alterations in capillary density shift curves horizontally. Arrow represents control blood flow under normal conditions. Pathway A is taken by vasodilator that increases oxidative metabolism. Pathway B is taken by vasodilator that does not affect metabolism or increase capillary density. Pathway C is taken by vasodilator that decreases capillary density. Pathway D is taken by vasodilator that decreases metabolism. Pathway E is taken by vasoconstrictor that decreases metabolism. Pathway F is taken by vasoconstrictor that decreases capillary density. Pathway G is taken by vasoconstrictor that does not affect metabolism or capillary density. Pathway H is taken by vasoconstrictor that increases capillary density. Pathway I is taken by vasoconstrictor that increases metabolism. (Diagram from Kvietys PR, Granger DN;[2] reproduced with permission.)

When vascular compromise develops in a gradual fashion due to atheromata or vasculitis, the formation of collateral channels is stimulated. These new vessels may not respond to standard physiologic stimuli, but adequately preserve intestinal blood flow. The angiographic demonstration of collateral vessels indicates that successful compensation for thrombosis has occurred, and by inference, that the occlusive lesion has been present for some time.

SIGNS AND SYMPTOMS OF INTESTINAL ISCHEMIA

Two distinct syndromes of intestinal ischemia are recognized, reflecting the rate at which the ischemia develops.

Acute Intestinal Ischemia

Acute intestinal ischemia produces an initial intense vasoconstriction with a transudation of fluid into the interstitium of the mucosa and submucosa, aided by the local accumulation of metabolites which attack the endothelial integrity. The immediate consequence of these events is a stimulation of bowel motility, soon followed by paralytic ileus when the muscle becomes impaired.

The patient experiences abdominal pain of crampy character as the proximal bowel responds to the focal ileus with distention. As the process continues, generalized ileus eliminates the cramping sensation and diffuse steady pain with rebound tenderness becomes apparent indicating inflammation of the peritoneum.

Within the segments of paralyzed bowel, bacterial replication occurs. As the bowel becomes devitalized, diapedesis of the mixed flora and endotoxin into the peritoneal cavity and the systemic circulation produces sepsis and may lead to septic shock and death. Surgical resection of the infarcted segment, control of sepsis, and restoration of the circulating blood volume must be achieved to reverse this process in most cases, although hypoperfusion syndromes of short duration may be reversed by early appropriate measures to restore the intestinal circulation.

Early changes in the mucosa follow a sequence of hypoxia, edema, hyperemia, and mucosal slough with ulceration. The absence of countercurrent exchange in the muscularis may help to preserve this relatively hardy tissue. Transient ischemia may thus produce segmental ulceration with subsequent repair and no permanent defect. When the episode is prolonged enough to damage the intestinal muscle, scarring and stricture develop with the potential for obstruction and intussusception. Intestinal webs and strictures discovered during childhood may be the result of vascular accidents during fetal development.

Serial abdominal radiographs may reveal the characteristic changes of focal ileus, mucosal edema ("thumbprinting") and ulceration with the separation of bowel loops providing indirect evidence of bowel wall edema. Identification of these changes is dependent upon intraluminal air or contrast and must be evaluated in the context of the patient's medical history (Figure 10-4).

Changes in hematologic and biochemical profiles generally occur when the ischemic event is well-advanced and reflect the pooling of fluid in the bowel and mesentery, the inflammatory response, and release of tissue proteins into the circulation. On one small series, elevated serum phosphate was the best biochemical indicator of bowel infarction. The passage of bloody stool indicates a significant breech of the mucosa and is an important sign. Occasionally gastrointestinal hemorrhage may not be grossly detectable, or in the case of rapidly developing ileus, may remain trapped in the paralyzed gut.

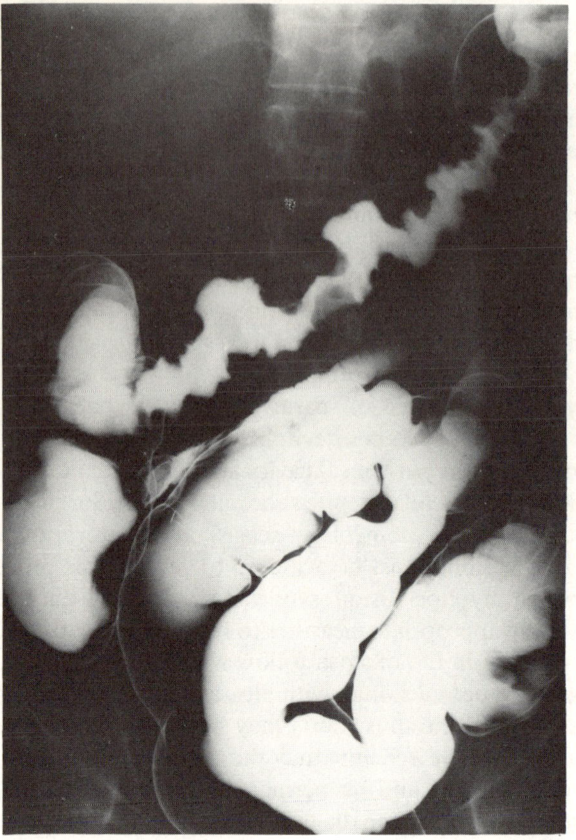

Figure 10-4 Air-contrast barium enema demonstrating segmental mucosal edema. Patient was a 57-year-old woman taking caffeine-ergotamine tartrate who developed abdominal pain and bloody diarrhea. Follow-up examination five months later was normal.

Abdominal ultrasound is helpful in detecting pancreatic edema or pseudocysts as well as biliary tract abnormalities which might mimic intestinal ischemia. Computed tomography (CT) of the abdomen may detect changes in the aorta that suggest the diagnosis of vascular disease. Scanning with technetium 99-labeled aggregates has been shown to indicate persistent uptake in the splanchnic bed. Nuclear magnetic resonance has not been evaluated to date.

Chronic Intestinal Ischemia

Chronic intestinal ischemia is a rare syndrome generally seen in patients with extensive atherosclerosis, abdominal aortic dissection or arteritis. The syndrome is characterized by postprandial abdominal pain produced by an inability of the blood vessels to augment blood flow in response to food in the small bowel. Typically pain occurs one to three hours after a meal, has a steady character, and subsides after several hours duration. Patients learn to reduce their food intake and therefore eliminate or minimize their discomfort. Such patients will often present with rapidly developing malnutrition and can easily be mistaken for patients with abdominal carcinomatosis.

The syndrome of chronic intestinal ischemia has unfortunately acquired the label "intestinal angina." The drug treatment for cardiac angina generally includes digoxin and vasodilators. These same drugs may precipitate intestinal infarction in a patient with marginal perfusion of the gut through shunting of blood to the extremities and digitalis-induced splanchnic vasoconstriction, and should therefore be used with great caution when the angina is below the diaphragm.

DIAGNOSIS

Establishing the correct diagnosis is the key to proper management. Any patient with congestive heart failure, vasculitis, atherosclerosis, atrial myxoma, arrhythmias, valvular heart disease, or hypotension is a prime candidate for mesenteric ischemia. The use of vasospastic drugs may induce the syndrome. Occasionally, therapeutic maneuvers become so focused on treatment for the primary process that abdominal symptoms are neglected. Once identified, general supportive measures with provision of adequate oxygenation, fluid replacement and control of underlying cardiac arrhythmias are indicated. Nasogastric suction will minimize bowel distention. Serial examinations to detect the development of peritoneal signs and serial radiographs to monitor the status of ileus and the development of free air are of prime importance (Figure 10-5). Proctoscopic examination may disclose rectal demarcation of ischemic areas. Blood cultures are essential to detect bacteremia and guide antibiotic therapy.

Barium studies may establish the characteristic mucosal changes early in the course of bowel ischemia, but they should be avoided when ileus or peritoneal signs have developed because of potential for perforation and abdominal contamination. Careful review of abdominal plain films will often make barium of Gastrografin studies superfluous.

Abdominal angiography might seem to be a logical method to evaluate arterial lesions. Its usefulness is somewhat limited because 30% of intestinal ischemia results from arteriolar lesions which cannot be identified by angiogram and many elderly people will have atherosclerotic occlusion of one or more splanchnic vessels with total compensation through long-standing collateral vessels. These considerations make the

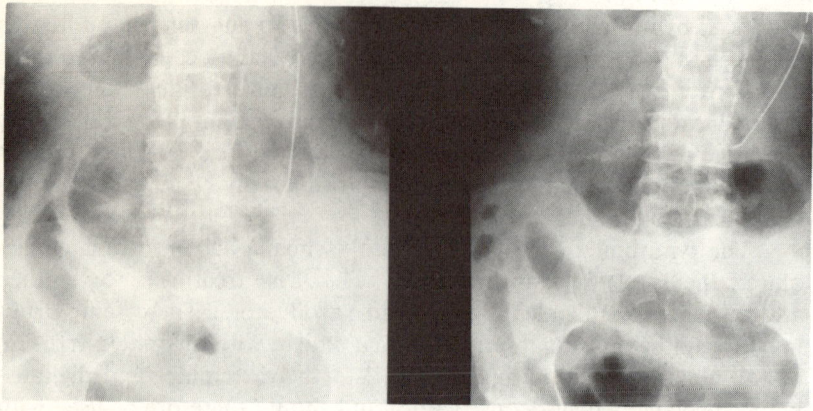

Figure 10-5 Serial abdominal films, taken five days apart, in an elderly woman with atrial fibrillation, who was admitted for abdominal pain and elevated amylase. At laparotomy, multiple emboli were found in the superior mesenteric artery with small bowel necrosis. The persistence of dilated loops of small bowel is compatible with ischemic injury.

angiogram of most use in the younger patient with chronic atrial fibrillation or suspected atrial myxoma who develops an acute abdomen (Figure 10-6). Angiographic findings of use are vascular occlusion or vasospasm, which may be manifest by beading or constriction of the superior mesenteric artery, narrowing of the intestinal arcades, or focal hypoperfusion of the intramural vessels (Figure 10-7). Protracted venous pooling may also be seen. If possible, digoxin and vasoactive drugs should be discontinued.

TREATMENT

Boley and coworkers have developed a protocol attempting to reduce ischemic vasoconstriction by the use of intra-arterial vasocilators such as papaverine, thereby limiting the zone of potential infarction.[3] Obliteration of the reactive vascular response permits continued perfusion through collaterals and enhances survival of the affected bowel (Figure 10-8). Preliminary reports are encouraging but widespread use of this technic has not taken hold.

Definitive treatment requires surgical intervention with resection of the ischemic area, embolectomy, and revascularization.[4] The findings at laparotomy may be misleading because the full extent of compromised bowel is not often demarcated, and reactive vasoconstriction may persist for several days after re-establishing arterial flow. In addition, if the patient cannot be stabilized by adequate fluid repletion, the changes in splanchnic blood flow induced by general anesthesia and laparotomy may extend the initial lesion. Many surgeons favor a "second look" exploration 24 to 48 hours after the initial resection to be sure that no compromised bowel has been left in situ.

Delay in laparotomy until gangrenous bowel has perforated and frank peritoneal soilage has occurred increases patient mortality several-fold. The decision to proceed with surgery is guided by the quality of pain and abdominal findings, the evolving changes on serial radiographic examinations, the character of the stool, and the patient's general condition.

PREVENTIVE MEASURES

Patients with chronic atrial fibrillation, particularly those with past evidence of embolic injury, should be anticoagulated with vitamin K antagonists on a routine basis. The use of low-dose aspirin, dipyridamole,

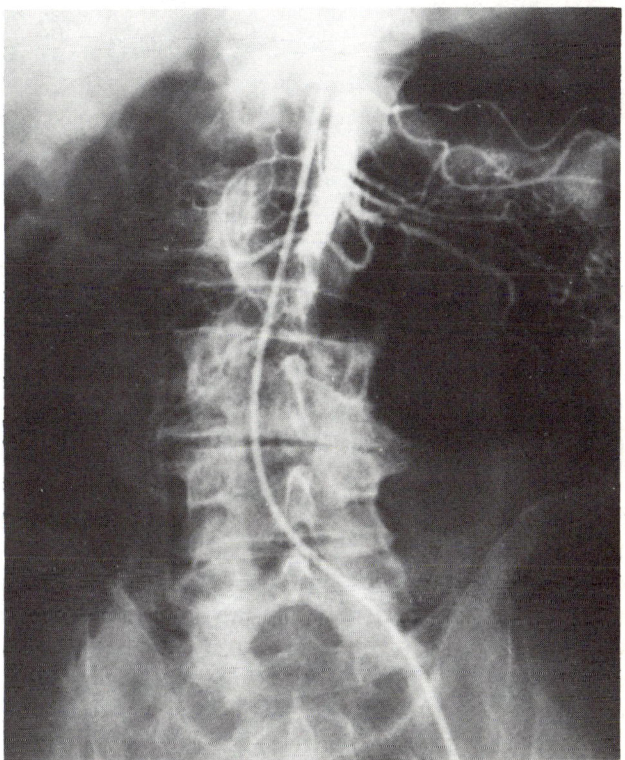

Figure 10-6   Angiogram of the superior mesenteric artery demonstrating embolic occlusion distal to the inferior pancreaticoduodenal arcade. The patient was a 58-year-old man who developed abdominal pain seven days after myocardial infarction.

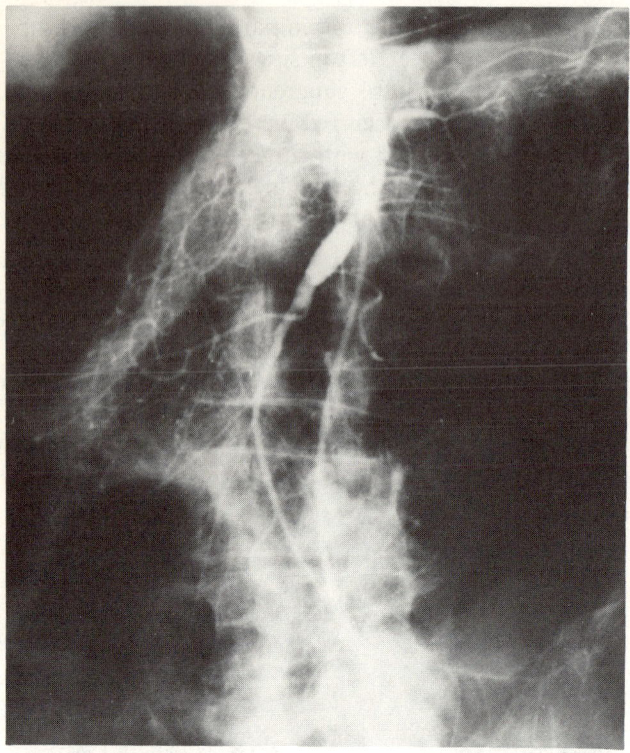

Figure 10-7 Same patient as Figure 10-6. Patient was being treated with dopamine hydrochloride for hypotension. Following embolectomy, marked vasoconstriction is seen of the main trunk of the superior mesenteric artery, the jejunal and ileal branches, and the middle colic artery. The vasoconstriction was attributed to patients' low cardiac output, dopamine therapy, and postembolic state.

and sulfinpyrazone has not been evaluated. Aspirin gastritis may be expected to confound evaluation of patients at risk.

Efforts to control cardiac arrhythmias and prevent endocardial thrombi are important. Patients with subacute bacterial endocartitis must be treated aggressively.

Early detection of abdominal aortic aneurysms with surgical repair may preempt atherosclerotic occlusion of the splanchnic vessels. Finally, one should be cautious in the diuresis of patients with congestive heart failure, for excessive dehydration may constrict the circulating blood volume in patients with partially occluded vessels and produce ischemia or infarction.

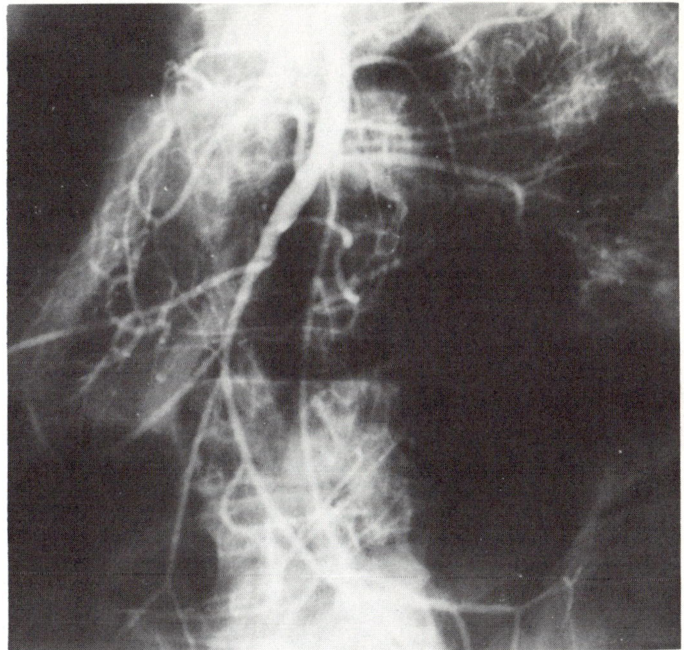

Figure 10-8   Same patient as Figure 10-6. Following intra-arterial infusion of iso-proterenol hydrochloride, the superior mesenteric arteriogram returns to normal.

ACKNOWLEDGMENT

The illustrations were drawn by Julie Newell, the radiographs supplied by Drs. Jerry Petasnick and Claire Smith, and secretarial assistance provided by Charlene Schwar.

REFERENCES

1. Jacobsen ED, Gallavan RH, Jr, Fondacaro JD: A model of the mesenteric circulation. *Am J Physiol* [Gastrointestinal and Liver Physiology] 1982;5: G541–546.
2. Kvietys PR, Granger DN: Vasoactive agent and splanchnic oxygen uptake. *Am J Physiol* [Gastrointestinal and Liver Physiology] 1982;6:G1–G9.
3. Boley SJ, Brandt LS, Veith FJ: Ischemic disorders of the intestine. *Curr Probl Surg* 1978;15:1.
4. Ockner RK: Vascular diseases of the bowel, in Sleisenger MH, Fordtran JS, (eds): *Gastrointestinal Disease*. Philadelphia, WB Saunders Co, 1978, pp 1889–1915.

11 *Thrombotic Thrombocytopenic Purpura*

Ennio C. Rossi

Thrombotic thrombocytopenic purpura (TTP) is a severe, frequently fatal, disease characterized by a diagnostic pentad composed of thrombocytopenia, hemolytic anemia, neurologic symptoms, renal involvement, and fever.[1] The first case of TTP was described in 1925 by Moschcowitz under the title 'An Acute Febrile Pleiochromic Anemia with Hyaline Thrombosis of the Terminal Arterioles and Capillaries; an Undescribed Disease.'[2] Ironically, we can only assume this patient exhibited thrombocytopenia because a platelet count was not performed. However, the report did include a description of the thrombi of terminal arterioles and capillaries which are characteristic of TTP. This new disease was defined with greater clarity 11 years later when Baehr et al reported four additional cases.[3] They documented thrombocytopenia and provided new insights concerning the nature of the thrombi. Moschcowitz had called the thrombi "hyaline" because they stained pink with hematoxylin-eosin, and had concluded that they were composed of agglutinated red blood cells. Baehr and his colleagues, on the other hand, noted that "by reducing the light through the condenser, the thrombotic material lost its homogeneous appearance and appeared granular. . . . The Giemsa stain brought out the morphology of agglutinated blood platelets."[3] Thus, Baehr et al were the first to suggest that the thrombi were composed primarily of platelets. Subsequently, the new disease went under a variety of names until Singer at al[4] coined the term thrombotic thrombocytopenic purpura. In 1962 Brain et al[5] drew attention to the prominence of fragmented red blood cells ("schistocytes") and introduced the term "microangiopathic hemolytic anemia" (MAHA) to describe the traumatic hemolysis that occurred in this disease. By 1958, 63 cases of TTP had been reported[6] and by 1966 the number had increased to 271.[1]

CLINICAL PRESENTATION

Amorosi and Ultmann[1] reviewed the first 271 cases of TTP and confirmed a triad of clinical features composed of thrombocytopenia, hemolytic anemia, and neurologic symptoms. They also noted a conspicuous prevalence of renal disease and fever, and suggested that these

219

findings should be included to form a pentad of clinical features. The anemia is microangiopathic in type with the number of schistocytes roughly proportional to disease severity.[7] Thrombocytopenia is severe with platelet counts usually less than $30,000/\mu l$. Neurologic manifestations are variable and may be transient in nature. Classically the patient complains of severe headache and mental confusion. As neurologic symptoms intensify, slurred speech, transient periods of aphasia and paresis, seizures, and coma may be observed. Renal manifestations include hematuria and proteinuria. If renal involvement is extensive, serum urea nitrogen and creatinine concentrations will increase, and the clinical picture may begin to resemble the hemolytic uremic syndrome (HUS) (see chapter 12). Although the clinical presentation is dominated by blood, renal, and central nervous system changes, the dissemination of thrombotic lesions to other organs can lead to other symptoms. Abdominal pain is not uncommon. Pancreatitis has been described as a presenting complaint in TTP[8] and mild pancreatitis could explain the abdominal pain experienced by many patients. Chest pain, anginal in type, has also been observed. These symptoms are concordant with autopsy reports which identify heart, brain, kidneys, pancreas, and adrenals as the organs where thrombi are most commonly found.[1]

Ridolfi and Bell[9] reviewed 275 cases of TTP reported between the years 1964–1980. Their analysis of clinical features substantially agreed with the previous study of Amorosi and Ultmann. Table 11-1 provides a resume of clinical findings from these two reviews.

Table 11-1
Signs and Symptoms of Thrombotic Thrombocytopenic Purpura

	Amorosi and Ultmann (1966)[1] (%)	Ridolfi and Bell (1981)[9] (%)
Pentad of Signs		
Microangiopathic hemolytic anemia	96	98
Thrombocytopenia	96	83
Neurologic signs	92	84
Renal involvement	88	76
Fever	98	59
Presenting Complaints		
Neurologic	60	52
Hemorrhagic	44	38
Malaise, weakness	25	29
Nausea, vomiting, diarrhea	24	24
Abdominal pain	11	14
Arthralgia, myalgia	7	6
Icterus	9	2.5

Adapted from Ridolfi RL, Bell WR.[9]

PATHOLOGY

The suggestion, made by Baehr et al,[3] that the "hyaline" thrombi of TTP were composed of aggregated platelets received early support from other investigators.[10,11] However, in 1957 Craig and Gitlin[12] challenged this conclusion. By using immunofluorescent techniques they demonstrated fibrin but not platelets in the thrombi of TTP. This observation suggested that TTP might be a reflection of disseminated intravascular coagulation (DIC), and led to the further suggestion that TTP was comparable to the generalized Shwartzman reaction.[13] However, convincing evidence for a coagulopathy in TTP has not been found.[14,15] Eventually electron microscopic studies[16-18] upheld Baehr's original suggestion and confirmed that the thrombotic lesion of TTP is indeed composed of aggregated platelets. However, the vascular determinant for platelet thrombus formation in TTP is not at all clear. Gore[9] discovered subendothelial deposits of "hyaline"-like material, which he termed a "pre-thrombotic" lesion, and postulated that this material eroded through the endothelial surface and served as a nidus for platelet aggregate formation. However, it is more likely that the hyalinized "pre-thrombotic" lesion represents an old thrombus that has undergone organization and re-endothelization. The arteriolar-capillary microaneurysms described by Orbison[20] are probably also secondary phenomena reflecting dilatation of vascular segments proximal to points of occlusion. Nonetheless, some as yet undescribed predisposing vascular abnormality seems necessary to explain platelet thrombus formation in TTP.

PATHOGENESIS

There are probably multiple etiologies for TTP. They could include either stimuli that induce platelet thrombosis, or defects in the protective mechanisms that should prevent them. Conceivably, each stimulus or defect could be evoked or uncovered in a specific clinical setting and establish its own unique pathway to the clinical end-point of TTP. Indeed, there is evidence to suggest that there may be several different pathogenic mechanisms.

When TTP occurs in a patient with SLE[21,22] an etiologic relationship to vasculitis or immunologic mechanisms is easily envisioned. Its documented association with other collagen vascular diseases such as rheumatoid arthritis,[23] Sjögren's syndrome,[24] and polymyositis[25] provides further evidence for the occurrence of TTP secondary to other diseases, and underscores the possibility that immune mechanisms could be responsible for at least some idiopathic cases. There is evidence to support this conclusion. Increased levels of platelet-associated IgG have been described in some patients[26,27] and circulating immune complexes

222

have been detected in at least one case.[28] TTP plasma has been shown to be cytotoxic to endothelial cells in vitro[29,30] and recently the sera from three patients with TTP were found to contain an antibody directed against endothelial cells.[31] Further details concerning possible immunologic mechanisms can be found in Neame's review of this subject.[32]

Infectious agents have been implicated, and Ridolfi and Bell[9] cite 18 instances in which the disease was preceded by a nonspecific viral-type respiratory infection. Coxsackie B virus was implicated in two cases,[33] *Mycoplasma* in one case,[34] and a Microtatobiote was isolated in two patients with HUS and one patient with TTP.[35] An infectious or environmental factor may explain the simultaneous occurrence of TTP in a husband and wife,[36] and two siblings sharing the same environment.[37]

The possibility that abnormalities in the mechanisms controlling platelet responsiveness might be critical to the pathogenesis of TTP is suggested by the respective *agonistic* and *antagonistic* effects of thromboxane (TxA_2) and prostacyclin (PGI_2) upon platelet aggregation.[38,39] The potential importance of balanced synthesis of these prostaglandins to thrombotic events was first expressed by Moncada and Vane.[40] The relevance of prostaglandins to TTP was subsequently suggested by the observation of Remuzzi et al[41] that TTP plasma lacked the capacity to stimulate prostacyclin elaboration by normal vessels. This observation was confirmed by others[42,43] and appears consistent with reports of decreased PGI_2 metabolites in TTP.[42,44] A genetic determinant may be suggested by the fact that a low level of plasma PGI_2–stimulating factor has been observed in the healthy family members of patients with TTP and HUS.[43,45]

An alternative mechanism for decreasing PGI_2 activity in TTP was suggested by the observation of Chen et al[46] that TTP plasma accelerated the degradation of PGI_2. This observation was confirmed by Remuzzi et al[47] and subsequently a nondialyzable "prostacyclin-stabilizing factor" was identified in normal serum by Wu et al.[48]

Alteration of TxA_2/PGI_2 balance may also play a role in the conspicuous incidence of TTP in pregnancy. Ridolfi and Bell[9] state that 9% of the reported cases of TTP occurred in pregnant or postpartum women. Pregnancy normally calls forth an increase in PGI_2 production.[49] This response is lacking in patients with preeclampsia.[50,51] Consequently, this disorder is associated with a shift in the PGI_2/TxA_2 balance which favors TxA_2 synthesis, vasoconstriction, and intravascular platelet aggregation. This is consistent with the reports of activated platelets[52] and shortened platelet life span[53] in preeclampsia, with a relative insufficiency of PGI_2 production in eclampsia,[54] and with the reduced fetal vascular PGI_2 activity observed in infants born of preeclamptic mothers.[55] The occurrence of microangiographic hemolytic anemia (MAHA) and thrombocytopenia in "severe" eclampsia,[56] the high incidence of TTP in pregnancy,[9] and the reports of TTP or HUS following use of oral contraceptives,[57,58] all suggest that pregnancy may stress the mechanisms controlling platelet activation, and that TTP in pregnancy may constitute a discrete clinical subset with its own unique pathogenic mechanism.

However, a dissenting note to the role of PGI_2 deficiency in TTP was recently sounded by Lee et al[59] when they reported normal plasma concentrations of 6-keto-PGI_1 alpha and thromboxane B_2 in two cases of TTP. This observation along with the relative ineffectiveness of PGI_2 in the treatment of TTP[44,59] suggests that a decrease in PGI_2 synthesis does not provide the answer in all cases of TTP.

Lian has reported that 20 to 30 plasma samples obtained from patients with TTP induced aggregation/agglutination of washed normal platelets.[60,61] This effect was inhibited by normal plasma but was not affected by cyclooxygenase or metabolic inhibitors.[62] Although the nature of this platelet aggregating factor (PAF) is unclear, it is interesting that the sera recently shown by Burns and Zucker-Franklin to contain antibodies directed against endothelial cells[31] also demonstrated PAF activity. Thus, the PAF activity of those samples could have an immunological basis. An alternative explanation consistent with the presence of PAF activity in TTP plasma was recently offered by Moake et al[63] who observed abnormally large VIIIR:VWF multimers in the plasma of four patients with chronic relapsing TTP in remission. During relapse, platelet agglutination was accompanied by a reduction in the quantity of the large VIIIR:VWF multimers, suggesting that they might play some role in mediating the platelet response. Interestingly, the fact that two of these plasmas were from patients with "congenital" TTP[64,65] suggests a possible genetic determinant for this abnormality. Further support for a genetic determinant in TTP is provided by reports of TTP-HUS in siblings,[66-68] and consecutive generations.[69]

It is difficult to imagine how a single pathogenic mechanism could accommodate all of the many observations that have been reported in TTP. At this point it is probably best to subscribe to the hypothesis of Umlas and Kaiser[70] that TTP is a syndrome rather than a disease with a unifying pathogenesis. This conclusion would also be consistent with the highly variable results that have been achieved with different forms of management.

MANAGEMENT OF TTP

Amorosi and Ultmann recorded only 27 survivals among the initial 271 cases of TTP.[1] By contrast, Ridolfi and Bell noted 127 survivals in the 275 patients reported since 1965.[9] The recent success is probably accounted for by the new modalities of treatment that have been employed,

224

as well as by earlier diagnosis and improved supportive care. Amorosi and Ultmann[1] concluded that splenectomy and steroids, the earlier forms of treatment, were probably ineffective. Other investigators have arrived at the same conclusion based upon more recent experience.[71-73] Cuttner,[74] on the other hand, stated that "splenectomy and corticosteroids remain a cornerstone of treatment" in her report of survival in TTP of 13 of 15 patients (87%) treated with splenectomy, corticosteroids, and dextran 70. However, Cuttner's series contained a total of 20 patients. Review of the therapy administered to the 7 patients who died indicates that only 2 of them received dextran. Thus the mortality among those who received dextran (2/15), compared to the mortality of those who did not (5/5), reveals that omission of dextran was associated with a significant increase in mortality ($P = 0.0135$; calculated by Fisher's exact test of χ^2 by Dr. Alan Dyer). Since all 20 patients received steroids and 18 underwent splenectomy, a potential beneficial effect of steroids and splenectomy can be neither proved nor disproved. However, this analysis does suggest that dextran 70, a known inhibitor of platelet function,[75] may have been the primary determinant for survival in the series reported by Cuttner.

Reports of survival in TTP began to appear more frequently after platelet aggregate formation was accepted as the fundamental pathophysiology, and inhibitors of platelet function were employed in treatment. Lerner et al were the first to report remission in TTP following the use of a drug (dextran) which was avowedly used for its inhibitory effect upon platelet function.[14] Subsequently, remissions were reported following the use of aspirin,[76] and aspirin in combination with dipyridamole.[77-81] The cumulative survival rate achieved with platelet function inhibitors has been approximately 50%.[71,72]

Reports of remarkable success have also accompanied the use of blood or plasma exchange. Remission following exchange transfusion was first reported in 1959 by Rubinstein et al.[82] However, exchange procedures were not employed with great frequency in TTP until Bukowski et al reported remission in seven of 13 patients following exchange transfusion,[83] and in two of two following plasmapheresis.[84] Subsequently, exchange procedures were associated with survival in an additional eight of 11,[85,86] and two of two[87,88] patients with TTP. In 1979 Taft[89] reported survival in three of four patients following plasmapheresis and noted that the likelihood of remission was directly proportional to the amount of plasma exchanged. The response to exchange procedures has been frequently dramatic and comatose patients may be fully alert within hours of completion of the procedures.[88] The reason why exchange procedures are beneficial is not at all clear. However, immunologic theories of pathogenesis suggest that its effectiveness could be related to the removal of immune complexes, endothelial antibodies, or other immunologic determinants. This was the prevailing wisdom until it was shown that remission could also be induced by plasma infusion alone.

In 1977 Byrnes and Khurana[90] reported a case of TTP in which plasma infusion was associated with remission. The importance of this observation resides in the fact that it stimulated thought concerning alternative pathogenic mechanisms, and raised, for the first time, the possibility that the effectiveness of exchange procedures might be related to the correction of plasma deficiencies, rather than the removal of circulating "toxins." This observation stimulated speculation that some cases of TTP may be related to a deficiency of prostacyclin, which remains an intriguing possibility. However, it had considerably lesser impact upon patient management. Although plasma infusion is apparently sufficient therapy in "congenital" TTP,[64,65] its inadequacy in the more common fulminant variety was quickly documented by others,[87,91] as well as by Byrnes and Khurana when a fulminant relapse in their patient required plasma exchange.[90] However, the relative ineffectiveness of plasma infusion in most cases of TTP does not invalidate the fascinating alternative pathogenic mechanisms that were suggested by the observation of Byrnes and Khurana. The effectiveness of exchange procedures may indeed be related in some cases to the correction of a plasma deficiency. When plasma infusion fails to achieve or sustain remission, it may reflect inadequate correction rather than faulty hypothesis.

A definitive evaluation of therapeutic measures in TTP is hampered by the anecdotal nature of reports and the variable pathogenesis. Over the past decade there have been occasional calls for multi-institutional, randomized, clinical trials to determine optimal therapy. Interestingly, none has ever been performed and it is unlikely that they ever shall be. The ethical imperatives that bind physicians[92] and the tests of "reasonableness" that clinical studies must pass[93] make it very difficult to design ethical clinical trials that could yield meaningful data. For this reason we must rely on past experience to formulate optimal treatment.

The encouraging and frequently dramatic response achieved with exchange procedures would seem to dictate that some form of plasma exchange should be employed as first line treatment in TTP, with antiplatelet drugs an important adjunctive measure. Both modalities are soundly based upon the current pathophysiologic concepts of TTP. Plasma exchange would simultaneously remove platelet activators and correct presumptive deficiencies, while antiplatelet drugs would suppress the platelet's ability to aggregate. Although both forms of treatment have been used alone successfully, their use in combination would increase the likelihood of success. There is no evidence that antiplatelet drugs operate at any level other than the suppression of platelet function. Conversely, plasmapheresis only alters the platelet's environment and may not reverse

226

the fundamental disease process. If the disease process remains active, the abnormal plasma environment may be gradually re-established. If the platelet count increases during that interim and antiplatelet drugs are not employed, a point may be reached at which the re-established abnormal plasma environment interacts with young, reactive platelet to produce a relapse. There are at least two cases in which this sequence of events may have occurred.[88,89] For this reason it is particularly important to maintain platelet function suppression following an apparent post-pheresis remission. The duration of maintenance therapy with anti-platelet drugs is not established but should probably continue for at least three months. The potential peril of reactive platelets in TTP carries the obvious corollary that platelet transfusions are contraindicated. Recent reports of sudden death,[94,95] clinical deterioration,[89] and decreased survival[86] following platelet transfusion dramatically demonstrate the potential risk of administering platelets to a patient with TTP.

The combination of plasmapheresis and antiplatelet drugs has been successfully used by Myers et al[96,97] and provides the framework for the best of present-day therapy. The patient with TTP should be treated with daily plasmapheresis. Aspirin 325 mg and dipyridamole 400 mg daily should provide adequate suppression of platelet function. In the comatose patient, dextran may be more feasible. Steroids and/or vincristine sulfate[98,99] could provide an immunosuppressive effect which might be beneficial in chronic forms of the disease that have an immunologic basis. However, it seems clear that steroids by themselves are not adequate. Finally, splenectomy is relatively ineffective, and is probably not justified in early treatment. These recommendations are based upon current knowledge and must be considered tentative. It is to be hoped that future studies provide more basic knowledge concerning etiology, and permit the development of therapeutic regimens that are tailored to specific pathogenic mechanisms.

REFERENCES

1. Amorosi EL, Ultmann JE: Thrombotic thrombocytopenic purpura: report of 16 cases and review of the literature. *Medicine* 1966;45:139–159.
2. Moschcowitz E: An acute febrile pleiochromic anemia with hyaline thrombosis of the terminal arterioles and capillaries: an undescribed disease. *Arch Intern Med* 1925;36:89–93.
3. Baehr G, Klemperer P, Schifrin A: An acute febrile anemia and thrombocytopenic purpura with diffuse platelet thromboses of capillaries and arterioles. *Trans Assoc Am Physicians* 1936;51:43–58.
4. Singer K, Bornstein FP, Wile SA: Thrombotic thrombocytopenic purpura. *Blood* 1947;2:542–554.
5. Brain MC, Dacie JV, Hourihane D O'B: Microangiopathic hemolytic anemia: the possible role of vascular lesions in pathogenesis. *Br J Haematol* 1962;8:358–374.

6. Antes EH: Thrombotic thrombocytopenic purpura: a review of the literature with report of a case. *Ann Intern Med* 1958;48:512–536.

7. Shumway CN Jr, Miller G: An unusual syndrome of hemolytic anemia, thrombocytopenic purpura and renal disease. *Blood* 1957;12:1045–1060.

8. Olsen H: Thrombotic thrombocytopenic purpura as a cause of pancreatitis. *Dig Dis* 1973;18:238–246.

9. Ridolfi RL, Bell WR: Thrombotic thrombocytopenic purpura: report of 25 cases and review of the literature. *Medicine* 1981;60:413–428.

10. Carter JR: Generalized capillary and arteriolar platelet thrombosis. *Am J Med Sci* 1947;213:585–592.

11. Trobaugh FE Jr, Markowitz M, Davidson CS, et al: An acute febrile illness characterized by thrombocytopenic purpura, hemolytic anemia, and generalized platelet thrombosis. *Arch Path* 1946;41:327–334.

12. Craig JB, Gitlin D: The nature of the hyaline thrombi in thrombotic thrombocytopenic purpura. *Am J Pathol* 1957;33:251–258.

13. Taub RN, Rodriguez-Erdmann F, Dameshek W: Intravascular coagulation, the Shwartzman reaction and the pathogenesis of thrombotic thrombocytopenic purpura. *Blood* 1964;24:775–779.

14. Lerner RG, Rapaport SI, Meltzer J: Thrombotic thrombocytopenic purpura; serial clotting studies, relation to the generalized Shwartzman reaction, and remission after adrenal steroid and dextran therapy. *Ann Intern Med* 1967;66:1180–1190.

15. Jaffe EA, Nachman RL, Merskey C: Thrombotic thrombocytopenic purpura: coagulation parameters in twelve patients. *Blood* 1973;42:499–507.

16. Feldman JD, Mardiney MR, Unanue ER, et al: The vascular pathology of thrombotic thrombocytopenic purpura; an immunohistochemical and ultrastructural study. *Lab Invest* 1966;15:927–946.

17. Neame PB, Lechago J, Ling ET, et al: Thrombotic thrombocytopenic purpura: report of a case with disseminated intravascular platelet aggregation. *Blood* 1973;42:805–814.

18. Neame PB, Hirsh J, Browman G, et al: Thrombotic thrombocytopenia purpura: a syndrome of intravascular platelet consumption. *Can Med Assoc J* 1976;19:1108–1112.

19. Gore I: Disseminated arteriolar and capillary platelet thrombosis: a morphologic study of its histogenesis. *Am J Pathol* 1950;26:155–175.

20. Orbison JL: Morphology of thrombotic thrombocytopenic purpura with demonstration of aneurysms. *Am J Pathol* 1952;28:129–143.

21. Beigelman PM: Variants of the platelet thrombosis syndrome and their relationship to disseminated lupus. *Arch Pathol* 1951;51:213–223.

22. Siegel BM, Friedman IA, Kessler S, et al: Thrombohemolytic thrombocytopenic purpura and lupus erythematosus. *Ann Intern Med* 1957;47:1022–1029.

23. Dunea G, Meuhrcke RC, Nakamoto S, et al: Thrombocytopenic purpura with acute anuric renal failure. *Am J Med* 1966;41:1000–1006.

24. Steinberg AD, Green WT, Talal N: Thrombotic thrombocytopenic purpura complicating Sjögren's syndrome. *JAMA* 1971;215:757–761.

25. McLeod BC, Wu KK, Knospe WH: Plasmapheresis in thrombotic thrombocytopenic purpura. *Arch Intern Med* 1980;140:1059–1060.

26. Morrison J, McMillan R: Elevated platelet-associated IgG in thrombotic thrombocytopenic purpura. *JAMA* 1977;238:1944–1945.

27. Kelton JG, Neame PB, Walker I, et al: Thrombotic thrombocytopenic purpura: mechanism for effectiveness of plasmapheresis. *Thromb Haemost* 1979;42:114.

28. Meister RJ, Sacher RA, Phillips T: Immune complexes in thrombotic thrombocytopenic purpura. *Ann Intern Med* 1979;90:717.
29. Wall RT, Harker LA, Quadracci LJ, et al: Immune-mediated endothelial cell injury in the pathogenesis of thrombotic thrombocytopenic purpura (TTP). *Clin Res* 1977;25:350A.
30. Foster PA, Andersen JC: Effects of plasma from patients with thrombotic thrombocytopenic purpura (TTP) on cultured human endothelial cells. *Blood* 1979;54(suppl 1):240a.
31. Burns ER, Zucker-Franklin D: Pathological effects of plasma from patients with thrombotic thrombocytopenic purpura on platelets and cultured vascular endothelial cells. *Blood* 1982;60:1030–1037.
32. Neame PB: Immunologic and other factors in thrombotic thrombocytopenic purpura (TTP). *Semin Thromb Hemostas* 1980;6:416–429.
33. Berberich FR, Cuene SA, Chard RL, et al: Thrombotic thrombocytopenic purpura: three cases with platelet and fibrinogen survival studies. *J Pediatr* 1974;84:503–509.
34. Reynolds PM, Jackson JM, Brine JAS, et al: Thrombotic thrombocytopenic purpura—remission following splenectomy. *Am J Med* 1976;61:439–447.
35. Mettler NE: Isolation of a microtatobiote from patients with hemolytic-uremic syndrome and thrombotic thrombocytopenic purpura and from mites in the United States. *N Engl J Med* 1969;281:1023–1027.
36. Watson CG, Cooper WM: Thrombotic thrombocytopenic purpura: concomitant occurrence in husband and wife. *JAMA* 1971;215:1821–1822.
37. Paz RA, Elijovich F, Barcat JA, et al: Fatal simultaneous thrombocytopenic purpura in siblings. *Br Med J* 1969;4:727–728.
38. Hamberg M, Svensson J, Samuelsson B: Thromboxanes: a new group of biologically active compounds derived from prostaglandin endoperoxides. *Proc Natl Acad Sci USA* 1975;72:2994–2998.
39. Moncada S, Gryglewski R, Bunting S, et al: An enzyme isolated from arteries transforms prostaglandin endoperoxides to an unstable substance that inhibits platelet aggregation. *Nature* 1976;263:663–665.
40. Moncada S, Vane JR: Unstable metabolites of arachidonic acid and their role in hemostasis and thrombosis. *Br Med Bull* 1978;34:129–135.
41. Remuzzi G, Misiani R, Mecca G, et al: Thrombocytopenic purpura—a deficiency of plasma factors regulating platelet-vessel-wall interaction? *N Engl J Med* 1978;299:311.
42. Machin SJ, Defreyn G, Chamone DAF, et al: Plasma 6-keto-PGF 1 alpha levels after plasma exchange in thrombotic thrombocytopenic purpura. *Lancet* 1980;1:661.
43. Jorgensen KA, Pedersen RS: Familial deficiency of prostacyclin production stimulating factor in the hemolytic uremic syndrome of childhood. *Thromb Res* 1981;21:311–315.
44. Hensby CN, Lewis PJ, Hilgard P, et al: Prostacyclin deficiency in thrombotic thrombocytopenic purpura. *Lancet* 1979;1:748.
45. Remuzzi G, Marchesi D, Misiani R, et al: Familial deficiency of a plasma factor stimulating vascular prostacyclin activity. *Thromb Res* 1979;16:517–525.
46. Chen Y-C, Hall ER, McLeod B, et al: Accelerated prostacyclin degradation in thrombotic thrombocytopenic purpura. *Lancet* 1981;2:267–269.
47. Remuzzi G, Imberti L, de Gaetano G: Prostacyclin deficiency in thrombotic microangiopathy. *Lancet* 1981;2:1422–1423.
48. Wu KK, Papp AC, Hall ER, et al: Reduction of serum prostacyclin binding in thrombotic thrombocytopenic purpura and its correction by a serum protein fraction. *Clin Res* 1982;30:332A.

49. Ferris TF: Toxemia of pregnancy and prostaglandins, in Wu KK, Rossi EC (eds): *Prostaglandins in Clinical Medicine: Cardiovascular and Thrombotic Disorders*. Chicago, Year Book Medical Publishers, 1982, pp 325–334.

50. Goodman RP, Killam AP, Brash AR, et al: Prostacyclin production during pregnancy: comparison of production during normal pregnancy and pregnancy complicated by hypertension. *Am J Obstet Gynecol* 1982;142:817–822.

51. Ylikorkala O, Makila U-M, Viinikka L: Amniotic fluid prostacyclin and thromboxane in normal, preeclamptic, and some other complicated pregnancies. *Am J Obstet Gynecol* 1981;141:487–490.

52. Whigham KAE, Howie PW, Drummond AH, et al: Abnormal platelet function in preeclampsia. *Br J Obstet Gynaecol* 1978;85:25–32.

53. Rakoczi I, Tallian F, Bagdany S, et al: Platelet life span in normal pregnancy and preeclampsia as determined by a non-radioisotope technique. *Thromb Res* 1979;15:553–556.

54. Lewis PJ, Sheperd GL, Ritter J, et al: Prostacyclin and preeclampsia. *Lancet* 1981;1:559.

55. Remuzzi G, Marchesi D, Mecca G, et al: Reduction of fetal vascular prostacyclin activity in preeclampsia. *Lancet* 1980;1:310.

56. Pritchard JA: Management of preeclampsia and eclampsia. *Kidney Int* 1980;18:259–266.

57. Brown CB, Clarkson AR, Robson JS, et al: Haemolytic uraemic syndrome in women taking oral contraceptives. *Lancet* 1973;1:1479–1481.

58. Vesconi S, Langer M, Rossi E, et al: Thrombotic thrombocytopenic purpura during oral contraceptive treatment. *Thromb Haemostas* 1978;40:563–564.

59. Lee SH, Wainscoat JS, Zeitlin H, et al: Prostacyclin and thromboxane A_2 in thrombotic thrombocytopenic purpura. *Br Med J Clin Res* 1981;283:1351–1352.

60. Lian EC-Y, Harkness DR, Byrnes JJ, et al: Presence of a platelet aggregating factor in the plasma of patients with thrombotic thrombocytopenic purpura (TTP) and its inhibition of normal plasma. *Blood* 1979;53:333–338.

61. Lian EC-Y: The role of increased platelet aggregation in TTP. *Semin Thromb Hemostas* 1980;6:401–415.

62. Lian EC-Y, Savaraj N: Effects of platelet inhibitors on the platelet aggregation induced by plasma from patients with thrombotic thrombocytopenic purpura. *Blood* 1981;58:354–359.

63. Moake JL, Rudy CK, Troll JH, et al: Unusually large plasma factor VIII: von Willebrand factor multimers in chronic relapsing thrombotic thrombocytopenic purpura. *N Engl J Med* 1982;307:1432–1435.

64. Schulman I, Pierce M, Lukens A, et al: Studies on thrombopoiesis. I. A factor in normal human plasma required for platelet production; chronic thrombocytopenia due to its deficiency. *Blood* 1960;16:943–957.

65. Upshaw JD Jr: Congenital deficiency of a factor in normal plasma that reverses microangiopathic hemolysis and thrombocytopenia. *N Engl J Med* 1978;298:1350–1352.

66. Wallace DC, Lovric A, Clubb JS, et al: Thrombotic thrombocytopenic purpura in four siblings. *Am J Med* 1975;58:724–734.

67. Fuchs WE, George JN, Dotin LN, et al: Thrombotic thrombocytopenic purpura: occurrence two years apart during late pregnancy in two sisters. *JAMA* 1976;235:2126–2127.

68. Hellman RM, Jackson DV, Buss DH: Thrombotic thrombocytopenic purpura and hemolytic-uremic syndrome HLA-identical siblings. *Ann Intern Med* 1980;93:283–284.

69. Kirchner KA, Smith RM, Gockerman JP, et al: Hereditary thrombotic

thrombocytopenic purpura: microangiopathic hemolytic anemia, thrombocytopenia, and renal insufficiency occurring in consecutive generations. *Nephron* 1982;30:28-30.

70. Umlas J, Kaiser J: Thrombohemolytic thrombocytopenic purpura (TTP); a disease or a syndrome? *Am J Med* 1970;49:723-728.

71. Amorosi EL, Karpatkin S: Antiplatelet treatment of thrombotic thrombocytopenic purpura. *Ann Intern Med* 1977;86:102-106.

72. Bukowski RM, Hewlett JS, Reimer RR, et al: Therapy of thrombotic thrombocytopenic purpura: an overview. *Semin Thromb Hemostas* 1981;7:1-8.

73. Bukowski RM: Thrombotic thrombocytopenic purpura: a review, in Spaet TH (ed.): *Progress in Hemostasis and Thrombosis.* New York, Grune & Stratton, 1982, vol 6, pp 287-337.

74. Cuttner J: Thrombotic thrombocytopenic purpura: a ten-year experience. *Blood* 1980;56:302-306.

75. Weiss HJ: The effect of clinical dextran on platelet aggregation, adhesion, and ADP release in man: in vivo and in vitro studies. *J Lab Clin Med* 1967;69:37-46.

76. Jobin F, Delage J-M: Aspirin and prednisone in microangiopathic haemolytic anemia. *Lancet* 1970;2:208-210.

77. Zacharski LR, Walworth C, McIntyre OR: Antiplatelet therapy for thrombotic thrombocytopenic purpura. *N Engl J Med* 1971;285:408-409.

78. Giromini M, Bouvier CA, Dami R, et al: Effect of dipyridamole and aspirin in thrombotic microangiopathy. *Br Med J* 1972;1:545-546.

79. Amir J, Krauss S: Treatment of thrombotic thrombocytopenic purpura with antiplatelet drugs. *Blood* 1973:42:27-33.

80. Rossi EC, Redondo D, Borges WH: Thrombotic thrombocytopenic purpura: survival following treatment with aspirin, dipyridamole, and prednisone. *JAMA* 1974;228:1141-1143.

81. Eckel RH, Crowell EB Jr, Waterhouse BE, et al: Platelet-inhibiting drugs in thrombotic thrombocytopenic purpura. *Arch Intern Med* 1977;137:735-737.

82. Rubinstein MA, Kagan BM, MacGillviray MH, et al: Unusual remission in a case of thrombotic thrombocytopenic purpura syndrome following fresh blood exchange transfusions. *Ann Intern Med* 1959;51:1409-1419.

83. Bukowski RM, Hewlett JS, Harris JW, et al: Exchange transfusions in the treatment of thrombotic thrombocytopenic purpura. *Semin Hematol* 1976; 13:219-232.

84. Bukowski RM, King JW, Hewlett JS: Plasmapheresis in the treatment of thrombotic thrombocytopenic purpura. *Blood* 1977;50:413-417.

85. Pisciotta AV, Garthwaite T, Darin J, et al: Treatment of thrombotic thrombocytopenic purpura by exchange transfusion. *Am J Hematol* 1977;3:73-82.

86. Gottschall JL, Pisciotta AV, Darin J, et al: Thrombotic thrombocytopenic purpura: experience with whole blood exchange transfusion. *Semin Thromb Hemostas* 1981;7:25-32.

87. Rossi EC, del Greco F: Treatment for thrombotic thrombocytopenic purpura with hemodialysis and exchange transfusions. *N Engl J Med* 1978;298:972.

88. Rossi EC, del Greco F, Kwaan HC, et al: Hemodialysis-exchange transfusion for treatment of thrombotic thrombocytopenic purpura. *JAMA* 1980;244: 1466-1468.

89. Taft EG: Thrombotic thrombocytopenic purpura and dose of plasma exchange. *Blood* 1979;54:842-849.

90. Byrnes JJ, Khurana M: Treatment of thrombotic thrombocytopenic purpura with plasma. *N Engl J Med* 1977;297:1386-1389.

91. Ansell J, Beaser RS, Pechet L: Thrombotic thrombocytopenic purpura fails to respond to fresh frozen plasma infusion. *Ann Intern Med* 1978;89:647–648.
92. Spodick DH: The randomized controlled clinical trial: scientific and ethical bases. *Am J Med* 1982;73:420–425.
93. Curran WJ: Reasonableness and randomization in clinical trials: fundamental law and governmental regulation. *N Engl J Med* 1979;300:1273–1275.
94. Harkness DR, Byrnes JJ, Lian EC-Y, et al: Hazard of platelet transfusion in thrombotic thrombocytopenic purpura. *JAMA* 1981;246:1931–1933.
95. Byrnes JJ: Plasma infusion in the treatment of thrombotic thrombocytopenic purpura. *Semin Thromb Hemostas* 1981;7:9–14.
96. Myers TJ, Wakem CJ, Ball ED, et al: Thrombotic thrombocytopenic purpura: combined treatment with plasmapheresis and antiplatelet agents. *Ann Intern Med* 1980;92:149–155.
97. Myer TJ: Treatment of thrombotic thrombocytopenic purpura with combined exchange plasmapheresis and anti-platelet agents. *Semin Thromb Hemostas* 1981;7:37–42.
98. Abramson N: Treatment for thrombotic thrombocytopenic purpura with vincristine. *N Engl J Med* 1978;298:971–972.
99. Gutterman LA, Stevenson TD: Treatment of thrombotic thrombocytopenic purpura with vincristine. *JAMA* 1982;247:1433–1436.

12 *The Hemolytic Uremic Syndrome*

Ennio C. Rossi

In 1955 Gasser et al[1] described a fatal disorder in five children characterized by hemolytic anemia, thrombocytopenia, and renal failure which they named the "hemolytic uremic syndrome" (HUS). In 1957, Allison[2] reported six additional cases and drew attention to fragmented erythrocytes, the hallmarks of microangiopathic hemolytic anemia (MAHA).[3] Subsequent reports confirmed the existence of the syndrome,[4-7] documented recurrent episodes,[4] and described a gastrointestinal prodrome.[5-7] Over the next decade, endemic foci of HUS were identified in Argentina,[8] France,[9] South Africa,[10] and California;[11] and "epidemic" outbreaks were recorded in North Wales[12] and Scotland.[13] These reports added several hundred cases to the literature and disclosed the highly variable severity of HUS. For example, HUS in Argentina[8] was severe with extrarenal manifestations and high mortality, while the disease in California[11] was milder and had a lower mortality rate. Prodromal symptoms suggested an infectious etiology. However, an analysis of familial occurrences also suggested possible genetic determinants. Kaplan et al[14] observed two distinct patterns in the reports of HUS in siblings. In the first pattern, illness occurred simultaneously (mortality rate, 19%) and implicated an environmental factor. In the second pattern, the illness occurred at distant intervals, carried a mortality rate of 68%, and suggested a possible genetic basis. The second group's lack of prodrome also favored a genetic etiology,[15] and its higher mortality rate agreed with a previous study which had shown an association between the absence of prodrome and poor prognosis.[16] Thus, Gasser's initial definition of the hemolytic uremic syndrome evolved to include a number of subtypes that were seemingly different.[15] This is not surprising since the initial report of a new syndrome usually describes fulminant, fatal disease with striking clinical signs. After the syndrome is accepted, it gradually acquires a more heterogeneous appearance as less severe cases are reported.[17] As concerns HUS, heterogeneity became even more obvious when it became apparent that the disease was not confined to children.

Although HUS remains much more common in children, it has also been described in adults,[18-28] particularly postpartum women,[29-43] and women taking oral contraceptives,[44-46] or estrogen preparations.[47] HUS

234

has also been described as a secondary event in patients with polyarthralgia,[21] scleroderma,[27] metastatic carcinoma,[48] and renal transplant rejection.[49,50] The occasional presence of a prodrome again invokes a possible infectious etiology. However, the report of fatal HUS in young and middle-aged men from three generations of the same family[25] suggests that genetic factors may lie dormant until adult life. In any event, HUS is not confined to the pediatric age group, and the recent description of the simultaneous occurrence of HUS in mother and child[51] illustrates this point.

CLINICAL PRESENTATION

The hemolytic uremic syndrome comprises a diagnostic triad of hemolytic anemia, thrombocytopenia, and renal failure.[52,53] The gastrointestinal prodrome is usually mild in both children and adults, but may, on occasion, be severe enough to warrant hospitalization. HUS becomes manifest either immediately thereafter or following a "latent" period with the appearance of anemia, thrombocytopenia, hypertension, and oliguria which may progress rapidly to anuria. The microangiopathic anemia is usually severe and the thrombocytopenia may also be quite marked. Fever and central nervous system signs have been prominent in reports from Argentina[8] and France,[54] and recently Bale et al[55] reported acute neurologic complications in 50% of 60 children with HUS in Utah. The addition of fever and central nervous system involvement to the triad of HUS fulfills the diagnostic pentad of thrombotic thrombocytopenia purpura (TTP)[56] (see chapter 11). A clinical distinction between these disorders can be preserved by emphasizing the predominance of renal failure in HUS, and the prevalence of neurologic signs in TTP.[57] However, the renal "involvement" of TTP, and the extrarenal complications of HUS[8,54,55,58] create an area of ambiguity which cannot be clarified by clinical criteria.[59]

The distinction between HUS and TTP has been ambiguous from the outset. One case with acknowledged similarities to "Moschcowitz's disease"[60] was included among the original five cases of HUS.[1] Allison's diagnosis in the second series of cases was "thrombotic thrombocytopenia of childhood." However, the survival of four of six children seemed inconsistent with the high mortality rate of TTP[56] and may explain why Allison's cases (two) have been considered examples of HUS. A survival/fatality criterion of definition may have been operative also in two reports of a young girl that defined her condition during life as HUS,[4] and following necropsy five years later, as TTP.[61] Heptinstall[62] has noted that patients with terminal renal failure[21] have been published as cases of TTP, while others easily categorized as TTP have been called HUS.[18] The lack of true distinction between these disorders is emphasized further by recent reports of TTP, or HUS, occurring in HLA-identical siblings,[63] and consecutive generations.[64] These experiences suggest that HUS and TTP may be variants of the same disease process, and that clinical distinctions may be more a matter of formulation than substantive difference. Their similarities in pathology, and their conceptual parallels in pathogenesis and management would seem to support this conclusion.

PATHOLOGY

The original five cases described by Gasser et al[1] all showed renal cortical necrosis at autopsy. In addition, one case showed extensive extrarenal thrombi suggestive of "Moshcowitz's disease," two showed "anemic infarcts" of the lung, and one demonstrated "arteriosclerosis of the spleen." Microvascular thrombi, largely composed of platelets, were found in the kidneys and other organs of the two fulminant cases described by Allison.[2] Platelet thrombi were also the predominant early lesions in renal biopsies of non-lethal HUS.[65] Electron microscopic studies by Courtecuisse et al[66] revealed a number of early glomerular lesions including platelet pseudopodia projecting through endothelial cell fenestrations, subendothelial platelet aggregate formation, and platelet debris lodged against and within the basement membrane. Similar lesions were observed two to three weeks following the onset of anuria by Franklin et al,[23] and Date et al.[67] Sequential biopsies in nonlethal HUS disclosed evolution of these early lesions, through various degrees of endothelial swelling and proliferative disease, to late changes indistinguishable from malignant nephrosclerosis. These findings were reminiscent of the evolutionary changes in renal pathology observed in rabbits following a single infusion of procoagulant material.[68] Consequently, Vitsky et al[69] concluded that the platelet thrombi usually associated with TTP and the proliferative changes more characteristic of HUS could be different stages of the same disease process, and Habib et al[70] affirmed that the renal lesions of HUS and TTP are fundamentally indistinguishable.

Thrombotic microangiopathy (TMA), a term originally proposed by Symmers,[71] accurately describes the anatomical changes seen in both HUS and TTP. Substitution of the terms renal and disseminated TMA for HUS and TTP would be appropriate because it emphasizes the only sure distinction that exists.

PATHOGENESIS

An immune response to an environmental factor is the most plausible etiology for HUS or TTP,[72] and several viruses have been implicated as causative agents. Sera from children with HUS have revealed evidence for infection with coxsackie[73] and echo[74] enteroviruses, and influenza[75] and respiratory[54] myxoviruses. Arthropod-borne arboviruses and have been implicated in Argentina,[8] and a mite-borne Microtatobiote[76] was indentified in the blood of two patients with HUS and one with TTP. HUS has also occurred in association with outbreaks of bacillary dysentery in India[67] and Bangladesh.[77] The higher incidence of HUS in children is unexplained but might be due, in part, to the greater likelihood that adults have acquired immunities to offending organisms. A unique immunologic predisposition in children may also explain HUS in association with thymic alymphoplasia[78] or following vaccination.[54,78,79]

Endothelial damage by antibodies or bacterial endotoxins may be the initial event in the pathogenetic process. An antibody directed against endothelial cells has been found in the sera of patients with TTP,[80] and conceivably could be present in patients with HUS. Alternatively, endotoxemia accurately predicted the occurrence of HUS during the epidemic of shigellosis in Bangladesh.[77] Regardless of the cause, extensive endothelial damage would activate hemostatic mechanisms and could lead to arteriolar and glomerular capillary occlusion. Coagulation studies in HUS have not revealed convincing evidence for disseminated intravascular coagulation.[81-83] However, animal experiments have shown that the vascular lesions induced by endotoxin infusion can be prevented by aspirin,[84] but not by heparin.[85] This suggests that the platelet may play a primary role in endotoxin-induced occlusive vascular disease.

In 1972, Harker and Slichter[86] demonstrated that patients with HUS and TTP had shortened platelet but normal fibrinogen survival times. These observations were confirmed by Katz et al.[87] Subsequently George et al[88] demonstrated that the shortened platelet survival time in HUS could be lengthened by dipyridamole, an inhibitor of platelet adhesiveness, but not by heparin. Further evidence for platelet activation in HUS includes descriptions of acquired platelet storage pool disorder,[89] reduced platelet aggregation,[90] and increased plasma concentrations of the platelet-specific proteins, beta thromboglobulin and platelet factor 4.[91] Since the adherence of platelets to the endothelium is mediated by the von Willebrand factor,[92] the increase in factor VIII antigen that occurs in uremia[93-95] may establish conditions particularly favorable to the accretion of platelets on damaged endothelium. The intense deposition of factor VIII antigen in the glomeruli of HUS[96] supports this conclusion, and the presence in platelets of a mitogenic factor that stimulates smooth muscle proliferation[97] could explain late nephrosclerotic changes. Thus, the occurrence of HUS could ultimately depend upon the integrity of the physiologic mechanisms that control platelet-endothelial interactions.[98]

Baumgartner and Muggli demonstrated that platelets form a monolayer of spread-out, degranulated platelets, or "pseudoendothelium," on de-endothelialized vascular surfaces.[99] Additional platelets did not adhere to this monolayer suggesting the existence of a physiologic mechanism that limited platelet-endothelial interaction. The discovery of prostacyclin (PGI_2),[100] a potent inhibitor of platelet aggregation, provided the probable mediator of this effect. Since activated platelets and thrombin stimulate the production of PGI_2 by cultured human endothelial cells,[101,102] it is reasonable to suspect that uncontrolled platelet aggregation leading to vascular occlusion could be due to defects in the elaboration of prostacylin by vascular endothelium. This suspicion was confirmed by the observation[103] that patients with HUS lacked a plasma factor required for prostacyclin elaboration by normal vessels. The recent demonstration of a familial deficiency of this factor could explain some cases of familial HUS,[104] while epidemic, endotoxemia-induced HUS[77] could be explained by an overwhelmed, but otherwise normal, prostacyclin system.[105] Since PGI_2 is a potent vasodilator, its deficiency may also contribute to hypertension, and the progressive demand for increased PGI_2 synthesis imposed by pregnancy (see chapter 11) could explain the increased risk of HUS that exists during late pregnancy and the postpartum period. Although other factors are undoubtedly involved, uncontrolled platelet-endothelial interaction in arterioles and glomerular capillaries appears to be a central event in the pathogenesis of HUS. This premise has led to several innovations in the management of HUS.

MANAGEMENT

The cornerstone of treatment in HUS is the effective management of renal failure. Gianantonio et al[106] analyzed the results of treatment in 678 cases of childhood HUS, and convincingly demonstrated the importance of dialysis in the care of these patients. The renal thrombotic lesion suggests that inhibitors of hemostatic mechanisms may also be beneficial, and heparin, thrombolytic agents, and antiplatelet drugs have all been used. However, an accurate assessment of their effectiveness is virtually impossible because of the improved survival attributable to dialysis,[106] the variability of disease severity in different countries,[15] and the inclination of clinicians to use hemostatic inhibitors in a variety of combinations. For these reasons, the usefulness of hemostatic inhibitors in HUS is the subject of continuing controversy.

Kaplan et al[10] and Vitacco et al[107] concluded that heparin was not helpful in the treatment of HUS in children. This parallels the experience in adult HUS where heparin, with few exceptions,[35,46] was similarly ineffective.[18,32,37] However, the frequent occurrence of chronic progressive disease[108] led Proesmans and Eeckels[109] to suggest that heparin therapy might reduce long-term sequelae. This conclusion has been challenged[110] and the controversy concerning heparin remains unresolved. The results with fibrinolytic agents have also been mixed. A favorable report from the Netherlands[83] may reflect, primarily, the milder form of disease found in that country.[11,15] Other reports[16,38] have been less encouraging; in a recent study the endarterial infusion of urokinase was considered ineffective and possibly detrimental.[111] Powell and Ekert[112] reported that a combination of heparin, streptokinase, and antiplatelet drugs appeared to prevent chronic renal sequelae more effectively than heparin alone. In view of the previous experiences with heparin, and heparin-streptokinase combinations, the favorable results reported by Powell and Ekert[112] may have been due to the addition of antiplatelet drugs.

The effectiveness of antiplatelet drugs in TTP[113] provides a rationale for their use in HUS.[114] A further justification is contained in reports of the beneficial effect of dipyridamole in renal transplant rejection,[115] and various forms of renal vascular disease.[116] Several other case reports also encourage this approach. Brown et al[44] noted that the only recovery in their series of five occurred in the patient who received dipyridamole. Similarly, Utting and Shreeve[24] achieved remission in HUS with aspirin and dipyridamole after employing streptokinase and heparin without success. Thorsen et al[26] demonstrated a relationship between aspirin dosage and the platelet count, while Ponticelli et al[28] reported survival in ten of 11 adult cases with a combination of heparin and antiplatelet drugs. Arenson and August[117] achieved beneficial effects in three children using the same combination, but O'Regan et al[118] reported inconclusive reports when antiplatelet drugs were used alone.

The limitation of hemostatic inhibitors in the treatment of thrombotic microangiopathy is discerned more easily in TTP than HUS. TTP, with its disseminated lesions, is a harsher test of hemostatic inhibitors and easily discloses the relative ineffectiveness of heparin[113] and fibrinolytic agents,[119] and the limitation of antiplatelet agents.[114] Conversely, in HUS, the favorable acute prognosis achieved by dialysis leaves long-term improvement, difficult to prove or disprove, as the only goal available to hemostatic inhibitors. However, plasma infusion or exchange have been extremely effective in TTP, and recent reports indicate that they are equally beneficial in HUS.[27,43]

The most important determinant of recovery in HUS is probably early diagnosis. This point is illustrated by our recent experience with a 19-year-old eclamptic patient who became comatose and anuric two days postpartum and whose mother had died of a similar illness following the patient's birth (unpublished data, January 1982). Twice daily plasmaphereses with intervening hemodialyses begun on the fourth post-partum day were followed by complete recovery six days later. This suggests that early diagnosis and the prompt institution of plasmapheresis[43] can reverse the disease process before renal damage becomes irreversible. Gianantonio et al[106] have noted an inverse relationship between prognosis and the duration of oligoanuria. Indeed, the better prognosis observed in HUS with prodrome may be due to the fact that patients with prodromal symptoms are more inclined to seek medical attention prior to the onset of anuria. Conversely, in the absence of prodrome, anuria may develop insidiously and renal damage may be already irreversible when the patient first seeks attention. Renal thrombi may have undergone organization, at which point it may be unreasonable to expect plasmapheresis or hemostatic inhibitors to affect greatly the outcome.

It is likely that interdictions established in the treatment of TTP are also valid for HUS. Harkness et al[120] have recently provided dramatic evidence of the hazard of platelet transfusion in TTP. Platelet transfusions during the early, thrombocytopenic, acute phase of HUS are also contraindicated because they would increase glomerular thrombi and augment renal damage.

In summary, the key to effective treatment of HUS is early diagnosis. Intensive plasmapheresis and hemodialysis may reverse the process and effect complete recovery if the stimulus is self-limited. If the stimulus is ongoing, the addition of plasmapheresis and antiplatelet agents to maintenance hemodialysis may stabilize the process, but reversal will probably depend upon identification and effective treatment of the underlying cause. If anuria is well-established the same measures should be employed. However, it may be necessary to scale down therapeutic expectations in inverse proportion to the duration of antecedent anuria. These recommendations, as in TTP, must be considered tentative. More basic knowledge must be obtained before we can devise therapeutic regimens that deal effectively with the highly variable clinical manifestations of HUS.

REFERENCES

1. Gasser C, Gautier E, Steck A, et al: Hämolytisch-urämische Syndrome: bilaterale Nierenrindennekrosen bei akuten erworbenen hämolytischen Anämien. *Schweiz Med Wochenschr* 1955;85:905–909.
2. Allison AC: Acute haemolytic anaemia with distortion and fragmentation of erythrocytes in children. *Br J Haematol* 1957;3:1–18.
3. Brain MC, Dacie JV, Hourihane D O'B: Microangiopathic hemolytic anemia: the possible role of vascular lesions in pathogenesis. *Br J Haematol* 1962;8:358–374.
4. Shumway CN Jr, Miller G: An unusual syndrome of hemolytic anemia, thrombocytopenic purpura and renal disease. *Blood* 1957;12:1045–1060.
5. Lamvik JO: Acute glomerulonephritis with hemolytic anemia in infants. *Pediatrics* 1962;29:224–236.
6. Gianantonio CA, Vitacco M, Mendilaharzu, J, et al: Acute renal failure in infancy and childhood. *J Pediatr* 1962;61:660–678.
7. Shumway CN, Terplan KL: Hemolytic anemia, thrombocytopenia, and renal disease in childhood: the hemolytic-uremic syndrome. *Pediatr Clin North Am* 1964;11:577–591.
8. Gianantonio C, Vitacco M, Mendilaharzu F, et al: The hemolytic-uremic syndrome. *J Pediatr* 1964;64:478–491.

9. Habib R, Mathieu H, Royer P: Le syndrome hémolytique et urémique de l'enfant. *Nephron* 1967;4:139–172.

10. Kaplan BS, Katz J, Krawitz S, et al: An analysis of the results of therapy in 67 cases of the hemolytic-uremic syndrome. *J Pediatr* 1971;78:420–425.

11. Tune BM, Leavitt TJ, Gribble TJ: The hemolytic-uremic syndrome in California: a review of 28 nonheparinized cases with long-term follow-up. *J Pediatr* 1973;82:304–310.

12. McLean MM, Jones CH, Sutherland DA: Haemolytic-uraemic syndrome: a report of an outbreak. *Arch Dis Child* 1966;41:76–81.

13. Ruthven IS, Fyfe WM: The haemolytic uraemic syndrome—an epidemic disease? *Scott Med J* 1968;13:162–165.

14. Kaplan BS, Chesney RW, Drummond KN: Hemolytic uremic syndrome in families. *N Engl J Med* 1975;292:1090–1093.

15. Dolislager D, Tune B: The hemolytic-uremic syndrome: spectrum of severity and significance of prodrome. *Am J Dis Child* 1978;132:55–58.

16. Stuart J, Winterborn MH, White RHR, et al: Thrombolytic therapy in haemolytic-uraemic syndrome. *Br Med J* 1974;3:217–221.

17. Brain MC: The haemolytic-uraemic syndrome. *Semin Hematol* 1969; 6:162–180.

18. Clarkson AR, Lawrence JR, Meadows R, et al: The haemolytic uraemic syndrome in adults. *Q J Med* 1970;39:227–239.

19. Giromini M, Laperrouza C: Prolonged survival after bilateral nephrectomy in an adult with haemolytic uraemic syndrome. *Lancet* 1969;2:169–170.

20. King LR, Wulsin JH, McAdams AJ: Hemolytic-uremic syndrome in older children and adults. *J Urol* 1969;101:273–275.

21. Dunea G, Muehrcke RC, Nakamoto S, et al: Thrombotic thrombocytopenic purpura with acute anuric renal failure. *Am J Med* 1966; 41:1000–1006.

22. Shapiro CM, Kanter A, Lopas H, et al: Hemolytic-uremic syndrome in adults. *JAMA* 1970;213:567–570.

23. Franklin WA, Simon NM, Potter EV, et al: The hemolytic-uremic syndrome. *Arch Pathol* 1972;94:230–240.

24. Utting JA, Shreeve DR: Haemolytic-uraemic syndrome in an adult with pericarditis and pleurisy. *Br Med J* 1973;2:591.

25. Karlsberg RP, Lacher JW, Bartecchi CE: Adult hemolytic-uremic syndrome:familial variant. *Arch Intern Med* 1977;137:1155–1157.

26. Thorsen CA, Rossi EC, Green D, et al: The treatment of the hemolytic-uremic syndrome with inhibitors of platelet function. *Am J Med* 1979; 66:711–716.

27. Remuzzi G, Misiani R, Marchesi D, et al: Treatment of the hemolytic uremic syndrome with plasma. *Clin Nephrol* 1979;12:279–284.

28. Ponticelli C, Rivolta E, Imbasciati E, et al: Hemolytic uremic syndrome in adults. *Arch Intern Med* 1980;140:353–357.

29. Robson JS, Martin AM, Ruckley VA, et al: Irreversible post-partum renal failure. *Q J Med* 1968;37:423–435.

30. Scheer RL, Jones DB: Malignant nephrosclerosis in women post-partum. *JAMA* 1967;201:600–604.

31. Wagoner RD, Holley KE, Johnson WJ: Accelerated nephrosclerosis and post-partum acute renal failure in normotensive patients. *Ann Intern Med* 1968;69:237–248.

32. Clarkson AR, Meadows R, Lawrence JR: Post-partum renal failure. The generalized Shwartzman reaction. *Australas Ann Med* 1969;18:209–216.

33. Rosenmann E, Kanter A, Bacani RA, et al: Fatal late post-partum intravascular coagulation with acute renal failure. *Am J Med Sci* 1969;257:259–273.

34. Churg J, Koffler D, Paronetto F, et al: Hemolytic uremic syndrome as a cause of post-partum renal failure. *Am J Obstet Gynecol* 1970;108:253–261.

35. Luke RG, Siegel RR, Talbert W, et al: Heparin treatment for post-partum renal failure with microangiopathic haemolytic anemia. *Lancet* 1970;2:750–752.

36. Ponticelli C, Imbasciati E, Tarantino A, et al: Post-partum renal failure with microangiopathic haemolytic anaemia. *Nephron* 1972;9:27–41.

37. Eisinger AJ: The post-partum haemolytic uraemic syndrome. *J Obstet Gynecol Br Commonw* 1972;79:139–143.

38. Calvert GD: Post-partum haemolytic uraemic syndrome: case report and brief review. *J Obstet Cynecol Br Commonw* 1972;79:244–249.

39. Finkelstein FO, Kashgarian M, Hayslett JP: Clinical spectrum of post-partum renal failure. *Am J Med* 1974;57:649–654.

40. Gomperts ED, Sessel L, du Plessis V, et al: Recurrent post-partum haemolytic uraemic syndrome. *Lancet* 1978;1:48.

41. Nissenson AR, Krumlovsky FA, del Greco F: Post-partum hemolytic uremic syndrome: late recovery after prolonged maintenance dialysis. *JAMA* 1979;242:173–175.

42. Brandt P, Jespersen J, Gregersen G: Post-partum haemolytic-uraemic syndrome treated with antithrombin-III *Nephron* 1981;27:15–18.

43. Spenser CD, Crane FM, Kumar JR, et al: Treatment of post-partum hemolytic uremic syndrome with plasma exchange. *JAMA* 1982;247:2808–2809.

44. Brown CB, Clarkson AR, Robson JS, et al: Haemolytic uraemic syndrome in women taking oral contraceptives. *Lancet* 1973;1:1479–1481.

45. Schoolwerth AC, Sandler RS, Klahr S, et al: Post-partum nephrosclerosis, and nephrosclerosis in women taking oral contraceptives. *Arch Intern Med* 1976;136:178–185.

46. Khanh BT, Bhathena D, Vazquez M, et al: Role of heparin therapy in the outcome of adult hemolytic uremic syndrome. *Nephron* 1976;16:292–301.

47. Ashouri OS, Marbury TC, Fuller TJ, et al: Hemolytic uremic syndrome in two postmenopausal women taking a conjugated estrogen preparation. *Clin Nephrol* 1982;17:212–215.

48. Lohrmann H-P, Adam W, Heymer B, et al: Microangiopathic hemolytic anemia in metastatic carcinoma. *Ann Intern Med* 1973;79:368–375.

49. Hutton MM, Prentice CRM, Allison ME, et al: Renal homotransplant rejection associated with microangiopathic hemolytic anemia *Br Med J* 1970;3:87–88.

50. Petersen VP, Olson TS: Late transplant failure due to the hemolytic-uremic syndrome. *Acta Med Scand* 1971;189:377–380.

51. Siegler RL: Simultaneous microangiopathic hemolytic anemia, thrombocytopenia, and acute nephropathy in mother and child. *Am J Dis Child* 1980;134:991–992.

52. Liberman E: Hemolytic-uremic syndrome. *J Pediatr* 1972;80:1–16.

53. Goldstein MH, Churg J, Strauss L, et al: Hemolytic-uremic syndrome. *Nephron* 1979;23:263–272.

54. Mathieu H, Leclerc F, Habib R, et al: Étude clinique et biologique de 38 observations de syndrome hémolytique et urémique. *Arch Fr Pediatr* 1969;26:369–390.

55. Bale JF Jr, Brasher C, Siegler RL: CNS manifestations of the hemolytic-uremic syndrome. *Am J Dis Child* 1980;134:869–872.
56. Amorosi EL, Ultmann JE: Thrombotic thrombocytopenic purpura: report of 16 cases and review of the literature. *Medicine* 1966;45:149–159.
57. Bukowski RM: Thrombotic thrombocytopenic purpura: a review, in TH Spaet (ed): *Progress in Hemostasis and Thrombosis*. New York, Grune & Stratton, 1982, vol 6, pp 287–337.
58. Burns JC, Berman ER, Fagre JL, et al: Pancreatic islet cell necrosis: association with hemolytic-uremic syndrome. *J Pediatr* 1982;100:582–584.
59. Kaplan BS, Drummond KN: The hemolytic-uremic syndrome is a syndrome. *N Engl J Med* 1978;298:964–966.
60. Moschcowitz E: An acute febrile pleiochromic anemia with hyaline thrombosis of the terminal arterioles and capillaries: an undescribed disease. *Arch Intern Med* 1925;36:89–93.
61. MacWhinney JB Jr, Packer JT, Miller G, et al: Thrombotic thrombocytopenic purpura in childhood. *Blood* 1962;19:181–199.
62. Heptinstall RH: *Pathology of the Kidney*. Boston, Little, Brown & Co., 1974, pp 675–711.
63. Hellman RM, Jackson DV, Buss DH: Thrombotic thrombocytopenia purpura and hemolytic-uremic syndrome in HLA-identical siblings. *Ann Intern Med* 1980;93:283–284.
64. Kirchner KA, Smith RM, Gockerman JP, Luke RG: Hereditary thrombotic thrombocytopenic purpura: microangiopathic hemolytic anemia, thrombocytopenia, and renal insufficiency occurring in consecutive generations. *Nephron* 1982;30:28–30.
65. Bartman J, Jacques M, Dustin P Jr: Anémie hémolytique, purpura thrombocytopénique et néphropathie aiguë chez un nourrisson. Étude au microscope électronique des lésions rénales. *Rev Belge Path Med Exp* 1964; 30:5–27.
66. Courtecuisse V, Habib R, Monnicr C: Nonlethal hemolytic and uremic syndromes in children: an electron-microscope study of renal biopsies from six cases. *Exp Mol Pathol* 1967;7:324–347.
67. Date A, Raghupathy P, Shastry JCM: Nephron injury in the haemolytic-uraemic syndrome complicating bacillary dysentery. *J Pathol* 1981;133:1–16.
68. Vassalli P, Simon G, Rouiller C: Electron microscopic study of glomerular lesions resulting from intravascular fibrin formation. *Am J Pathol* 1963; 43:579–617.
69. Vitsky BH, Suzuki Y, Strauss L, et al: The hemolytic-uremic syndrome: A study of renal pathologic alterations. *Am J Pathol* 1969;57:627–639.
70. Habib, R, Courtecuisse V, Leclerc F, Mathieu H, Royer P: Étude anatomo-pathologique de 35 observations de syndrome hémolytique et urémique de l'enfant. *Arch Fr Pediatr* 1969;26:391–416.
71. Symmers WStC: Thrombotic microangiopathic haemolytic anaemia (thrombotic microangiopathy). *Br Med J* 1952;2:897–903.
72. Brain MC, Neame PB: Thrombotic thrombocytopenic purpura and the hemolytic uremic syndrome. *Semin Thromb Hemostas* 1982;8:186–187.
73. Ray C, Tucker VL, Harris DJ, et al: Enteroviruses associated with the hemolytic-uremic syndrome. *Pediatrics* 1970;46:378–388.
74. Peil C: Hemolytic-uremic syndrome. *Pediatr Clin North Am* 1966;13: 295–314.
75. Chan JCM, Eleff MG, Campbell RA: The hemolytic-uremic syndrome in non-related adopted siblings. *J Pediatr* 1969;75:1050–1053.
76. Mettler NE: Isolation of a microtatobiote from patients with hemolytic-

uremic syndrome and thrombotic thrombocytopenic purpura and from mites in the United States. *N Engl J Med* 1969;281:1023–1027.

77. Koster F, Levin J, Walker L, et al: Hemolytic-uremic syndrome after shigellosis—relation to endotoxemia and circulating immune complexes. *N Engl J Med* 1978;298:927–933.

78. Dubilier LD, Chadwick JA, Leddy JP: Thymic alymphoplasia associated with the hemolytic-uremic syndrome. *J Pediatr* 1968;73:714–724.

79. Dosik H, Tricario F: Haemolytic-uraemic syndrome following mumps vaccination. *Lancet* 1970;1:247.

80. Burns ER, Zucker-Franklin D: Pathological effects of plasma from patients with thrombotic thrombocytopenic purpura on platelets and cultured vascular endothelial cells. *Blood* 1982;60:1030–1037.

81. Avalos JS, Vitacco M, Molinas F, Penalver J, Gianantonio C: Coagulation studies in the hemolytic-uremic syndrome. *J Pediatr* 1970;76:538–548.

82. Katz J, Lurie A, Kaplan BS, Krawitz S, Metz J: Coagulation findings in the hemolytic-uremic syndrome of infancy: similarity to hyperacute renal allograft rejection. *J Pediatr* 1971;78:726–734.

83. Monnens L, Kleynen F, van Munster P, et al: Coagulation studies and streptokinase therapy in the haemolytic-uraemic syndrome. *Helv Paediatr Acta* 1972;27:45–54.

84. Evans G, Mustard JF: Inhibition of the platelet-surface reaction in endotoxin shock and the generalized Schwartzman reaction. *J Clin Invest* 1968;47:31a.

85. Gaynor E, Bouvier C, Spaet TH: Vascular lesions: possible pathogenetic basis of the generalized Schwartzman reaction. *Science* 1970;170:986–988.

86. Harker LA, Slichter SJ: Platelet and fibrinogen consumption in man. *N Engl J Med* 1972;287:999–1005.

87. Katz J, Krawitz S, Sacks PV, et al: Platelet, erythrocyte, and fibrinogen kinetics in the hemolytic-uremic syndrome of infancy. *J Pediatr* 1973;83: 739–748.

88. George CRP, Slichter SJ, Quadracci LJ, et al: A kinetic evaluation of hemostasis in renal disease. *N Engl J Med* 1974;291:1111–1115.

89. Pareti FI, Capitanio A, Mannucci L, et al: Acquired dysfunction due to the circulation of "exhausted" platelets. *Am J Med* 1980;69:235–240.

90. Kaplan BS, Fong JSC: Reduced platelet aggregation in hemolytic-uremic syndrome. *Thromb Haemost* 1980;43:154–157.

91. Appiani AC, Edefonti A, Bettinelli A, et al: The relationship between plasma levels of the factor VIII complex and platelet release products (β-thromboglobulin and platelet factor 4) in children with the hemolytic-uremic syndrome. *Clin Nephrol* 1982;17:195–199.

92. Weiss HJ, Baumgartner HR, Tschopp TB, et al: Correction by factor VIII of the impaired platelet adhesion to subendothelium in von Willebrand disease. *Blood* 1978;51:267–269.

93. Ruggeri ZM, Ponticelli C, Mannucci PM: Factor VIII and chronic renal failure. *Br Med J* 1977;1:1085.

94. Remuzzi G, Livio M, Roncaglioni MC, et al: Bleeding in renal failure: Is von Willebrand factor implicated? *Br Med J* 1977;2:359–361.

95. Warrel RP Jr, Hultin MB, Coller BS: Increased factor VIII/von Willebrand factor antigen and von Willebrand factor activity in renal failure. *Am J Med* 1979;66:226–228.

96. Hoyer JR, Michael AF, Hoyer LW: Immunofluorescent localization of antihemophilic factor antigen and fibrinogen in human renal disease. *J Clin Invest* 1974;53:1375–1384.

97. Ross R, Glomset J, Kariya B, et al: A platelet-dependent serum factor that stimulates the proliferation of arterial smooth muscle cells in vitro. *Proc Natl Acad Sci USA* 1974;71:1207–1210.
98. Rossi EC, Carone FA, del Greco F: Platelets and the hemolytic-uremic syndrome. *Ann Clin Lab Sci* 1981;11:269–273.
99. Baumgartner HR, Muggli R: Adhesion and aggregation: morphological demonstration and quantitation in vivo and in vitro, in Gordon JL (ed): *Platelets in Biology and Pathology*. Amsterdam, Elsevier/North Holland, 1976, pp 23–60.
100. Moncada S, Gryglewski R, Bunting S, et al: An enzyme isolated from arteries transforms prostaglandin endoperoxides to an unstable substance that inhibits platelet aggregation. *Nature* 1976;263:663–665.
101. Weksler BB, Marcus AJ, Jaffe EA: Synthesis of prostaglandin I$_2$ (prostacyclin) by culture human and bovine endothelial cells. *Proc Natl Acad Sci USA* 1977;74:3922–3926.
102. Weksler BB, Ley CW, Jaffe EA: Stimulation of endothelial cell prostacyclin production by thrombin, trypsin, and the ionophore A 23187. *J Clin Invest* 1978;62:923–930.
103. Remuzzi G, Misiani R, Marchesi D: Hemolytic-uremic syndrome: deficiency of plasma factor(s) regulating prostacyclin activity. *Lancet* 1978;2:871–872.
104. Jorgensen KA, Pedersen RS: Familial deficiency of prostacyclin production stimulating factor in the hemolytic uremic syndrome of childhood. *Thromb Res* 1981;21:311–315.
105. Rossi EC, Carone FA, del Greco F: Hemolytic-uremic syndrome and platelet-endothelial interactions, in Remuzzi G, Mecca G, de Gaetano G (eds): *Hemostasis, Prostaglandins, and Renal Disease*. New York, Raven Press, 1980, pp 321–329.
106. Gianantonio CA, Vitacco M, Medilaharzu F, et al: The hemolytic-uremic syndrome. *Nephron* 1973;11:174–192.
107. Vitacco M, Avalos JS, Gianantonio CA: Heparin therapy in the hemolytic-uremic syndrome. *J Pediatr* 1973;83:271–275.
108. Gianantonio CA, Vitacco M, Medilaharzu F, et al: The hemolytic-uremic syndrome: renal status of 76 patients at long-term follow-up. *J Pediatr* 1968;72:757–765.
109. Proesmans W, Eeckels R: Has heparin changed the prognosis of the hemolytic-uremic syndrome. *Clin Nephrol* 1974;2:169–173.
110. Kaplan BS, Thomson PD, de Chadarevian J-P: The hemolytic-uremic syndrome. *Pediatr Clin N Am* 1976;23:761–777.
111. Jones RWA, Morris MC, Maisey MN, et al: Endarterial urokinase in childhood hemolytic uremic syndrome. *Kidney Int* 1981;20:723–727.
112. Powell HR, Ekert H: Streptokinase and anti-thrombotic therapy in the hemolytic-uremic syndrome. *J Pediatr* 1974;84:345–349.
113. Amorosi EL, Karpatkin S: Antiplatelet treatment of thrombotic thrombocytopenic purpura. *Ann Intern Med* 1977;86:102–106.
114. Rossi EC, Green D, del Greco F: The use of inhibitors of platelet function in thrombotic microangiopathy, in Remuzzi G, Mecca G, de Gaetano G (eds): *Hemostasis, Prostaglandins, and Renal Disease*. New York, Raven Press, 1980, pp 413–422.
115. Kincaid-Smith P: Modifications of the vascular lesions of rejection in cadaveric renal allografts by dipyridamole and anticoagulants. *Lancet* 1969;2: 920–922.

116. Kincaid-Smith P: Coagulation and renal disease. *Kidney Int* 1972;2: 183–190.
117. Arenson EB, August CS: Preliminary report: treatment of the hemolytic-uremic syndrome with aspirin and dipyridamole. *J Pediatr* 1975;86: 957–961.
118. O'Regan S, Chesney RW, Mongeau J-G, et al: Aspirin and dipyridamole therapy in the hemolytic-uremic syndrome. *J Pediatr* 1980;97:473–476.
119. Kwaan HC, Gallo G, Potter EV, et al: The nature of the vascular lesion in thrombotic thrombocytopenic purpura. *Ann Intern Med* 1968;68:1169.
120. Harkness DR, Byrnes JJ, Lian E C-Y, et al: Hazard of platelet transfusion in thrombotic thrombocytopenic purpura. *JAMA* 1981;246:1931–1933.

13 *Disseminated Intravascular Coagulation*

Kenneth K. Wu

DEFINITION

Disseminated intravascular coagulation (DIC) is a clinicopathologic condition characterized by diffuse microvascular thrombosis, consumption of coagulation factors, and hemorrhage. It is not a disease entity but an intermediate pathologic mechanism that may occur in association with a number of diseases. Although intravascular coagulation was produced in experimental animals by infusion of erythrocyte lysates and tissue extracts more than 100 years ago,[1,2] recognition of the human syndrome and elucidation of its pathophysiology are of recent history. Human subjects with snake bite exhibited unclottable blood. Mellanby discovered in 1909 that the coagulation defects induced by snake venom were due to hypofibrinogenemia secondary to disseminated intravascular coagulation.[3] This finding stimulated interest in snake venom research with the subsequent discovery of several important venom proteins. In 1957, Krevans et al reported that DIC could be triggered by intravascular hemolysis due to mismatched blood transfusions.[4] This observation paved the way for the subsequent treatise by Lasch et al, which stressed the multiple causes for DIC.[5] The monograph by McKay gave detailed descriptions of clinical manifestations and clinicopathologic correlations of DIC.[6] Subsequent developments of techniques for detection of fibrin degradation products by Merskey et al[7] and Hawiger et al[8] facilitated the diagnosis of DIC. Clinical manifestations, laboratory abnormalities, and clinical course of DIC are extremely variable. Several terms have been utilized in an attempt to provide some useful classification of the various clinical stages. *Compensated DIC* refers to an early phase of DIC where increased production of the consumable coagulation factors overcompensates for the loss of these factors. Hence, the factors may be elevated rather than reduced. *Decompensated DIC* then refers to the drop of these factors. Based on the onset and clinical course, DIC is divided into *acute*, *subacute*, and *chronic* stages. Distinction of these stages is difficult because the underlying diseases that trigger DIC often exert a tremendous influence over the clinical presentation of DIC. On the basis of severity, DIC may be *low-grade* (mild), *moderate*, or *severe*. These criteria for distinguishing them have not been developed and the division is at best arbitrary.

ETIOLOGY

Any disease that can trigger the activation of intravascular coagulation may cause DIC. There exist several mechanisms by which DIC occurs in association with these disorders (Table 13-1).

Table 13-1
Pathogenetic Mechanisms of DIC

Mechanisms	Representative Disorders
Release of tissue thromboplastin	Massive tissue injuries and burns Obstetric complications (placenta previa, abruptio placentae, dead-fetus syndrome and amniotic fluid embolism)
Release of procoagulants	Mucus-producing tumors (pancreas, prostate, lung and stomach) Acute leukemia (acute promyelocytic leukemia, acute myelocytic leukemia, rarely acute lymphocytic leukemia) Chronic myelocytic and monocytic leukemia
Liberation of proteolytic enzymes	Snake bite Acute pancreatitis
Damage to endothelium	Gram-positive and negative bacterial infections Rickettsial infections (Rocky Mountain spotted fever) Viral infections (rubella, rubeola, varicella, influenza) Immune complex disorders (rare)
Impaired clearance of activated coagulation factors	Liver diseases
Localized consumption	Hemangioma (Kasabach-Meritt syndrome) Aortic aneurysm
Acidosis and hypoxia	Shock Cardiac arrest
Miscellaneous	Prothrombin complex preparations TTP Renal-homograft rejection

1. *Release of tissue thromboplastin.* Tissue factor (or thromboplastin) exists in most tissues. Massive tissue injury leads to the release of a large quantity of tissue thromboplastin into the circulation which activates the extrinsic coagulation pathway, resulting in fibrin formation. Head injury and severe burns are the common examples in this category.

The other common source of tissue thromboplastin is fetal-placental tissues. Normal parturition is considered to be associated with transient intravascular coagulation because of release of fetoplacental tissues into the maternal circulation.[9] These tissues are thromboplastic and capable of activating the extrinsic coagulation pathway. In obstetric complications such as abruptio placentae, placenta previa, and dead-fetus syndrome, the fetal and placental tissues released into the circulation become markedly increased to induce significant intravascular coagulation and consumption coagulopathy.[10] Amniotic fluid embolism is due to the leaking of amniotic fluid with its fetal debris into the circulation. The fetal debris may plug the pulmonary arteries, causing acute respiratory distress. Moreover, the tissue thromboplastin present in the amniotic fluid triggers the activation of coagulation and causes the typical manifestations of DIC. Lysis of blood cells due to mismatching of ABO or Rh blood groups during blood transfusion invariably causes DIC. Red cell stroma is thromboplastic, which is considered to be the major mechanism by which mismatched blood transfusions induce DIC. Antigen-antibody complexes and their damage to vascular endothelium also play an important role in triggering intravascular coagulation.

2. *Release of procoagulant substances.* Many solid tumor and leukemic cells can release procoagulant substances either by secretory processes or by rapid cell breakdown.[11] A procoagulant isolated from cell culture appears to possess the action of activating factor X.[12] On the other hand, the coarse granules present in the promyelocytes of acute promyelocytic leukemia contain thromboplastin-like activity.[13] Thus, the procoagulant substances are probably heterogeneous in their chemical structures and functional properties. Once their release into the circulation reaches a critical level, intravascular coagulation occurs. Solid tumors that are commonly associated with DIC include the mucus-producing adenocarcinoma, notably pancreatic, prostate, lung, and stomach adenocarcinomas.[14] Among the acute leukemias, DIC is invariably noted in the course of acute promyelocytic leukemia.[15] Chemotherapy may at times precipitate or aggravate the course and severity of DIC. DIC has also been reported in patients with acute myelocytic leukemia[16] and chronic myelocytic and monocytic leukemias.[17] DIC has also been described in acute lymphocytic leukemia but its incidence is extremely low.

3. *Liberation of proteases.* Snake bite by vipers and rattlesnakes may produce a syndrome similar to DIC.[18,19] The venom of these snakes contains proteolytic enzymes which can directly activate factor X or prothrombin, leading to fibrin formation. Acute pancreatitis, particularly the hemorrhagic type, is often associated with liberation from the pancreas of potent proteolytic enzymes into the circulation.[20] These proteases can activate coagulation and fibrinolysis and produce DIC.

4. *Damage to the endothelium.* Normal endothelium provides a

natural barrier preventing blood coagulation factors and platelets from activation. Exogenous agents such as endotoxins, viruses, and immune complexes may cause damage to the endothelium and break the barrier. Subendothelial tissues, notably collagen and possibly proteoglycans, initiate the activation of several interwoven systems in the blood. Factor XII is activated, leading to the rapid procession of intrinsic cascade and fibrin formation. Activated factor XII also converts prekallikrein into kallikrein, which in turn converts high molecular weight kininogen into bradykinin. Bradykinin production accounts for hypotension observed in the majority of patients with DIC. Kallikrein in combination with high molecular weight kininogen digests factor XII into fragments which are capable of activating prekallikrein and fibrinolysis. Kallikrein can also activate the complement system. In addition to its effect on the plasma proteins, collagen induces platelet adhesion, release reaction, and aggregate formation. The activated platelets provide the active membrane surface for acceleration of the coagulation cascade. Thus, damage to the endothellium results in fibrin formation, platelet aggregation, fibrinolysis, kinin formation, and complement activation. Activated complements promote granulocyte migration, vessel wall permeability and platelet aggregation.

DIC caused by infectious agents is considered to be mediated by endothelial damage.[21,22] Gram-negative bacterial infections represent the most common form of endotoxemia-induced DIC. DIC can also be caused by gram-positive bacterial infections (pneumococcal, streptococcal, and staphylococcal), rickettsial (Rocky Mountain spotted fever), viral (dengue hemorrhagic fever, varicella, variola rubella, rubeola, and influenza), protozoan, and fungal infections. The mechanisms by which the nonendotoxin-producing agents induce DIC are not entirely clear but probably are due to their direct damage to the endothelial cells.

Although immune complexes cause endothelial damage, directly activate platelets and complements, the occurrence of DIC in immune complex disorders is rare.

5. *Impaired clearance of activated coagulation factors*. The reticuloendothelial cells (RE) in the liver and other organs rapidly clear activated coagulation factors as a defense mechanism against unnecessary clot formation. Once the RE function is impaired, as in hepatic failure, activated factors are accumulated and intravascular coagulation may occur.

6. *Localized activation of coagulation*. Giant hemangiomas and aortic aneurysms can cause a bleeding diathesis similar to DIC.[23,24] Strictly speaking, these conditions do not cause disseminated but rather localized intravascular coagulation. However, because of the profound effects of the local blood stasis on the coagulation system, consumption coagulopathy occurs which is often indistinguishable from that caused by other conditions.

7. *Shock.* Regardless of its origins, shock is a common cause of DIC.[25] Mechanisms by which shock induces DIC are multiple but the most important are acidosis and hypoxia. Acidosis enhances the activation of the coagulation cascade and hypoxia may induce vascular injury. Occlusion of the microvessels leads to further tissue hypoxia and blood stasis and thus perpetuates a vicious cycle.

8. *Miscellaneous causes.* Transfusions of prothrombin complex preparations may cause DIC because of the presence of activated coagulation factors in these preparations.[26] DIC is also a rare complication of thrombotic thrombocytopenic purpura.[27] DIC is often seen in renal homograft rejection.[28]

PATHOGENESIS

Symptomatology and coagulation abnormalities of DIC are attributable to several factors: (1) microsvascular fibrin deposition, (2) consumption of coagulation factors, (3) secondary fibrinolysis, and (4) kinin productions (Figure 13-1). Interplay of these factors renders the syndrome variable. As described above, once the coagulation system is turned on, activated coagulation factors are generated and the final activated coagulation factor of the cascade, thrombin, acts on fibrinogen in a stepwise fashion. First, it removes two small peptides, fibrinopeptide A and B, from α- and β-chains of fibrinogen molecules, respectively. Secondly, the remaining fibrinogen molecules, termed fibrin monomers, are polymerized. The polymers are finally cross-linked by factor XIII. The fibrin thrombi formed in the circulation are eventually lodged in the small blood vessels. Alternatively, multiple fibrin clots may be formed on the damaged vascular wall of the microcirculation. These clots block the blood flow in the microcirculation leading to tissue hypoxia and organ malfunction. Moreover, reduced vascular calibers along with rough vascular wall causes damage to red blood cells and produce various forms of fragmented red cells (schistocytes). When the degree of intravascular hemolysis has reached a critical level, microangiopathic hemolytic anemia may occur. Fibrin may be deposited in any organ, but its deposition in kidneys, skin, lungs, brain, and gastrointestinal (GI) tract produces clinical symptoms. In autopsy studies, fibrin thrombi are most often observed in kidneys.[29] Renal involvement affects primarily the afferent capillaries and arterioles of glomeruli. Glomerular filtration is reduced and azotemia is noted. Eventually acute cortical neurosis may occur. Similar morphologic pictures may be observed in the dermal, pulmonary, cerebral, and mesenteric vessels which produce a variety of clinical symptoms, to be discussed below.

Coagulation factors are consumed following disseminated fibrin formation. However, not all the factors are equally consumable. In acute DIC, fibrinogen, factors V, VIII:coagulant activity (VIII:C), and XIII

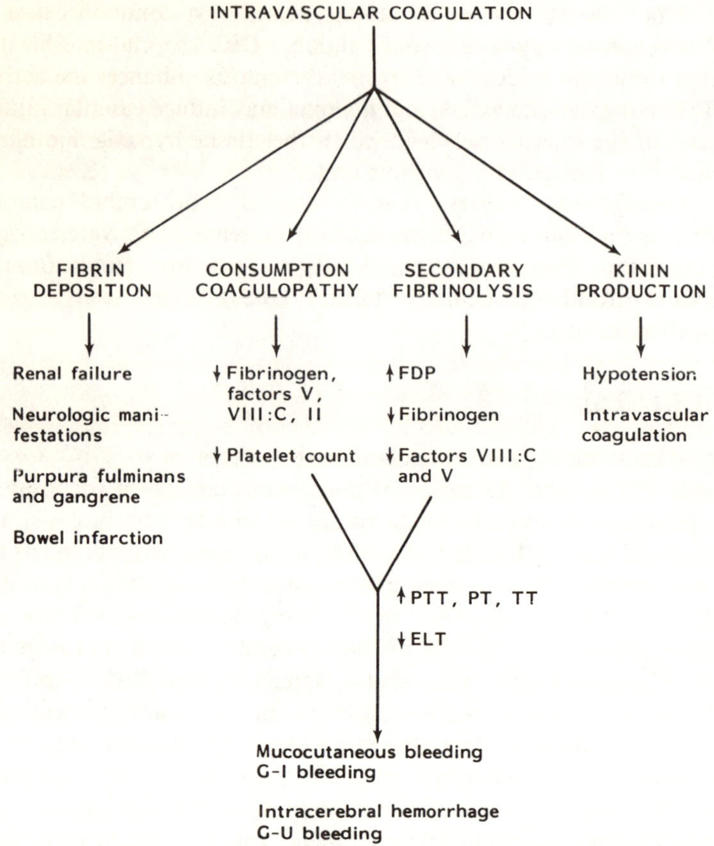

Figure 13-1 Pathophysiology of DIC. Abbreviations: Factor VIII:C = factor VIII procoagulant activity; FDP = fibrin degradation products; PTT = activated partial thromboplastin time; PT = prothrombin time; TT = thrombin time; ELT = euglobulin lysis time.

are most consumable. Prothrombin is partially consumed while factors VII, IX, X, XI, and XII are only mildly or not consumed at all. Fibrinogen is the ultimate substrate in the coagulation cascade and its consumption for fibrin formation is anticipated. Factors V and VIII:C are cofactors in the coagulation cascade and therefore are vulnerable to be used up. Factors XII, XI, X, and IX are zymozines and once they are activated the active enzymes catalyze the coagulation reaction. After the reaction is completed, the enzymes are dissociated from the reaction complex and act on new molecules. Hence, it is understandable that these factors are not consumed. Although prothrombin is also a proenzyme, it is converted to thrombin which may be bound to its natural inhibitor, ie, antithrombin III (AT-III), and be removed. The plasma AT-III is often depressed in DIC for the same reason. Thrombocytopenia is accompanied by increased megakaryocytes in the bone marrow. It has been implied that thrombocytopenia is due to consumption of platelet during thrombus formation. However, it is not entirely clear whether this is the major mechanism. It is possible that platelets are damaged passing through the microcirculation and the damaged platelets are removed by the RE cells in the system.

Fibrinolysis represents an important defense mechanism against excessive thrombus formation. Intravascular coagulation can trigger the activation of fibrinolytic system by several mechanisms. As mentioned earlier, activated factor X and fragments of factor XII can directly convert plasminogen into plasmin. Kallikrein which is generated during intravascular coagulation can also activate plasminogen. Plasmin is a potent serine protease which digests fibrin and, unfortunately, fibrinogen as well into several degradation products.[30] Plasmin cleaves fibrin-fibrinogen to fragment X, which is digested into fragments D and E. Hence, fragments X and Y are high molecular weight fibrin degradation products (FDP) and D and E fragments are low molecular weight FDP. FDP interfere with fibrin polymerization and hence retard the coagulation process.[31] Moreover, FDP inhibit platelet function.[32] FDP are cleared primarily by the RE system. Their blood levels are the net of the difference between production and clearance. In addition to its effects on fibrin-fibrinogen, plasmin can also digest factors V and VIII:C, further aggravating the pathologic reduction of these two factors.

In summary, plasmin is generated during DIC to remove fibrin thrombi. However, it digests fibrinogen and factors V and VIII:C, further compromising the coagulation defects. The degradation products are anticoagulatory and platelet-aggregatory and hence enhance the bleeding tendency.

Byproducts of intravascular coagulation have profound vascular effects which contribute to the clinical symptoms. Bradykinins which are generated from kininogens are vasodilators and cause hypotension. Activated complements induce chemotaxis and increase vascular permeability. These substances can cause inflammatory responses. Neutrophils and monocytes that are attracted to thrombotic sites are capable of releasing tissue thromboplastins, further promoting the fibrin thrombi.

CLINICAL MANIFESTATIONS

The cardinal symptoms are the paradoxical coexistence of bleeding and thrombosis. The extent and severity of bleeding and thrombosis are determined by the balance between coagulation, cg, thrombin activity, and fibrinolysis, ie, plasmin activity. The intricate relationship between the two systems and the interplay of important factors render the clinical manifestations quite variable and unpredictable. The onset of DIC may be abrupt or insidious depending on the underlying diseases and rate of coagulation and fibrinolysis. The clinical course may range from fulminant to chronic. Gram-negative septicemia and obstetric complications tend to cause acute fulminant DIC, whereas malignancy is usually associated with chronic indolent DIC. There are many exceptions to this generalization. It is prudent to consider each patient individually.

Because of a high degree of awareness of DIC in certain diseases, coagulation tests are routinely performed and diagnosis of DIC is often based on the abnormal coagulation tests without clinical evidence of hemorrhage or thrombosis. Coagulation abnormalities at this stage tend to be mild and hence the term low-grade DIC.

Bleeding is due to the combination of several mechanisms, ie, reduction of coagulation factors due to consumption and fibrinolytic digestion, inhibition of fibrin polymerization due to FDP, and thrombocytopenia. Spontaneous bleeding into the skin, GI tract, genitourinary tract (hematuria), and brain (cerebral hemorrhage) is the most common. The mucocutaneous bleeding may range from petechiae and mucosal oozing to massive mottling changes and ecchymosing lesions. The extreme form is purpura fulminans which is usually caused by streptococcal infections and is characterized by severe cutaneous bleeding and superficial gangrene as well as thrombotic lesions in the internal organs.[33,34] Massive GI bleeding and intracerebral hemorrhage are the most serious bleeding manifestations of DIC. Although a direct correlation between coagulation and platelet defects and bleeding manifestations has not been documented, it is the author's experience that severe reductions of fibrinogen level to less than 50 mg/dl and platelet count to less than 20,000/μl herald severe bleeding complications. Trauma and surgical procedures induce excessive bleeding. Even minor procedures such as venepuncture cause excessive oozing from the puncture site. Arterial puncture may lead to devastating subcutaneous and intramuscular bleeding and is absolutely contraindicated in severe DIC.

Microvascular thrombosis is most often noted in the kidneys. The initial stage of glomerular capillary thrombosis is presented with reduced creatinine clearance, increased serum creatinine, and urea nitrogen. Hematuria is common. The severe form may be presented by acute cortical necrosis and acute renal shutdown. Digital ischemic pain and gangrene are due to occlusion of the terminal digital arterioles by microthrombi. Microvascular thrombosis of the brain is manifested by confusion, disorientation, and seizure. Localizing signs are unusual but may occur. Severe occlusion may lead to acute thrombotic stroke. Mesenteric thrombosis may cause bowel necrosis. Pulmonary function may be impaired because of diffuse microvascular thrombosis in the lungs, giving rise to a clinical picture similar to acute respiratory distress syndrome. Severe sepsis may cause a fulminant DIC syndrome known as Waterhouse-Friderichsen syndrome.[35,36] This syndrome, which most frequently occurs in memingococcemia, is, aside from other organ involvement, due to hemorrhagic necrosis of the adrenal gland and hence has the manifestations of adrenal insufficiency.

It should be emphasized that bleeding and thrombotic manifestations may occur concurrently in the same patient. There exists a wide spectrum of symptomatology which may be masked by the underlying disease. Diagnosis of DIC often requires confirmation by laboratory tests.

LABORATORY FINDINGS

The major laboratory findings reside in the coagulation tests (Table 13-2). The earliest coagulation changes are the presence in the circulation of thrombin and other activated factors. These activated factors may be measured directly but their measurement requires specialized technics which are often cumbersome and not suitable for routine diagnostic use. To circumvent this, one can measure the early products of thrombin. As mentioned earlier, thrombin acts on fibrinogen first by removing fibrinopeptides A and B. Fibrin monomer then forms polymers but can also form fibrin monomer complex with fibrinogen. Hence, plasma fibrinopeptide A, fibrinopeptide B, and fibrin monomer complexes are expected to be elevated in DIC. Fibrinopeptides A and B can be accurately measured by radioimmunoassay.[37,38] Both products are found to be

Table 13-2
Rationale for Abnormalities of Coagulation Tests in DIC

Mechanisms	Laboratory Tests	
Early fibrinogen products	↑ Fibrinopeptide A	
	↑ Fibrinopeptide B	
	↑ Fibrin monomer complexes	
Consumption	↓ Fibrinogen	↓ Platelet count
	↓ Factor V	
	↓ Factor VIII:C, ↓ AT-III	
Fibrinolysis	↑ FDP (latex-particle, TRCHII, staphylococcal clumping)	
	↓ ELT	
Multiple factors	↑ aPTT, ↑ PT, ↑ TT	
Others	↓ Fibronectin	

Abbreviations: Factor VIII:C = factor VIII procoagulant activity; AT-III = antithrombin III; FDP = fibrin degradation products; TRCHII = tanned red cell hemagglutination inhibition test; ELT = euglobulin lysis time; aPTT = activated partial thromboplastin time; PT = prothrombin time; TT = thrombin time; ↑ denotes increased, ↓ reduced.

elevated in DIC and are considered to be the sensitive and specific tests for intravascular coagulation. It is to be noted, however, that they have a short half-life and their values have already declined when DIC is still active. Since fibrinopeptides A and B are equally affected, measurement of one product is sufficient. At the present time, fibrinopeptide A measurement is favored. Several technics are available for measurement of fibrin monomer complexes. The ethanol gelation test is based on the determination of ethanol-induced gel formation when fibrin monomer complex is present.[39] The protamine sulfate titration test is based on the rationale that fibrin monomer complexes precipitate on the addition of protamine sulfate solution.[40] The larger the quantity of fibrin monomer, the higher the titer of protamine sulfate. These tests are neither sensitive nor specific and falsely positive and negative results are encountered. Hence, their values in the diagnosis of DIC are considered to be inadequate. Fibrin monomer complexes can also be measured by more specialized biochemical technics such as gel exclusion chromatography[41] and immune precipitates[42] but their diagnostic values have not been established. Moreover, these procedures are time-consuming and generally considered to be unsuitable for diagnostic use.

Serum FDP are a sensitive index of DIC. These products can be screened by the latex agglutination test,[43] where latex particles are coated with antibodies reacting with fibrinogen and FDP. Since serum does not contain fibrinogen, the quantity detected in the serum represents FDP. For rapid screening purposes, the results are expressed as < 10 μg/ml, which is the normal range; 10–40 μg/ml; and > 40 μg/ml. The test is equally sensitive for fragments X, Y, D, and E. To be more precise, the tanned red cell hemagglutination inhibition (TRCHII) test may be used.[7] This test is probably more sensitive than the latex method, although both are based on a similar immunologic principle. Like the latex method, the TRCHII test detects all the fragments with equal sensitivity. By contrast, the staphylococcal clumping method, which is based on the interaction between staphylococcal proteins and FDP, is more sensitive in detecting high molecular weight products X and Y, and less sensitive for fragments D and E.[44] Elevation of FDP is an essential component for diagnosis of DIC. A normal level of FDP should raise the question of whether the diagnosis of DIC is correct. High FDP by themselves, however, are not diagnostic for DIC because they may be present in a number of clinical conditions other than DIC. The serum FDP level is elevated in renal failure, pneumonia, deep vein thrombosis, pulmonary embolism, liver disease, etc.[45]

Systemic fibrinolysis is enhanced in DIC. Fibrinolysis can be measured by screening laboratory tests such as whole blood lysis and euglobulin lysis time, the latter being a more refined test than the former.

Both tests are based on the determination of time lapse for clot lysis. Euglobulin lysis time (ELT) is relatively more sensitive than whole blood lysis time, although neither test is considered to be sufficiently sensitive. Euglobulin is a fraction of plasma prepared by acidification of plasma with acetic acid. The precipitated euglobulin is rich in fibrinogen, plasminogen, and plasminogen activators. Under normal circumstances, it takes longer than three hours for a euglobulin clot to be lysed. Shortened ELT, ie, less than three hours, is indicative of enhanced systemic fibrinolysis. As just mentioned, this test is insensitive, though. It does, however, have diagnostic value when it is shortened. Shortened ELT may be observed more frequently in conditions that are associated with primary fibrinolysis.

In severe DIC, plasma fibrinogen, prothrombin, factors V, and VIII:C are subnormal because of consumption and plasmin digestion. These factors can be measured routinely by standard procedures based on the general principle of determining the ability of patient's plasma in correcting plasma that is devoid of a given factor to be tested. Caution should be taken in interpreting a single determination of these factors. Of particular importance is the plasma fibrinogen level. Fibrinogen is an acute-phase reactant and is elevated in many acute conditions which can also trigger DIC. The basal value prior to DIC may be extremely elevated, say, 900 mg/dl (normal 200–450 mg/dl). Following DIC, the value may drop to 250 mg/dl, which represents a substantial reduction, and yet if only a single determination is obtained, it is still within the normal range. Under these circumstances, serial determinations of these factors are extremely helpful in discerning whether consumption coagulopathy has occurred. In the early phase of DIC, the factor consumption may be compensated by an increased production of these consumable factors. As a matter of fact, fibrinogen and factor VIII:C may be elevated in the "compensated" phase of DIC. Because of the wide spectrum of coagulation abnormalities in DIC, activated partial thromboplastin time (aPTT) and prothrombin time (PT) are likewise variable in DIC. They may be extremely prolonged in severe DIC but may be completely normal. Hence, their diagnostic usage is of secondary importance. On the other hand, they may be useful indicators of the severity of DIC. Thrombin time, which measures the conversion of fibrinogen to fibrin, is usually prolonged because FDP are potent inhibitors of fibrin polymerization.

Regardless of the methods used for its measurement, be it radial immunodiffusion, thrombin time, or chromogenic substrate assay, antithrombin III is often reduced in severe DIC. However, this finding is not specific since deep vein thrombosis, liver disease, and heparin usage are also associated with reduced levels of AT-III.[46]

258

In addition to thrombocytopenia, microangiopathic hemolytic anemia may occur in DIC. In a prospective study, significant schistocytosis was noted in about one third of patients with DIC.[47] Platelet function has been reported to be abnormal due to acquired storage pool deficiency.[48]

Fibronectin is a cold-sensitive protein with wide distribution and broad biologic function. Its serum level has been shown to be reduced in DIC.[49] The pathophysiologic significance and diagnostic value of this observation remain to be explored.

Other laboratory findings pertaining to organ dysfunction are typical abnormalities of that organ system and will not be discussed here.

DIAGNOSIS

Diagnosis of decompensated DIC is based on the following criteria: (1) presence of an underlying disease that triggers DIC, (2) evidence of hypofibrinogenemia, (3) increased fibrin degradation products, and (4) thrombocytopenia. When the clinical picture is less clear because of multifactorial influence, the following additional criteria should be sought to support the diagnosis: (5) consumption of factors V and VIII:C, (6) elevated fibrinopeptide A and/or fibrin monomer complexes, and (7) schistocytosis. Diagnosis of a typical decompensated DIC is usually easy. It should be emphasized that although clinical manifestations such as bleeding and microvascular thrombosis are important as far as treatment and prognosis are concerned, they are not essential for the diagnosis of DIC.

Diagnosis of compensated DIC is often more difficult and should be based on the following criteria: (1) presence of an underlying disease, (2) evidence of intravascular coagulation, ie, elevated fibrinopeptide A and/or fibrin monomer complex, and (3) elevated serum fibrin degradation products. It should be emphasized that fibrinogen and VIII:C may be elevated or normal and platelet counts and other coagulation factors are normal in compensated DIC.

The separation of DIC into acute, subacute, and chronic DIC is based primarily on clinical judgment and somewhat arbitrary. No rigid criteria are available for the clinical distinction.

There are no completely satisfactory criteria for categorizing the severity of DIC. We have relied heavily on the fibrinogen level, platelet count, and symptoms to judge the severity of DIC. DIC is usually mild or low-grade when the fibrinogen level is > 100 mg/dl, platelet count $> 50,000/\mu l$. DIC is considered to be severe when fibrinogen is < 50 mg/dl and platelet count $< 20,000/\mu l$, and moderate when the fibrinogen level is 50–100 mg/dl and platelet count 20,000 to 50,000/μl. Severe DIC is usually associated with brisk or imminent bleeding and/or thrombotic presentations. It is our experience that screening tests such as aPTT, PT, thrombin time (TT), and other factors are less reliable for determining the severity of DIC.

DIFFERENTIAL DIAGNOSIS

DIC should be differentiated from thrombotic thrombocytopenic purpura (TTP), conditions associated with enhanced fibrinolysis ("primary" fibrinolysis), coagulopathy due to chronic liver disease, and conditions with complex, multifactorial coagulation abnormalities. The major points for differential diagnosis are summarized in Table 13-3, and described briefly below.

TTP is a syndrome characterized by diffuse platelet deposition on the microvascular endothelium. Patients with TTP present with an acute onset of fever, microangiopathic hemolytic anemia and thrombocytopenia, fleeting neurologic manifestations, and renal failure. Hence there exist some similar features between TTP and DIC. In most cases, the differential diagnosis is simple because coagulation defects such as reduced coagulation factors and prolonged PTT and PT, which are the hallmark of DIC, occur only in approximately 25% of TTP. Schistocytosis and microangiopathic hemolytic anemia can be detected in virtually all patients with TTP and is noted in only a small number of DIC patients. Fleeting neurologic manifestations occur only rarely in DIC. TTP tends to appear in otherwise healthy individuals without underlying diseases.

Primary fibrinolysis refers to an enchancement of systemic fibrinolysis due to an increased release of plasminogen activators as in prostate disorders or their reduced clearance, as in liver diseases.

Table 13-3
Differential Diagnosis Between DIC and TTP

	DIC	TTP
Underlying diseases	Always present	May be idiopathic
Consumption coagulopathy	Always present	Present in < 25% cases
Microangiopathic morphology	Present in < 30% cases	Always present
aPTT, PT	Usually prolonged	Usually normal
Plasma fibrinogen	↓	N
Factors V, VIII:C	↓	N
FDP	↑↑↑	↑
Schistocytes	↑	↑↑↑
Platelet count	↓↓	↓↓
Neurologic symptoms	±	+ + +

Abbreviations: DIC = disseminated intravascular coagulation; TTP = thrombotic thrombocytopenic purpura; N normal, + + + almost always present. See also footnote, Table 13-2.

Fibrinolysis may be activated when blood comes in contact with a foreign surface such as a cardiopulmonary bypass device. Primary fibrinolysis is characterized by reduction in coagulation factors, predominantly fibrinogen, factors V and VIII:C, and high levels of FDP which may lead to severe bleeding. Platelet counts are unaffected and schistocytes are notably absent.

Diagnosis of DIC either due to chronic liver failure or coexisting with liver disease because of shock is a challenging problem. As the liver plays a pivotal role in maintaining the homeostasis of coagulation and fibrinolysis, multiple coagulation defects occur when liver function fails. Coagulation factors, except factor VIII:C, are reduced. FDP are increased because of impaired synthesis. Serum FDP levels are increased because of enhanced fibrinolysis. As the liver removes activated coagulation factors, its failure is theoretically associated with some degree of intravascular coagulation. However, overt consumption coagulopathy is lacking in the majority of liver diseases because factor VIII:C is often markedly elevated and the platelet count is normal. When severe consumption occurs, factor VIII:C becomes reduced. We have found that serial measurements of VIII:C are probably the most reliable way of ascertaining the diagnosis of DIC. It should be stressed that as the basal VIII:C level can be extremely elevated, a single VIII:C value may not be reliable unless the value has dropped below the normal range.

Complex coagulopathy secondary to multiple contributing factors is common in severely ill patients with septic shock. Coagulopathy may be related to liver disease and vitamin K deficiency. Thrombocytopenia may be due to bone marrow suppression and/or septicemia-induced immune thrombocytopenia. To differentiate between DIC and the multiple coagulopathy requires the prudent use of clinical and laboratory skills. The task may be impossible to accomplish at times, even in the hands of the most experienced coagulation specialists.

TREATMENT

Once the diagnosis of DIC is established, the therapeutic strategies should be aimed at prompt elimination of the underlying causes and providing general supportive care. These two measures are adequate in controlling DIC in the majority of patients with DIC. However, in severe cases, particularly when bleeding and/or thrombotic presentations are imminent, specific anticoagulant therapy in conjunction with specific factor replacement are indicated.

Treatment of the underlying diseases represents the most important therapeutic strategy. In obstetric complications, evacuation of the uterus to remove the residual fetal and placental tissues is often sufficient to abate the DIC. Likewise, surgical removal of angiomas and repair of aortic aneurysms are effective measures in controlling DIC causes by these localized disorders. Microorganisms that cause septicemia should be identified and promptly treated with proper antibiotics. Solid tumors and leukemia should be managed by surgery, radiotherapy, chemotherapy, or combination modality therapy. It should be emphasized that the cancer therapy may induce rapid tumor cell breakdown and aggravate DIC. Snakebite should be treated promptly with appropriate antivenoms. Acute hemorrhagic pancreatitis should be managed by medical measures, including fluid and electrolyte replacement and blood transfusions to maintain a normal water and electrolyte balance. Similarly, shock, burns, and injuries should be treated with standard surgical and medical measures.

Certain general precautions are valuable. Arterial punctures and biopsy procedures should be avoided. Surgery should be postponed. Aspirin and other drugs that inhibit platelet function should not be given to patients with DIC. Patients should be examined frequently to identify early bleeding and thrombotic presentations. Vital signs should be monitored frequently. Laboratory tests, particularly coagulation and hematologic tests, should be obtained frequently to assess the progress of DIC. Water and electrolyte imbalance should be promptly corrected. Anemia should be corrected by red cell transfusion. Causes of fever should be investigated and proper antibiotics should be promptly administered when secondary infections are evident.

Despite a prolonged history of using heparin in the control of intravascular coagulation, its efficacy remains controversial. Evaluation of its efficacy is hampered by the difficulty in conducting prospective controlled studies and by the variability of the clinical course of the disorder. The rationale for using heparin in the treatment of DIC is based on the fact that heparin acts as a cofactor of a natural inhibitor, AT-III.[50] In the presence of heparin, AT-III effectively inhibits thrombin as well as factors Xa, IXa, XIa, and XIIa, and hence the intravascular coagulation. Heparin was first employed successfully in treating a patient with purpura fulminans,[51] but subsequent conflicting results failed to convincingly substantiate its therapeutic value.[52-54] Hence, heparin use should be considered as being empirical and limited to certain selected cases. In our opinion, the indications for administering heparin include the following two subgroups of DIC: (1) predominant thrombotic presentations such as digital gangrene and purpura fulminans, and (2) severe DIC with devastating bleeding. Since the original report of successful treatment of purpura fulminans with heparin, several other studies have supported this observation which may be extended to other DIC subgroups with predominant clinical manifestations of overt thrombosis. Patients should be given a bolus of 5,000 to 10,000 IU heparin injection followed by approximately of 1000 IU/h continuous infusion. Consumed factors should be replaced with cryoprecipitates (or fresh frozen plasma) and platelet concentrates. Coagulation tests and platelet counts should be frequently performed to determine the efficacy of therapy and the adequacy (or overdose) of heparin. Treatment of DIC patients with devastating bleeding with heparin is more controversial. The major question is the dosage of heparin. It has been our experience that the "therapeutic" dose frequently exacerbates bleeding complications because of further disruption of normal hemostasis by the relatively high-dose heparin. We therefore have designed a protocol to determine the efficacy of minidose heparin along with cryoprecipitate the platelet concentrate transfusions in controlling bleeding in this group of patients. Heparin at 3 IU/kg body weight/h is infused continuously by an infusion pump. The dose may be escalated to 5 IU/kg/h in the next 24 hours depending on the coagulation responses. One hour following the initiation of heparin, five bags of cryoprecipitates are administered. Platelet concentrates (4 units) are administered when platelet counts are less than $20,000/\mu$l. Amounts of blood loss are monitored. Coagulation tests (aPTT, PT, TT, fibrinogen, and FDP) and hematologic tests (hemoglobin, hematocrit, platelet count) are obtained at 4, 12, and 24 hours, and then once or twice daily. Once the heparin has been infused for one hour, which is presumably effective in reducing the intravascular coagulation activity, we feel that it is important to replace the consumed coagulation factors. Since cryoprecipitates are rich in fibrinogen, factors V, VIII:C, and XIII, we prefer cryoprecipitates to fresh frozen plasma. We have treated several patients at Rush–Presbyterian–St. Luke's Medical Center by this protocol and the preliminary results suggest that this regimen is effective in controlling life-threatening bleeding accompanied by objective improvement of the coagulation parameters. These preliminary data must be further confirmed. The duration of heparin therapy depends on how rapidly the underlying causes can be eliminated. It may require a short-term therapy, ie, 24 hours just to cover the acute phase of DIC in obstetric complications and once the uterus has been evacuated, anticoagulant therapy may be discontinued shortly afterward. On the other hand, long-term therapy up to weeks may be required to control DIC due to a chronic disease, eg, malignancy.

Although secondary fibrinolysis is often quite overt in DIC and undoubtedly plays an important part in contributing to bleeding, antifibrinolytic agents such as epsilon aminocaproic acid (EACA) do not have a place in the treatment of DIC. Secondary fibrinolysis represents a defense mechanism. Blocking of this defense mechanism leads to more profound fibrin deposition and its subsequent detrimental effects.[55] Coumarins have no place in the treatment of DIC, either, because they do not have specific effects on rapid inhibition of intravascular coagulation.

As mentioned above, replacement of the consumed factors and

platelets is valuable when these preparations are used in conjunction with heparin. Heparin inhibits intravascular coagulation and hence allows the transfused factors to remain in the circulation without being further consumed for fibrin thrombus formation. Several preparations are available. Cryoprecipitates are rich in factors I, V, VIII, and XIII, while fresh frozen plasma contains equal amounts of all the coagulation factors. The advantage of cryoprecipitates lies in its low volume and therefore can replace a large quantity of these factors without fluid overload. The disadvantage is that it does not contain factor II (prothrombin), which may at times be severely depleted. Hence, selection of these preparations depends on the coagulation factor abnormalities. If the major purpose is to maintain a safe range of fibrinogen, cryoprecipitates will be preferred. On the other hand, if multiple factors are equally and severely depressed, fresh frozen plasma will be the treatment of choice. The other consideration is the replacement of AT-III. Preliminary data indicate that transfusion of AT-III concentrates may have an effect on DIC,[56] but further investigations are needed to substantiate this observation. It should be stressed that replacement of coagulation factors and platelets without the initial use of heparin may aggravate the intravascular coagulation and fibrin deposition and therefore should not be used alone.

In summary, treatment of the majority of DIC without devastating thrombotic and/or bleeding presentations requires proper therapy of the underlying disease and general support measures. Heparin in conjunction with platelet and cryoprecipitate infusions is indicated in patients with predominant thrombotic manifestations and in severe DIC associated with life-threatening bleeding.

PROGNOSIS

The prognosis of DIC is determined by the treatability of the underlying diseases. In disorders where the triggering causes can be promptly eliminated, DIC is transient and the prognosis is excellent. By contrast, DIC tends to be progressive and severe when the underlying diseases such as septic shock are refractory to multiple antibiotic therapy. The prognosis may be influenced by the severity of DIC. Cerebral and massive gastrointestinal hemorrhage, renal failure, and thrombotic stroke are grave prognostic signs.

The clinical course of DIC depends on the primary cause as well. The majority of the underlying diseases are associated with an acute clinical course. However, DIC due to malignancy and chronic liver failure may have a protracted, chronic clinical course. The coagulation abnormalities may fluctuate in accordance with the condition of the underlying diseases.

264

REFERENCES

1. Nauyn B: Untersuchungen über Blutgerrinnung im lebenden Tiere and ihre Folgren. *Arch Exp Pathol Pharmakol* 1873;1:1.
2. Foā P, Pellacani P: Sul fermento fibrinogeno. Sulle azioni tossiche, esercitate da alcuni organi freschi. *Arch Sci Med* 1884;7:113.
3. Mellanby J: The coagulation of blood. Part 2. The actions of snake venoms, peptone and leech extract. *J Physiol* 1909;38:441.
4. Krevans JR, Jackson DP, Conley CL, et al: The nature of the hemorrhagic disorders accompanied by hemolytic transfusions in man. *Blood* 1957;12:834.
5. Lasch HG, Krecke HJ, Rodriques-Erdman R, et al: Verbrauch-Koagulopathie (Pathogenese und Therapie). *Folia Haematol* 1961:61:325.
6. McKay DG: *Disseminated Intravascular Coagulation.* New York, Harper & Row, 1965.
7. Merskey C, Kleiner GJ, Johnson AJ: Quantitative estimation of split products of fibrinogen in human serum. Relation to diagnosis and treatment. *Blood* 1966;28:1.
8. Hawiger J, Niewiarowski S, Gurewich V, et al: Measurement of fibrinogen and fibrin degradation products in serum by staphylococcal clumping test. *J Lab Clin Med* 1970;75:93.
9. Kleiner GJ, Merskey C, Johnson AJ, et al: Defibrination in normal and abnormal parturition. *Br J Haematol* 1970;19:159.
10. Graeff H, Kuhn W: *Coagulation Disorders in Obstetrics. Pathobiochemistry, Pathophysiology, Diagnosis, Treatment.* Stuttgart, Georg Thieme Verlag, 1980.
11. Slichter SJ, Harker LA: Hemostasis in malignancy. *Ann NY Acad Sci* 1974;230:252.
12. Gordon SG, Franks C, Lewis B: Cancer procoagulant A: A factor X activating procoagulant from malignant tissue. *Thromb Res* 1975;6:127.
13. Gralnick HR, Abrell E: Studies of the procoagulant and fibrinolytic activity of promyelocytes in acute promyelocytic leukaemia. *Br J Haematol* 1973;24:89.
14. Sack GH, Levin J, Bell WR: Trousseau's syndrome and other manifestations of chronic disseminated coagulopathy in patients with neoplasms: Clinical pathologic, and therapeutic features. *Medicine* 1977;56:1.
15. Gralnick HR, Sultan C: Acute promyelocytic leukaemia: Haemorrhagic manifestation and morphologic criteria. *Br J Haematol* 1975;29:373.
16. Baker WG, Bank NU, Nachman RL, et al: Hypofibrinogenemic hemorrhage in acute myelogenous leukemia treated with heparin. With autopsy findings of widespread intravascular clotting. *Ann Intern Med* 1964;61:116.
17. German HJ, Smith JA, Lindenbaum J: Chronic intravascular coagulation associated with chronic myelocytic leukemia. Use of heparin in connection with a surgical procedure. *Am J Med* 1976;61:547.
18. Fainaru M, Eisenberg S, Manny N, et al: The natural course of defibrination syndrome caused by *Echis colorata* venom in man. *Thromb Diath Haemorrh* 1974;31:420.
19. Warrell DA, Pope HM, Prentice CRM: Disseminated intravascular coagulation caused by the carpet viper (*Echis carinatus*): Trial of heparin. *Br J Haematol* 1976;33:335.
20. Franza BR, Aronson DL, Finlayson JB: Activation of human prothrombin by procoagulant factor from the venom of *Echis carinatus*. *J Biol Chem* 1975;250:7057.
21. Gaynor E, Bouvier C, Spaet TH: Vascular lesions: Possible pathogenetic

basis of the generalized Shwartzman reaction. *Science* 1970;170:986.

22. Yoshikawa T, Tanaka KR, Guze LB: Infection and disseminated intravascular coagulation. *Medicine* 1971;50:237.

23. Good TA, Carnazzo SF, Good RA: Thrombocytopenia and giant hemangioma in infants. *Am J Dis Child* 1955;90:260.

24. ten Cate JW: Timmers H, Becker AE: Coagulopathy in ruptured dissecting aortic aneurysms. *Am J Med* 1975;59:171.

25. Krug H, Raszeja-Wanic B, Wochowiak A: Intravascular coagulation in acute renal failure after myocardial infarction. *Ann Intern Med* 1974;81:494.

26. White GC II, Roberts HR, Kingdon HS, et al: Prothrombin complex concentrates: Potentially thrombogenic materials and clues to the mechanism of thrombosis in vivo. *Blood* 1977;49:159.

27. Jaffe EA, Nachman RL, Merskey C: Thrombotic thrombocytopenic purpura — coagulation parameters in twelve patients. *Blood* 1973;42:499.

28. Starzl TE, Boehmig HJ, Ameniya H, et al: Clotting changes, including disseminated intravascular coagulation during rapid renal-homograft rejection. *N Engl J Med* 1970;283:383.

29. Bleyl U: Morphologic diagnosis of disseminated intravascular coagulation: histologic, histochemical and electron microscopic studies. *Semin Thromb Hemostas* 1977;3:247–267.

30. Verstraet M: Biochemical and clinical aspects of thrombolysis. *Semin Hematol* 1978;15:35.

31. Marder VJ, Shulman NR: High molecular weight derivatives of human fibrinogen produced by plasmin. II. Mechanism of their anticoagulant activity. *J Biol Chem* 1969;244:2120.

32. Stachurska J, Lopacink S, Gerdin B, et al: Effect of proteolytic degradation products of human fibrinogen and factor VIII on platelet aggregation and vascular permeability. *Thromb Res* 1979;15:663–672.

33. Chambers WN, Holyoke JB, Wilson RJ: Purpura fulminans. Report of two cases following scarlet fever. *N Engl J Med* 1952;247:933.

34. Hall WH: Purpura fulminans with Group B β-hemolytic streptococcal endocarditis. *Arch Intern Med* 1965;116:594.

35. Rich AR: A peculiar type of adrenal cortical damage associated with acute infections, and its possible relation to circulatory collapse. *Bull Johns Hopkins Hosp* 1944;74:1.

36. Ferguson JH, Chapman OD: Fulminating meningococcic infections and the so-called Waterhouse-Friderichsen syndrome. *Am J Pathol* 1948;24:763.

37. Nossel HL, Yudelman I, Canfield RE, et al: Measurement of fibrinopeptide A in human blood. *J Clin Invest* 1974;54:43.

38. Bilezikian SB, Nossel HL, Butler VP, et al: Radioimmunoassay of human fibrinopeptide B and kinetics of fibrinopeptide cleavange by different enzymes. *J Clin Invest* 1975;56:438.

39. Breen FA, Tullis JL. Ethanol gelation: A rapid screening test for intravascular coagulation. *Ann Intern Med* 1968;69:1197.

40. Lipinski B, Worowski K: Detection of soluble fibrin monomer complexes in blood by means of protamine sulfate test. *Thromb Diath Haemorrh* 1968;20:44.

41. Fletcher AP, Alkjaerig NK: Blood hypercoagulability, intravascular coagulation and thrombosis: New diagnostic concepts. *Thromb Diath Haemorrh* 1971;45 (suppl):389–394.

42. Kisker CT, Plummer G, Taylor B, et al: A method for measurement of fibrin monomer with the use of immune precipitate of fibrinogen. *J Lab Clin Med* 1977;89:653–658.

43. Marder VJ, Cruz GO, Schumer BR: Evaluation of a new antifibrinogen-coated latex particle agglutination test in the measurement of serum fibrin degradation products. *Thromb Haemost* 1977;37:183.
44. Carvalho CA, Ellman LL, Colman RW: A comparative study of the staphylococcal clumping test and an agglutination test for detection of fibrinogen degradation products. *Am J Clin Pathol* 1974;62:107.
45. Wilner GD: Molecular basis for measurement of circulating fibrinogen derivatives. *Prog Hemost Thromb* 1978;4:211–248.
46. Abildgaard U: Antithrombin and related inhibitors of coagulation. *Recent Adv Blood Coag* 1981;3:151–174.
47. Jacobson RJ, Jackson DP: Erythrocyte fragmentation in defibrination syndromes. *Ann Intern Med* 1974;81:207.
48. Pareti FI, Capitanio A, Mannucci PM: Acquired storage pool disease in platelets during disseminated intravascular coagulation. *Blood* 1976;48:511.
49. Mosher DF, Williams EM: Fibronectin concentration is decreased in plasma of severely ill patients with disseminated intravascular coagulation. *J Lab Clin Med* 1978;729–735.
50. Schipper HG, Lamping R, Kahle L, et al: Antithrombin III infusion in disseminated intravascular coagulation. *Lancet* 1978;2:854.
51. Little JR: Purpura fulminans treated successfully with anticoagulation. *JAMA* 1959;169:36.
52. Allen DM: Heparin therapy of purpura fulminans. *Pediatrics* 1966;38:211.
53. Hjort PF, Rapaport SI, Jørgensen L: Purpura fulminans: Report of a case successfully treated with heparin and hydrocortisone: Review of 50 cases from the literature. *Scand J Haematol* 1964;1:169.
54. Green D, Seeler RA, Allen N, et al: The role of heparin in the management of consumption coagulopathy. *Med Clin North Am* 1972;56:193.
55. Ratnoff OD: Epsilon aminocaproic acid—A dangerous weapon. *N Engl J Med* 1969;180:1124.
56. Schramm W, Marx R: Zur Behandlung thrombophiler Diathesen-Substitution mid Antithrombin-III-Konzentrat. *Blut* 1980;40:68-69.

14 *Peripheral Venous Thrombosis*

Richard M. Jay
Russell D. Hull

Venous thrombosis is a serious and potentially fatal disorder which frequently complicates the course of our hospitalized patients but also occurs in ambulant, otherwise healthy individuals. The clinical diagnosis of venous thrombosis is inaccurate due both to the low sensitivity and specificity of clinical findings.[1-5] Clinical diagnosis is insensitive because many potentially dangerous thrombi produce no clinical manifestations since they neither obstruct venous outflow nor are they associated with vessel wall or perivascular tissue inflammation. Clinical diagnosis is nonspecific because none of the symptoms and signs of venous thrombosis is unique to this condition and all may be caused by nonthrombotic disorders. The exception to the rule is the patient with phlegmasia cerula dolens in whom the diagnosis of massive ileofemoral thrombosis is clinically obvious. This syndrome occurs in fewer than 1% of patients with symptomatic venous thrombosis. In the vast majority of patients who present with clinically suspected venous thrombosis, the symptoms and signs are nonspecific and in more than 50% of these patients, the clinical suspicion of venous thrombosis is not confirmed by objective testing.[1-3] It should also be emphasized that patients with relatively minor symptoms and signs may have extensive, potentially dangerous, venous thrombi.

The differential diagnosis in patients who present with clinically suspected venous thrombosis include disorders of muscles, subcutaneous tissues, joints, periarticular soft tissues, lymphatics, bones, and nerves. It is frequently not possible to determine an alternative diagnosis at the time of referral but in our experience, having ruled out venous thrombosis by objective testing, it is often possible to determine underlying alternative diagnoses by careful follow-up (Table 14-1). In some patients, however, the cause of pain, tenderness, and swelling remains uncertain even after careful follow-up and is presumably due to inflammation of other soft tissues of the leg.

This work was supported by grants from the Province of Ontario and from the Canadian and Ontario Heart Foundation.

Table 14-1
Alternate Diagnosis in Consecutive Patients
with Negative Venograms

Diagnosis*	No. of Patients (%)
Muscle strain associated with unaccustomed exercise	21 (24)
Direct twisting injury to leg	9 (10)
Leg swelling in paralyzed leg	8 (9)
Venous reflux	6 (6)
Lymphangitis, lymphatic obstruction	6 (6)
Muscle tear	5 (5)
Baker's cyst	4 (4)
Cellulitis	3 (3)
Internal derangement of knee	2 (2)
Unknown	23 (26)
Total	87

*Diagnosis made postvenography with knowledge of the negative venogram result.

OBJECTIVE DIAGNOSIS OF DEEP VEIN THROMBOSIS

Because of its nonspecificity and insensitivity, clinical diagnosis is no longer adequate for management decisions in patients with suspected venous thrombosis. The potential disadvantages of investigating all patients with clinically suspected venous thrombosis are the expense of investigation, the inconvenience to the patient, and the possible morbidity of the tests. All of these potential disadvantages are outweighed by the advantages of investigating all patients. The cost and inconvenience of investigation are substantially less than the cost and inconvenience of unnecessary hospital admission or prolongation of hospital stay and of unnecessary anticoagulation in patients who are incorrectly diagnosed. Though there is some morbidity associated with diagnostic testing by venography, there is virtually none associated with noninvasive tests, which can be used as an alternative for venography in the majority of patients with clinically suspected venous thromboembolism. In addition, even the morbidity from venography is far less than the morbidity associated with anticoagulant therapy.

Venography

Venography is generally accepted as the standard objective method for the diagnosis of venous thrombosis.[6,7] However, venography is not readily repeatable and is therefore not a suitable screening test for subclinical venous thrombosis. With good technic, ascending venography will outline the entire deep venous system of the lower extremities, including the external and common iliac arteries in most patients. However, common femoral or iliac venography may be needed if the external and common iliac veins are not properly visualized by the ascending technic or if the inferior vena cava must also be outlined.

Normal anatomy of venous system   Accurate interpretation of venography requires knowledge of the normal anatomy of the venous system and its variation. The venous system in the leg consists of three pairs of deep calf veins, the posterior tibial, the peroneal, and the anterior tibial veins; the soleal and gastrocnemius plexus of veins; and the superficial venous system. The soleal plexus drains into the posterior tibial vein, the gastrocnemius plexus drains into the popliteal vein, and the three pairs of deep calf veins converge to form the popliteal vein. The popliteal vein becomes the superficial femoral vein at the junction of the proximal part of the popliteal fossa and the adductor canal in the thigh. The superficial femoral vein is joined by the deep femoral vein in the upper thigh to form the common femoral vein which, in turn, becomes the external iliac vein at the level of the inguinal ligament. The external iliac vein is joined by the internal iliac vein in the pelvis to form the common iliac vein, and the two common iliac veins converge to form the inferior vena cava. The superficial venous system consists of two major veins, the long and short saphenous veins, which drain into the common femoral and popliteal veins respectively. The superficial system is connected with the deep system by a series of communicating veins which contain valves that direct flow from the superficial into the deep system. A number of variations of the deep venous system have been recognized, the most common of which are the bifid popliteal veins and the bifid superficial femoral veins.

Criteria for the diagnosis of venous thrombosis   A number of venographic abnormalities have been defined as criteria for the diagnosis of acute deep vein thrombosis. The most reliable of these is the presence of an intraluminal filling defect, which is constant in all films and seen in a number of projections. Other, less reliable, criteria include (a) nonfilling of a segment of the deep venous system with abrupt termination of the column of contrast medium at a constant site below the segment and reappearance of the contrast medium at a constant site above that segment, and (b) nonfilling of the deep venous system above the knee despite adequate venographic technic. The likelihood that these appearances are due to venous thrombosis is increased if the abnormality is associated with the presence of abnormal collaterals. The presence of a constant filling defect is usually considered to represent an acute venous thrombosis, while the other two abnormalities may be caused by old venous thrombi or may represent technical artifacts caused by incomplete mixing of contrast medium with blood, by external compression on a vein, or by injecting the contrast medium too far proximal in the dorsal vein of the foot.

Pitfalls of venography   Venography is a difficult technic requiring considerable experience to execute and interpret properly. Unless care is taken to inject the dye into the distal dorsal foot vein, there may be nonfilling of calf veins which may be incorrectly interpreted as caused by thrombus because the vein is not filled or as normal because a filling defect is not visualized. The common femoral, external iliac, and common iliac veins may not be adequately filled by ascending venography. All too frequently an incorrect diagnosis is made because of an attempt to interpret the results of an inadequate venogram. Two errors that are commonly made are (1) failure to detect even large nonobstructive thrombi in the common femoral vein because flow into the external iliac or common iliac vein appears to be adequate, although filling of the common femoral vein is suboptimal, and (2) the incorrect diagnosis of venous thrombosis due to misinterpretation of a streaming effect in the common femoral or iliac vein caused by inadequate opacification. Misinterpreting an inadequate venogram (usually in the direction of a false-positive diagnosis) is becoming an important problem with the increasing use of venography in centers lacking expertise in this technic. These pitfalls can be minimized or avoided if radiologists and clinicians are sensitive to these problems and are prepared to repeat the test when the result is inadequate.

Side-effects of venography Venography is an invasive procedure which may produce pain in the foot while the dye is being injected or delayed pain in the calf one to two days after injection. The procedure may be complicated by superficial phlebitis and even deep-vein thrombosis in a small percentage of patients who have normal venography. In our experience, 3% to 4% of the patients with negative venography developed a positive fibrinogen leg scan after venography and about 1% to 2% developed clinically significant venous thrombosis. The hyperosmolar radiopaque contrast medium has been shown to damage endothelial cells and both the early and delayed pain associated with the injection is probably related to direct damage of the venous endothelium with contrast medium.

Other less common complications of venography include hypersensitivity reactions to the radiopaque dye and local skin and tissue necrosis due to extravasation of contrast at the site of injection.[8]

Many of these side-effects can be avoided by careful attention to technic. Care should be taken to ensure that the needle is firmly implanted in the vein and that the contrast should not be injected under pressure. Local pain can be reduced if lidocaine is mixed with the radiopaque material and postvenography phlebitis can be minimized if the leg is elevated after venography and the dye is washed out with an infusion of 150 to 250 ml of normal or heparinized saline. Recent evidence suggests that phlebitis can be reduced if the standard radiopaque material (60%) is diluted to 40% or if an isotonic radiopaque material is used. At present, the high cost of the isotonic preparations currently available makes widespread use prohibitive although less expensive preparations are now undergoing clinical trial. Patients with a history of hypersensitivity to radiopaque dye should not have venography performed, but should undergo objective testing with an alternative diagnostic test (see below).

Noninvasive Tests for the Diagnosis of Venous Thrombosis

In recent years, noninvasive tests have been developed as a replacement for venography because they have produced less discomfort and are both more convenient and versatile than venography. Of these, only three have been extensively evaluated. These are fibrinogen I 125 leg scanning,[9,10] impedance plethysmography,[11-14] and Doppler ultrasound.[15-18] Each of these tests has different applications depending on whether the patient has clinically suspected venous thrombosis or is being screened because of a high risk of developing venous thrombosis. Other diagnostic technics that have been evaluated to a limited extent include other forms of plethysmography,[19] thermography,[20] and various isotope technics.[21,22] Sensitive blood tests to detect intravascular fibrin formation and lysis are also undergoing clinical evaluation and may be of value. The most promising of these is the assay for fragment E.

Fibrinogen I 125 scanning

Principles   The diagnosis of venous thrombosis by radioiodine-labeled fibrinogen scanning depends upon the incorporation of circulating labeled fibrinogen into the thrombus. The increase in overlying surface radioactivity due to uptake of the radiofibrinogen into the thrombus is detected by a radioisotope detector, which is compact and portable allowing the test to be done at the patient's bedside.

Fibrinogen I 125 scanning can be used expectantly for screening medical and surgical patients who are at high risk of developing venous thrombosis or can be used to complete impedance plethysmography in symptomatic patients to confirm or exclude the diagnosis of clinically suspected venous thrombosis. The use of radiofibrinogen carries a theoretical risk of transmitting serum hepatitis but this risk has been eliminated for all practical purposes by preparing fibrinogen from a small number of carefully selected donors who have not transmitted hepatitis during years of frequent blood donations and who are hepatitis B-surface antigen–free.

Scanning technic   Patients are screened with an isotope detector probe with their legs elevated at 15 degrees above horizontal to minimize venous pooling in the calf veins. Readings are taken over both legs and recorded as a percentage of surface radioactivity measured over the heart. The surface radioactivity is recorded over the femoral vein at 7- to 8-cm intervals starting below the inguinal ligament and then at similar

272

intervals over the medial and posterior aspects of the popliteal fossa and calf. Venous thrombosis is suspected if there is an increase in the radioactive reading of more than 20% at any point compared with readings over adjacent points of the same leg, over the same point on the previous day, or over the corresponding point of the opposite leg. Venous thrombosis is diagnosed if the scan remains abnormal upon repeated examination and if the abnormality persists for more than a 24-hour period. The technic is simple and rapid, so that up to 20 patients can be screened daily by one technologist. The scanning time is limited by the in vivo survival of fibrinogen so that after a single injection of 100 μCi counting is possible for about seven days. The thyroid gland is blocked with potassium iodide (100 mg/daily), given orally in order to prevent excessive uptake of radioactive iodide. If the patient is still at risk for developing venous thrombosis after seven days, the injections can be repeated at intervals to extend the scanning time for the period of high risk.

Potential limitations of fibrinogen I 125 tests: The test is insensitive to thrombi in the pelvic veins,[23,24] because fibrinogen I 125 is a relatively low energy gamma emitter, and is unreliable in the upper thigh because of proximity to the bladder, which frequently contains radioactive urine, and because of the presence of large veins and arteries in the pelvis which produce an increase in the background count. This is not an important limitation in most patients since the thrombi rarely start in this region without concurrent thrombosis in the calf veins, but it is in patients with clinically suspected venous thrombosis and in patients undergoing hip surgery. The fibrinogen I 125 test is contraindicated during pregnancy and lactation and should not be used in young patients unless very definite indications exist.

Dosimetry: Following injection of 100 μCi of fibrinogen I 125, approximately 200 mrem is delivered to the blood, 20 mrem to soft tissues, and 5 mrem to kidneys. This is less than the acceptable total body absorbed radiation dose (500 mrem/year) recommended for the general population by the British National Council on Radiation Protection.[25]

Fibrinogen I 125 crosses the placenta and a small amount may enter the fetal circulation.[25] A study performed in postpartum women has demonstrated that radioactivity also appears in the breast milk.[25]

Causes of discrepancy between the results of leg scanning and venography

Abnormal Scan–Normal Venogram: Leg scan abnormalities in the presence of a normal venogram may be due to hematoma, inflammation, uptake of the radioactive fibrinogen by the surgical wound, or nonvisualization of thrombus by venography.

Normal Scan–Abnormal Venogram: A false-negative scan may occur in patients with an old venous thrombus that is no longer taking up fibrinogen if (1) thrombus forms after most of the radioactive fibrinogen has been cleared from the circulation, (2) the thrombus is too small to be detected by leg scanning, or (3) the thrombus is isolated in a common femoral or iliac vein.

Impedance plethysmography

Principles Plethysmography is a noninvasive method that detects volume changes in the leg. Several plethysmographic technics including impedance plethysmography, strain-gauge plethysmography, and air-cuff plethysmography have been used to detect venous thrombi, but impedance plethysmography has been the most thoroughly evaluated (Table 14-2).

Impedance plethysmography (IPG) is sensitive and specific for thrombosis of the popliteal, femoral, or iliac veins (proximal veins), but is relatively insensitive to calf vein thrombosis. This method is based on the principle that blood volume changes in the calf produced by inflation or deflation of a pneumatic thigh cuff results in changes in electrical resistance (impedance). These changes are reduced in patients with thrombosis of the popliteal or more proximal veins. The original method,[11] which required maximum respiratory effort, had shortcomings because sick patients were frequently unable to cooperate sufficiently for the test to be reliable. The test was therefore modified by using a pneumatic thigh cuff to temporarily occlude the venous outflow (occlusive impedance plethysmography).[12,13] This modified test is sensitive and specific for the diagnosis of proximal vein thrombosis.

Technic Occlusive impedance plethysmography is performed with the patient supine and the lower limb elevated 25 to 30 degrees, the knee flexed 10 to 20 degrees, and the ankle elevated to 15 cm higher than the knee. A pneumatic cuff 15 cm in width is applied to the mid-thigh and inflated to 45 cm of water, thereby occluding venous return. After a

Table 14-2
Occlusive Impedance Plethysmography — Correlations with Venography in Patients with Clinically Suspected Deep Vein Thrombosis (DVT)

Investigator	Year	Correlation with Normal Venograms (Specificity)	Correlation with Recent Proximal DVT (Sensitivity)
Hull	1976	97% (386/397)	93% (124/133)
Hull	1977	95% (108/114)	98% (59/60)
Toy	1978	100% (9/9)	94% (15/16)
Hull	1978	96% (304/317)	92% (155/169)
Flanigan	1978	95% (93/98)	96% (52/54)
Cooperman	1979	96% (72/75)	87% (20/23)
Gross	1979	95% (32/34)	100% (9/9)
Wheeler	1980	92% (191/208)	98% (88/90)
Hull	1981	98% (157/160)	95% (74/78)

274

predetermined period of time (see below), the cuff is rapidly deflated and the changes in the electrical resistance (impedance) resulting from alterations in blood volume distal to the cuff are detected by circumferential calf electrodes and recorded on ECG paper strip. The changes in impedance during cuff inflation and deflation are measured and both the total rise during cuff inflation and the fall occurring during the first three seconds of deflation are plotted on a two-way impedance plethysmograph. The graph includes a "discriminate line" which was developed by a discriminate function analysis to provide optimal separation of impedance plethysmograph results into a normal and abnormal for proximal vein thrombosis (Figure 14-1).[13]

The accuracy of impedance plethysmography is critically dependent on obtaining maximal venous filling during the temporary occlusion of venous outflow. The occlusive cuff technic, as originally performed, used only a 45-second occlusion time. This frequently resulted in suboptimal venous filling which compromised the accuracy of the test. Venous filling is improved by prolonging the period of cuff occlusion from 45 seconds to two minutes and by the introduction of repeated sequential testing. Prolongation of the occlusion time to 120 seconds ensures that maximal venous filling occurs for any single test and repeated sequential testing produces a further increase in venous capacity by stretching the vessel wall, a property known as stress relaxation of the vessel wall. These maneuvers increase both venous filling and therefore the sensitivity and

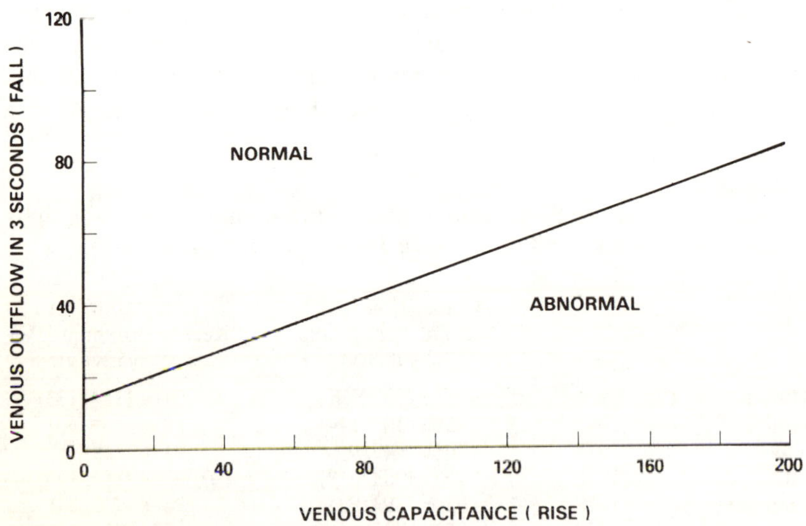

Figure 14-1 Impedance plethysmography scoring graph: The numbers on the horizontal and vertical axes refer to impedance units. (Reproduced from Hull et al[26] with permission of the American Heart Association, Inc.)

specificity of the test. As venous filling increases, there is a corresponding increase in venous emptying in normal legs. When a proximal vein thrombosis is present, however, increased venous filling is not associated with a proportional increase in venous emptying (because of the obstruction) so that the regression lines relating venous filling and emptying (see Figure 14-2) in legs negative and positive for proximal vein thrombosis diverge progressively as filling increases ($P < 0.001$). Thus, increased venous filling increases the separation between normal and abnormal impedance plethysmograph results and enhances the accuracy of the tests.[26]

Unrecognized contraction of leg muscles in patients who are apprehensive or have postoperative pain is a recognized cause of false-positive impedance plethysmograph results. The inexperienced technician may have difficulty in distinguishing an abnormal impedance plethysmograph result caused by venous thrombosis from that caused by isometric muscle contracture, which can be detected directly by electromyography. The use of electromyography in conjunction with impedance plethysmography is clinically feasible and appears to be a helpful addition for accuracy of detection.[27]

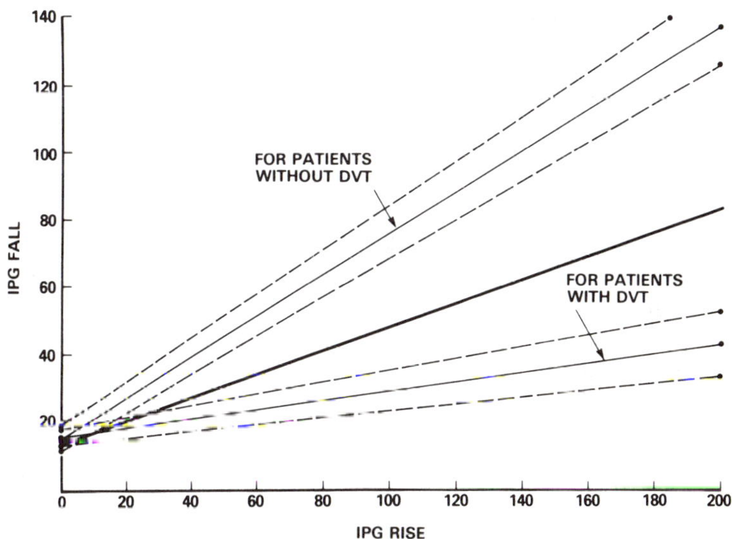

Figure 14-2   The relationship between venous filling (IPG rise) and venous emptying (IPG fall) in patients with and without proximal vein thrombosis. Venous filling is associated with a comparable increase in venous emptying in legs without thrombosis. In contrast, when there is obstruction, progressive venous filling produces relatively smaller changes in venous emptying.

276

Causes of discrepancy between impedance plethysmography and venography

Positive Venography–Negative Impedance Result: Impedance plethysmography only detects thrombi that produce obstruction to venous outflow and therefore will not detect most calf vein thrombi since they do not obstruct the main outflow track, and it may not detect small nonocclusive proximal vein thrombi. However, if optimal venous filling is used, it detects the majority of large nonocclusive thrombi. The test frequently becomes negative in patients with long-standing proximal vein thrombosis either because large collaterals develop or because the thrombus recanalizes.

Positive Impedance–Negative Venography: The impedance test does not distinguish between thrombotic and nonthrombotic obstruction to venous outflow. Thus false-positive results may be obtained if the patient is positioned incorrectly, or inadequately relaxed with constriction of the veins by contracting leg muscles if the vein is compressed by an extravascular mass, or if the venous outflow is impaired by raised central venous pressure. Reduced arterial inflow to the limb caused by severe obstructive arterial disease also compromises venous filling and may produce a false-positive result.

Doppler ultrasound

Principle   The Doppler ultrasound flowmeter examination is a noninvasive method used to measure flow in vessels; it has been evaluated as a diagnostic test in patients with clinically suspected deep vein thrombosis. In expert hands, Doppler ultrasound is a sensitive method for detection of proximal vein thrombosis, but it is less sensitive to calf vein thrombi.

The Doppler ultrasound flow velocity detector contains an oscillator which activates a piezo-electrical crystal in a hand-held probe, so that it emits an ultrasound beam at a frequency of 5 MHz. This beam is directed percutaneously at the underlying vein where it is reflected from the blood cells. If the blood is stationary, the frequency of the reflected beam is identical to that of the incident beam and no sound is recorded. If the particles of blood are moving, then the beam is reflected at a changed frequency (the Doppler shift) which is proportional to the velocity of flow. This difference in frequency between the incident and the reflected ultrasound beam is received by a second piezo-electrical crystal in the probe and amplified into an audible signal or flow sound.[17,18]

Technic of examination   The Doppler examination is performed with the patient lying comfortably in bed in a semiupright position. Care should be taken to remove garments that constrict venous outflow, because this would interfere with venous return.

The common femoral vein is located by placing the probe over the common femoral artery, which can be easily identified, and then moving the probe medially until a low-pitched sound typical of venous flow is heard. The intensity of this low-pitched sound changes with respiration and has been typically described as a "wind storm." When the abdomen is compressed above the inguinal ligament, this respiratory variation in the flow sound is abolished. Upon release of abdominal compression, there is an augmented sound as blood flow in the veins suddenly increases. The thigh and calf are gently squeezed, each producing an augmented sound due to the sudden acceleration of venous flow. Patency of the superficial femoral vein can be demonstrated by moving the probe distally along this vein and repeating calf and distal thigh compression. Augmentation of flow is also produced by sudden release of compression of the thigh proximal to the probe. The probe is then place over the posterior tibial vein which is located by identifying the posterior tibial artery. Augmentation of flow is produced by squeezing the foot and by suddenly releasing proximal calf compression.

The positive Doppler examination: The Doppler flowmeter technic is high sensitive to occluding thrombi in the popliteal and more proximal veins but is less sensitive to nonocclusive proximal thrombi and to calf vein thrombi. Obstruction to venous outflow may result in loss of phasicity of the venous signal and may produce a continuous venous sound due to loss of the normal respiratory fluctuation. In addition, augmentation of the venous signal, which normally occurs as a result of compression of the limb distal to the probe, or release of the compression proximal to the probe, may be diminished, high-pitched and of short duration, or absent.

Causes of discrepancy between Doppler ultrasound and venography The Doppler flowmeter method has many of the limitations of impedance plethysmography. It is relatively insensitive to calf vein thrombosis and may fail to detect partly occluding proximal vein thrombi. Though the technic is relatively simple and rapid, the performance of Doppler ultrasonography and its interpretation is much more dependent on the experience of the examiner. The results are subjective and may be less accurate than impedance plethysmography, except in expert hands. False-positive results may occur if the underlying vein is obstructed by compressing it with the transducer or if compression over the femoral vein or calf is carried out when the limb is drained of blood. False-positive results may also result from incorrect positioning of the patient, since this leads to the absence or decrease of the augmentation sound.

Other technics for the diagnosis of venous thrombosis A number of other diagnostic technics have been less intensively evaluated for the diagnosis of venous thrombosis. These include phleborrheography (aircuff plethysmography),[28] strain-gauge plethysmography,[19] thermography,[20] radionuclide venography,[21,22] and blood tests that reflect intravascular fibrin formation and fibrin breakdown. Preliminary studies with phleborrheography suggest that this technic is sensitive to proximal vein thrombosis. Its sensitivity to calf vein thrombosis is less well defined but may not be better than that achieved by impedance plethysmography or Doppler ultrasound. The main disadvantage of phleborrheography is that its interpretation is subjective. Promising initial results have been reported with thermography but further studies are required before its value and limitations can be adequately assessed. Radionuclide venography requires more adequate evaluation before its practical use can be determined. Sensitive tests for intravascular fibrin formation and fibrinolysis are promising but are technically difficult. These include radioimmunoassays of fibrinopeptide A and a fragment E of fibrin. Such tests can detect acute venous thrombosis but by their very nature are nonspecific.

The application of noninvasive tests with the diagnosis of clinically suspected venous thrombosis The objective, noninvasive diagnostic tests that have been adequately evaluated in patients with clinically suspected venous thrombosis are impedance plethysmography, fibrinogen I 125 leg scanning, and Doppler ultrasonography. None of these tests used alone is as accurate as venography for diagnosis. However, when used in appropriate combinations, these tests can replace venography in the majority of patients with clinically suspected venous thrombosis. Venography may still be required when the patient has a clinical condition known to produce false-positive results with one of the noninvasive tests (eg: arterial insufficiency; congestive heart failure, which can produce false-positive impedance plethysmography; or trauma to the legs, which may produce a false-positive fibrinogen leg scan).

Impedance plethysmography With the development of optimal venous filling,[26] occlusive cuff impedance plethysmography has evolved into a precise, highly reproducible test that is both highly sensitive and specific for proximal vein thrombosis. The results of multiple studies are shown in Table 14-2. The cumulative sensitivity is 95% and the specificity is 96%. The sensitivity reflects the proportion of positive impedance plethysmograph results in patients with proximal vein thrombosis diagnosed by venography, and the specificity reflects the proportion of patients with a negative impedance plethysmograph result in patients with negative venography. Impedance plethysmography has a potential disadvantage in that it is insensitive to calf vein thrombosis and detects only 20% of these thrombi. Thus, in patients with clinically suspected venous thrombosis a positive impedance plethysmograph result can be used to make therapeutic decisions in the absence of clinical conditions known to produce false-positive results, eg, in congestive cardiac failure, severe peripheral vascular disease, and local leg muscle tension. A normal result essentially excludes a diagnosis of occlusive proximal vein thrombosis but does not exclude the diagnosis of a calf vein thrombosis. In patients with a proximal vein thrombosis, as partial recanalization of the vessel occurs, or as the obstruction is lessened by the development of adequate collaterals, the impedance plethysmograph result becomes normal. A recent study in the Hamilton region demonstrated that of 131 consecutive patients with abnormal impedance plethysmograph results and venographically confirmed proximal vein thrombosis, 78 (63%) returned to normal by impedance plethysmography during the three-month period of long-term anticoagulation following the acute episode of proximal vein thrombosis.[29] Thus, performing an impedance plethysmograph evaluation at the end of long-term therapy is of practical value as a base line for future comparison.

Plethysmography as a screening test for venous thrombosis in high-risk patients: Impedance plethysmography as a screening test in high-risk patients is of clinical value in patients with a relatively high rate of proximal vein thrombosis, especially when used in combination with fibrinogen I 125 leg scanning. Such patient groups include patients having elective and emergency hip surgery and patients suffering spinal cord injury.

Doppler ultrasound   The advantages of this technic are that it can be performed more conveniently and rapidly than impedance plethysmography. The chief disadvantage of Doppler ultrasound is that its interpretation is subjective and the test requires considerable skill and experience to perform reliably. However, in skilled hands, it is almost as sensitive to symptomatic proximal vein thrombosis as impedance plethysmography and is a little more sensitive to symptomatic calf vein thrombi since it detects approximately 50% of such thrombi. Doppler ultrasound is more reliable than impedance plethysmography for detecting proximal vein thrombosis in patients with raised central venous pressure or arterial insufficiency. It has the advantage that it can be used in patients who have their legs in plaster or who are in traction.

Fibrinogen I 125 leg scanning   Fibrinogen I 125 leg scanning detects calf vein thrombi and thrombi in the distal half of the thigh that are accreting fibrin at the time of injection of the isotope. False-positive results occur if scanning is performed over a hematoma, over an area of inflammation, or if there is extensive edema; but in the absence of these conditions, leg scanning is both sensitive and specific for acute calf and lower thigh vein thrombosis.

Diagnostic fibrinogen I 125 leg scanning in patients with clinically suspected deep vein thrombosis: The sensitivity of diagnostic leg scanning depends upon the deposition of radiofibrinogen into or around an established thrombus, or incorporation into a new thrombus if extension occurs. The leg scan result becomes abnormal in approximately 70% of patients with established acute thrombus and thus fails to detect thrombus in up to 30% of symptomatic patients. The test result is frequently positive at 24 hours but may not become positive for up to 72 hours. Because of this, and failure to detect isolated thrombi in the upper thigh and pelvis, leg scanning should never be used alone in patients with clinically suspected venous thrombosis. However, because it is highly sensitive to calf vein thrombosis, it is a valuable diagnostic test to complement impedance plethysmography (which is highly sensitive to proximal vein thrombosis). Indeed, the combined approach of impedance plethysmography and leg scanning provides an alternative to venography in patients with clinically suspected venous thrombosis.

Expectant fibrinogen I 125 leg scanning as a screening test in high-risk patients: In high-risk medical and general surgical patients, leg scanning detects over 90% of acute calf vein thrombi, but it is less sensitive to proximal vein thrombi where only 70% of popliteal vein and 65% of femoral vein thrombi are detected. Leg scanning is a useful test in general surgical patients because in the majority of these patients proximal vein thrombosis is associated with calf vein thrombosis for which leg scanning is sensitive.

Leg scanning has special limitations when it is used to screen patients for thrombosis after surgery to the legs. This is because extravascular isotope accumulation in the hematoma and healing wound invariably leads to scan abnormality over the site of the surgery so that thrombi near the wound cannot be detected. This is a major limitation[30] in patients having hip surgery because up to 20% of thrombi may develop as isolated thrombi in the femoral vein under the surgical wound. Consequently, leg scanning has a sensitivity of only 50% when used expectantly in hip surgery patients. Leg scanning combined with impedance plethysmography, however, provides a clinically useful combined screening test (see below). In patients undergoing elective knee surgery, the leg scan is uninterpretable in the lower thigh, popliteal, and upper calf regions due to extravascular accumulation of isotope postoperatively. Furthermore, leg scanning is often performed through a plaster cast or bulky postoperative dressing which often further hinders the accuracy of this test. Used as a screening test in patients undergoing elective knee surgery, the sensitivity of leg scanning is about 75%.

Noninvasive tests in patients with clinically suspected venous thrombosis The noninvasive tests can be used singly or in combination to confirm or exclude the clinical suspicion of venous thrombosis (Figure 14-3). Both impedance plethysmography and Doppler ultrasound are sensitive methods for detecting proximal vein thrombosis but are insensitive for calf vein thrombi. If the results of either of these tests are positive for proximal vein thrombosis, in the absence of conditions that are known to produce false-positive results, a diagnosis of venous thrombosis can be confidently made and the patient treated appropriately. If, however, the results of Doppler ultrasound are positive only with the probe placed over the posterior tibial vein, confirmation should be obtained by venography since this test is relatively nonspecific at this site. If the results of impedance plethysmography or Doppler ultrasound are

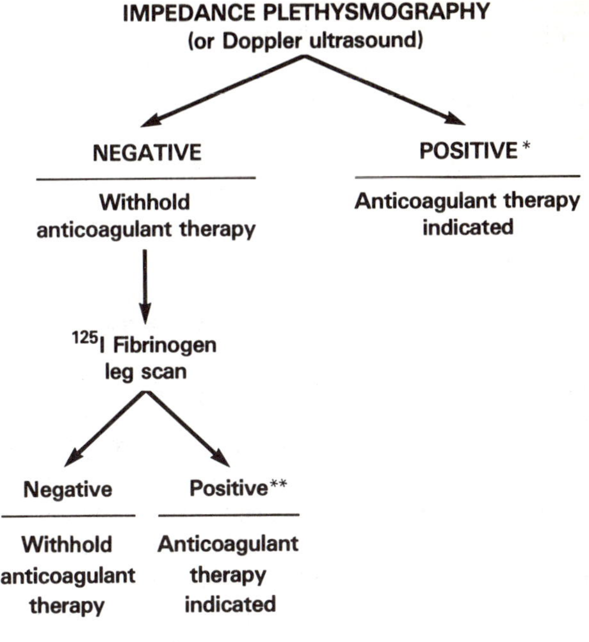

Figure 14-3 Practical noninvasive approach to diagnosis of patients with clinically suspected first episode of acute deep vein thrombosis.

negative, the clinician is faced with three alternatives; (1) repeated examinations with serial impedance plethysmography or Doppler ultrasound at intervals to detect extension of calf vein thrombosis; (2) venography; (3) fibrogen I 125 leg scanning to detect calf vein thrombosis.

Repeat examination of impedance plethysmography or Doppler ultrasound This approach has been used by a number of experienced clinical investigators with apparent safety. However, documentation of the safety of this approach awaits formal prospective study. The rationale for this approach is based on the philosophy that calf vein thrombi are clinically important only when they extend into the proximal veins at which point detection with impedance plethysmography or Doppler ultrasound is possible. Thus, by performing repeated examinations, it is possible to identify patients with extension of calf vein thrombi into the proximal veins who then can be treated appropriately. Extension is known to occur in approximately 20% of the immobilized patients and may also occur in a small percentage of the ambulant population.

Venography Venography following negative results from impedance plethysmography defeats the purpose of noninvasive testing and results in the performance of venography on 70% of symptomatic patients. For this reason, it is considered the least desirable of the three approaches.

Fibrinogen I 125 leg scanning This test is positive in most untreated patients with acute calf vein thrombosis even through there may be no extension of the thrombus since the radioactive fibrinogen diffuses into the thrombus and is laid down as radioactive fibrin. The fibrinogen I 125 is injected after negative results of impedance plethysmography and screening is performed within 24 hours and repeated at 72 hours[29,31] (see below).

Doppler ultrasound Doppler ultrasound has similar but somewhat lower sensitivity and specificity as impedance plethysmography for proximal vein thrombosis. Although its sensitivity for calf vein thrombosis is slightly higher, it could possibly be used instead of impedance plethysmography in combination with fibrinogen I 125 leg scanning, but such an approach would require formal testing before it could be recommended.

Combined use of impedance plethysmography and fibrinogen I 125 leg scanning as an alternative to venography We, in the Hamilton Regional Thrombosis Programme, have evaluated the combined use of impedance plethysmography and fibrinogen I 125 leg scanning in prospective studies in patients with clinically suspected venous thrombosis. The details of these studies are published elsewhere.[29,31] This approach detected all patients with proximal vein thrombi and the majority of patients with calf vein thrombi. The safety of combined impedance plethysmography and leg scanning was also tested by withholding treatment in patients who were negative by these noninvasive tests, irrespective of the results of venography. They were then followed up long-term; no patient died or developed clinical pulmonary embolism during a three-month follow-up period. Furthermore, none of the patients died or developed symptoms or signs of pulmonary embolism while awaiting a definitive diagnosis even though this took up to three days in some patients with calf vein thrombi. Thus, it appears safe to delay treatment in patients with a negative impedance plethysmograph result while awaiting the outcome of leg scanning. It is evident from these findings that the combined approach provides a safe replacement for venography in the majority of patients with clinically suspected deep vein thrombosis. The use of repeated impedance plethysmography alone is also advocated and appears to be safe. The use of serial impedance plethysmography alone or the combined approach of impedance plethysmography and leg scanning has a number of advantages over venography. Noninvasive testing is more versatile because it can be readily performed at the patient's bedside, in the outpatient clinic, or in an emergency room. It is particularly useful if outpatient venography cannot be performed at short notice since it also avoids the inconvenience and expense of unnecesary hospital admission in up to 50% of the ambulant symptomatic patients who were negative by objective testing.

Our current approach to the diagnosis of clinically suspected venous thrombosis is to perform impedance plethysmography immediately upon referral. If this test is positive in the absence of clinical conditions that are known to produce false-positive results, the diagnosis of venous thrombosis is established and the patient is treated accordingly. If the result of the initial impedance plethysmography is negative, the patient is either injected with fibrinogen I 125 and both leg scanning and impedance plethysmography are repeated 24 and 72 hours later, or the patient is followed by impedance plethysmography alone with evaluations being repeated on days one, three, five, and seven. If the results became positive in the absence of conditions known to produce a false-positive result, the patient is treated. If on follow-up the results remain negative, anticoagulant therapy is withheld, as for practical purposes deep vein thrombosis has been excluded from the differential diagnosis.

Cost effectiveness of clinical diagnosis, venography and noninvasive testing of patients with symptomatic deep vein thrombosis Our studies evaluating noninvasive testing in patients with clinically suspected venous thrombosis provided us with an opportunity to perform a cost-effectiveness analysis in 516 patients referred with clinically suspected venous thrombosis.[32] All were evaluated by three diagnostic approaches: clinical diagnosis, venography (which was the diagnostic reference method), and the combination of impedance plethysmography and leg scanning. Cost-effectiveness analysis is an economic tool that makes it possible to rank alternative approaches in terms of both cost and effectiveness. In this setting, the desired effect is measured in terms of the number of symptomatic patients with deep vein thrombosis who are correctly identified so that a distinction can be made between those who need hospital admission and/or treatment and those who do not.

The results are shown in Table 14-3a,b. Clinical diagnosis is clearly the least cost-effective approach. More than half the patients with the clinical diagnosis of deep vein thrombosis proved negative by objective testing. Thus, management based on the clinical diagnosis of deep vein thrombosis exposes more than 50% of patients to unnecessary admission to hospital and anticoagulant therapy. Venography is more cost-effective than clinical diagnosis, particularly when used as an outpatient investigation. When used in this way it prevents the unnecessary hospital admission (for two to three days) of the 50% of patients with clinically suspected venous thrombosis who do not have this diagnosis confirmed

Table 14-3a
Total Costs and Results of Alternative Strategies to Diagnose Deep Vein Thrombosis

Diagnostic Approach	No. of Correct Diagnoses	Cost	
		Canadian $	*American $*
Clinical diagnosis	201	$ 1,270,046	$986,508
Venography			
Outpatient	201	570,863	646,215
Elective inpatient	201	785,538	845,004
Impedance plethysmography			
Alone	142	395,359	321,488
Combined impedance plethysmography and leg scanning	184	550,046	456,504
Impedance plethysmography plus outpatient venography if impedance plethysmography is negative	201	577,609	603,552

Table 14-3b
Total Costs of Alternative Strategies for Each Patient with Venous Thrombosis Correctly Managed

Diagnostic Approach	Total Cost per Patient with Correct Diagnosis and Treatment Proximal Vein Thrombosis
	American $*
Clinical Diagnosis	$7,098
Venography	
Outpatient	4,649
Elective Inpatient	6,080
Impedance Plethysmography	
Alone	2,436
Plus Leg Scanning	3,308
Plus Venography	4,342

*United States dollar cost in an urban New England hospital.

by venography. In many centers, however, outpatient venography is not readily available, and patients with clinically suspected venous thrombosis are usually admitted to hospital, commenced on anticoagulant therapy, and then have the diagnosis confirmed or excluded at a later day by elective venography. For the reason discussed above, this approach is less cost-effective than outpatient venography. The combined use of impedance plethysmography and leg scanning is essentially as cost effective as venography. Impedance plethysmography alone is the least expensive of the approaches, and its effectiveness (used on a repeated basis) is currently under investigation.

The cost of admitting a patient to the hospital for diagnostic testing is likely to remain a major cost item. Therefore emphasis should be placed on outpatient diagnosis.

TREATMENT OF VENOUS THROMBOEMBOLISM

Objectives of Treatment

The main objectives of treating patients with venous thrombosis is to prevent the immediate and long-term complications of this disorder. These complications are pulmonary embolism, recurrent venous thrombosis, the morbidity of the acute event, and long-term postphlebitic syndrome. It should be emphasized that effective prophylaxis against venous thrombosis is now available for most high-risk patients. The use of primary prophylaxis in patients at high risk (see below) is much more effective for preventing morbidity and death due to venous thromboembolism than is confining intervention to treatment of the established event.

A number of different therapeutic approaches are available at the present time, but none are free from side-effects and all are relatively expensive. Because of this, it is important to ensure that the diagnosis of venous thromboembolism is confirmed by objective testing before embarking on treatment. The therapeutic approaches available are either directed at removing the obstruction by enzymatic means (thrombolytic therapy), preventing its extension by inhibiting blood coagulation (anticoagulant therapy), or preventing the occurrence of pulmonary embolism from leg vein thrombosis by interrupting the inferior vena cava. Although removing the thromboembolic obstruction is the most desirable theoretically, this is often not possible and, in practice, most patients are treated with anticoagulants. Anticoagulant therapy is highly effective and prevents death from pulmonary embolism in over 95% of patients who present with venous thromboembolic disease. Heparin may also prevent the postphlebitic syndrome in patients with calf vein thrombosis by preventing propagation of thrombi, but is less effective in patients with proximal vein thrombosis at presentation. Total lysis is infrequent with heparin. Instead, the thrombus usually becomes recanalized and organized, and the resulting valvular incompetence in turn leads to venous hypertension and, if severe, not uncommonly to the postphlebitic syndrome.

In theory, the most effective way of preventing postphlebitic syndrome in patients with proximal vein thrombosis would be to remove the thrombus either by surgical or enzymatic means. Thrombectomy is usually complicated by earlier recurrence. Thrombolytic therapy is associated with a higher risk of bleeding than heparin therapy and is contraindicated in patients who have had major surgery or trauma within ten days of the thrombotic event. This would exclude a large percentage of otherwise eligible patients. Furthermore, thrombolytic therapy may not prevent postphlebitic syndrome if the valves are damaged and become incompetent. Complete lysis with thrombolytic agents is uncommon if the thrombus has been present for 96 hours or longer, because the thrombus becomes more resistent to lysis as it ages. Most patients with pulmonary embolism, including those with major pulmonary emboli, recover completely if treated with heparin. A small number of these patients remain unresponsive to conservative measures, however, and die during the first few days after the embolic event, unless the pulmonary embolic obstruction can be rapidly removed either by thrombolytic therapy or specialized embolectomy. The application of thrombolytic therapy requires considerable experience and clinical judgment, since it is associated with a higher frequency of complications than heparin therapy alone.

Anticoagulant Therapy

Heparin is the treatment of choice in the initial management of many, if not most patients with acute venous thromboembolism. Heparin therapy is relatively safe and is effective for preventing extension venous thrombosis and both nonfatal and fatal pulmonary embolism.

Low doses of heparin, which are effective in preventing venous thromboembolism, are not effective in preventing the extension of established thromboembolism. The difference in dose requirements between prevention and treatment of venous thromboembolism probably reflects the biologic amplification of the coagulation cascade with each successive step in the activation process. Therefore, much more heparin is required to inhibit extension of established thrombi than is required to prevent thrombus formation.

Heparin Heparin is a heterogeneous material which is produced in mast cells. Its anticoagulant properties were first reported in 1916 and it became commercially available in 1935. Heparin is an anionic glycosaminoglycan (mucopolysaccharide) of highly variable molecular weight. The anticoagulant activity of heparin is influenced by its molecular weight, by its degree of n-sulfation, and by the sequence of the saccharide units. The anticoagulant activity of heparin resides in approximately one-third of the molecules of *United States Pharmacopeia* heparin and the most active fraction, in terms of antithrombin-III (AT-III) binding, is present in a fraction representing less than 10% of its bulk. There is a close relationship between the affinity of heparin to antithrombin III and its anticoagulant properties.

Following intravenous injection, heparin distributes throughout the plasma volume and is cleared with a half-life that varies considerably among individuals. In plasma, heparin is completely bound to proteins. After intravenous injection, there is an initial rapid disappearance of approximately 40% of the injected heparin in five minutes followed by a more gradual clearance with a mean heparin half-life of 60 minutes in normal persons. The initial rapid clearance is probably due to adsorption of heparin onto endothelial cells and possibly its diffusion into the extravascular tissues; the slower clearance is due to its elimination from the plasma. The clearance of heparin is more rapid in patients with pulmonary embolism than in venous thrombosis. The plasma half-life of heparin is slightly prolonged in renal failure.

Subcutaneous heparin therapy, in therapeutic doses, has the advantage of having a substantially prolonged plasma half-life. A therapeutic dose of subcutaneous heparin results in a circulating anticoagulant effect of 10 hours or more.[33]

Because heparin inhibits a number of activated clotting factors, coagulation tests can be used to measure its presence and concentration in the blood. A commonly used test for monitoring the heparin effect is the activated partial thromboplastin time (aPTT).

Heparin protocol Heparin is given as an initial intravenous bolus of 5000 IU followed by a maintenance infusion of 25,000 IU 24 hours. Activated partial thromboplastin time (aPTT) monitoring is performed four to six hours after the initial intravenous injection and then on a daily basis to ensure that an adequate response is obtained. Sufficient heparin should be administered for 24 hours to maintain the aPTT at 1½ to two times the preheparin control value. This anticoagulant response is equivalent to 0.3 to 0.4 IU/ml of heparin using protamine sulfate titration. If the aPTT response is above the therapeutic range, the dose of heparin should be reduced by between 2000 to 4000 IU for 24 hours, depending on the degree of prolongation, and the test repeated four to six hours later. If the result of the aPTT is below the therapeutic range, the 24-hour intravenous dose should be augmented by 2000 to 4000 IU for 24 hours; if the aPTT shows no or little prolongation, then to obtain an immediate effect a heparin bolus of 2000 to 4000 IU can be given. After the initial 72 hours of heparin administration, the most common causes of fluctuation in the heparin response are errors in the rate of infusion or laboratory error rather than variations in the rate of heparin clearance.

Heparin therapy should be continued for seven to ten days and overlapped for four to five days with oral anticoagulant therapy. Heparin therapy is discontinued once oral anticoagulant therapy has resulted in a full therapeutic effect.

Long-term therapy of oral anticoagulants should be continued for six to 12 weeks.[33,34] Moderate doses of subcutaneous heparin can be used instead of oral anticoagulants in patients in whom oral anticoagulants are contraindicated, in patients who have an increased risk of bleeding, or in patients in whom oral anticoagulant control is difficult or impractical (see below).

Alternate methods of administration of heparin include intermittent intravenous heparin injections and subcutaneous (therapeutic dose) heparin administration. Intermittent intravenous heparin infusion has been associated with a higher risk of bleeding than continuous intravenous infusion; a possible explanation for this is the observation that the 24-hour heparin dose tends to be higher with intermittent intravenous heparin. The intermittent heparin regimen has the advantage of simplicity but the patient's blood is incoagulable for a period of time after each injection. A practical regimen is the use of 5000 IU every four hours for a total dose of 30,000 IU/day.

Subcutaneous heparin therapy in an initial dose of 10,000 IU every 12 hours offers an alternative approach in patients in whom an intravenous administration is not possible due to lack of access or difficulty in monitoring. The heparin dose is adjusted according to the PTT taken at six-hour intervals between doses and is adjusted by 1000 and 2000 IU per dose, depending on whether the PTT response is below or above the therapeutic range. Although this approach would offer advantages with respect to simplicity and shortening hospital stay, its safety and efficacy for initial therapy require further investigation. This approach is more effective than the use of oral anticoagulants in long-term therapy.

Monitoring of heparin therapy Ideally, the amount of heparin given to a patient with venous thromboembolism should be the smallest dose that prevents thrombus extension. Unfortunately, the laboratory tests in routine use measure the effect of heparin on coagulation rather than its effect on thrombus extension. When heparin is given in a standard dose adjusted to the patient's weight, the response in terms of heparin level or aPTT varies greatly from patient to patient. Because of this, most centers use laboratory tests to monitor the anticoagulant effect of heparin. The value of these tests is related to their ability to predict that heparin is exerting its antithrombotic effect without exposing the patient to increased risk of bleeding. There is experimental evidence that the extension of venous thrombosis can be prevented if heparin is administered by continuous infusion in a dose that maintains the plasma heparin level above 0.3 IU/ml, or the aPTT at a level that is twice pretreatment value. This has led to the concept of the "therapeutic range." However, the validity of the therapeutic range has never been demonstrated by randomized clinical trials. A number of descriptive studies indicate that recurrent thromboembolism during treatment is associated with a relatively poor anticoagulant response measured either by the whole blood clotting time or by the aPTT. The evidence for the relationship between the results of coagulation tests during heparin therapy and an increased risk of bleeding is conflicting. There is indirect evidence that a relationship may exist between the dose of heparin administered over 24 hours and the risk of bleeding. But other factors, including age, sex, recent surgery or trauma, or the use of associated drugs such as aspirin are also important. A number of coagulation tests are used to monitor the anticoagulant effect of heparin treatment. Of these, the clotting time and activated clotting time are performed on whole blood while the aPTT, PTT, factor X_a inhibitor assay, thrombin clotting time (TT), and protamine titration heparin assay are performed on platelet-poor plasma. Tests performed on whole blood or platelet-rich plasma have the theoretical advantage that they are influenced by the antiheparin activity contained in the patient's platelets. However, tests using platelet-poor plasma can be performed in batches with an automatic clot timer and there is no evidence that they are less sensitive to the antithrombotic effect of heparin.

It is important to ensure that any coagulation test chosen to monitor heparin treatment is sensitive to at least 0.1 IU/ml of plasma and the results of the test are reproducible. The aPTT and TT are the tests most widely used to monitor the heparin dose and are the two tests that have been evaluated most extensively. However, there is no reason why they should be preferred over many of the other tests that are sensitive to heparin. If the aPTT is used, it is crucial that the reagent used is sensitive to heparin.

Adverse effects of heparin   The side-effects of heparin include bleeding, thrombocytopenia, arterial thromboembolism, hypersensitivity to heparin, and osteoporosis. Bleeding is the most important side-effect. The frequency of bleeding is affected by dose and by the underlying disorders that predispose the patient to bleeding. In the Hamilton region, major bleeding is relatively infrequent, occurring in 6% to 9% of patients receiving intravenous therapeutic doses of heparin. Patients at particular risk are the elderly, those with an underlying hemostatic defect, those treated with aspirin, and patients who have been exposed to recent surgery or trauma. The method of administration of heparin may influence bleeding being more common in patients who receive heparin by intermittent intravenous injections. The bleeding risk appears to increase with the total dose of heparin over a 24-hour period.

Heparin-induced thrombocytopenia is a now well-recognized complication of heparin therapy. Its frequency varies from center to center and, in our experience, occurs in approximately 4% of patients. Heparin-induced thrombocytopenia is more common in patients receiving beef lung heparin than porcine gut heparin. The mechanism of heparin-induced thrombocytopenia is unknown at present.

Arterial thromboembolism has been reported as a rare complication of heparin therapy. This life-threatening complication usually occurs about ten days after the initiation of therapy and occurs more frequently in the elderly. Clinical episodes of arterial ischemia are associated with thrombocytopenia. This devastating complication requires immediate withdrawal of heparin.

Hypersensitivity to heparin is very uncommon and may take the form of a skin rash or, less commonly still, an anaphylactic reaction.

Osteoporosis occurs rarely in patients receiving long-term subcutaneous therapy. This complication has been observed in patients receiving more than 15,000 IU of heparin a day for more than six months. Patients with this complication usually present clinically with a spontaneous fracture of the vertebral ribs.

Alopecia has been reported as a rare complication of heparin. Serum transformiminase levels may be moderately raised. Rarely, a blue discoloration of the toes associated with a burning sensation has been reported.

Antidote to heparin   The anticoagulant effect of heparin can be immediately neutralized by injection of protamine sulfate intravenously. The appropriate neutralizing dose depends on the dose of heparin, its route of administration, and the time at which it was given. If protamine sulfate is used within minutes of the intravenous heparin injection, then a full neutralizing dose—1 mg protamine/100 IU heparin—should be given. An occasional hypotensive response of protamine sulfate has been reported so that it must be injected slowly over a ten- to 30-minute period. Because the plasma half-life of intravenously administered heparin is approximately 60 minutes, an injection of protamine sulfate in a bolus of more than 50 mg is seldom required. Treatment with protamine sulfate may be repeated since protamine is cleared from the blood more rapidly than heparin. After a subcutaneous injection of heparin, protamine sulfate should be given in a dose equivalent to approximately 50% of the last heparin dose. This may have to be repeated because of the prolonged absorption from the subcutaneous depot.

Effectiveness of heparin therapy   The use of therapeutic doses of heparin with the aPTT maintained in the therapeutic range (1½ to two times the control value) is associated with a very low frequency of recurrent venous thromboembolism. The frequency of recurrent venous thromboembolism is less than 2% during therapy, but failure to follow heparin therapy with long-term anticoagulant therapy exposes the patient to the risk of a very high rate of recurrence. Recent data indicate that failure to follow the initial course of heparin therapy with adequate long-term therapy exposes the patient with proximal vein thrombosis (venous thrombosis involving the popliteal or more proximal veins) to a 40% to 50% risk of recurrent venous thrombosis and pulmonary embolism. The risk of recurrent venous thromboembolism is greatest in the first month after the initial event and then gradually subsides over the next three to five months.

Oral anticoagulant therapy for three months is the standard long-term anticoagulant approach. Subcutaneous heparin in therapeutic doses can also be used long-term and offers an alternative approach in patients who are pregnant or at high risk of bleeding.

Long-term treatment

Oral anticoagulant therapy: Experimental studies have demonstrated that it takes seven to ten days for a thrombus to become adherent to the vein wall. For this reason, it is generally recommended that heparin be continued for this period of time. It is standard practice to follow heparin therapy with oral anticoagulants for a period of three to six months. This approach is based largely on a retrospective study which demonstrated that, in patients not treated with oral anticoagulants, the risks of recurrent thromboembolism was greatest in the first month after the initial event and then gradually subsided over the next three to five months. Treatment with oral anticoagulants for six to 12 weeks after the initial course of heparin apparently reduced the risk of recurrence over the three- to five-month period but offered little benefit beyond this time. These observations are supported by the findings of recent randomized trials.[33,34]

The coumarins and indanedione derivatives produce their anticoagulant effect indirectly; unlike heparin, they are not direct anticoagulants and do not inhibit coagulation if they are added in vitro. These agents inhibit the effect of vitamin K on the hepatic synthesis of factors, II, VII, IX, and X. Oral anticoagulant therapy leads to synthesis of biologically inactive forms of these clotting proteins. The anticoagulant effect of these drugs is delayed until the normal clotting factors are cleared from the circulation. Thus, the peak inhibitory effect on the synthesis of biologically active vitamin K–dependent clotting factors occurs 36 to 72 hours after drug administration. With a 40-mg loading dose, factor VII levels usually fall rapidly to less than 20% of normal and sometimes to less than 10% of normal for up to three to four days. In some patients, however, suppression of factor VII to this level is seen within 24 hours. Sick patients with impaired liver function or reduced vitamin K stores are particularly susceptible to large loading doses. Equilibrium levels of factors II, IX, and X are not reached until about one week after initiation of therapy. The use of a small loading dose and initial daily dose tends to avoid overdose, especially in patients who are sensitive to warfarin, and this is the preferred approach. Recent randomized trials have demonstrated that warfarin sodium therapy is effective in the long-term treatment of patients with venous thromboembolism. The rate of recurrent venous thromboembolism is reduced to less than 2% during long-term therapy with warfarin sodium.

Recent prospective randomized studies[33-35] have provided more definitive information about the need for secondary prophylaxis and its monitoring in patients with venous thrombosis.

In one study,[33] patients were treated with full-dose heparin for 14 days and then randomized into groups receiving low-dose subcutaneous heparin (5000 IU every 12 hours) or full doses of oral anticoagulants. Subcutaneous heparin was not monitored but oral anticoagulants were adjusted to maintain the prothrombin time at 1½ times the control value. Patients with calf vein thrombosis were given secondary prophylaxis for six weeks and those with proximal vein thrombosis prophylaxis for three months. There were no recurrences in either group of patients who had calf vein thrombosis. However, there was a 40% rate of venographically confirmed recurrent venous thrombosis in patients with proximal vein thrombosis who received low-dose heparin. In contrast, the frequency of recurrent venous thrombosis was less than 2% in those patients receiving a full course of oral anticoagulants. In the second study,[34] a regimen in which an adjusted dose of subcutaneous heparin replaced the fixed low-dose heparin, the subcutaneous heparin dose was adjusted at onset to maintain the PTT at 1½ times control six hours after subcutaneous injection. On achieving this PTT response, the dose was fixed and no further monitoring was performed. The frequency of recurrent deep venous thrombosis was low (less than 4% in both groups) but there was statistically and clinically significant less bleeding in the adjusted heparin group. These findings indicate adequate long-term anticoagulant therapy is mandatory; low-dose heparin is ineffective for treating proximal vein thrombosis. Adjusted-dose subcutaneous heparin is an effective alternative to warfarin sodium and its use is associated with less bleeding. The findings suggest that patients with calf vein thrombi, however, can be safely treated with low-dose heparin for a period of six weeks.

In the third study,[35] patients with proximal vein thrombosis were treated with long-term warfarin therapy and randomized to receive less intense anticoagulant therapy monitored by Manchester comparative time (frequently used in Europe) or more intense anticoagulant therapy monitored by Simplastin prothrombin time (frequently used in North America). Two of the 47 patients (4%) suffered hemorrhagic complications compared with 11 of 49 patients (22%) in the more intensely anticoagulated group (P = .009). The frequency of recurrent venous thromboembolism was low in both groups (2%). These findings indicate that there is a causal relationship between the intensity of anticoagulant effect and hemorrhage. Our findings suggest that the dose of oral anticoagulants for patients with proximal vein thrombosis should be monitored to provide a less intensive anticoagulant effect than is presently used in North America. This could be achieved by using a more sensitive thromboplastin reagent or achieving a Simplastin prothrombin time of 15 to 16 seconds.

Oral anticoagulant protocol: Warfarin sodium is administered in an initial dose of 10 mg/day for the first two days and the daily dose is then adjusted according to the prothrombin time (PT). Heparin therapy is discontinued on the fourth or fifth day at which time the PT is prolonged into the therapeutic range (PT 1½ to two times the control value). There is experimental evidence that the maximal antithrombotic effect of oral anticoagulant therapy is delayed for up to five days, even though the anticoagulant effect, reflected by an increase in PT (due mainly to a fall in factor VII), may be evident within two to three days. For this reason, it is important to overlap oral anticoagulant therapy with heparin therapy for four to five days even though the PT may be prolonged into the therapeutic range after two to three days. Once the patient's condition is stable, PT is monitored weekly throughout the course of oral anticoagulant therapy. However, if there are factors which can produce an unpredictable response to warfarin (eg, concomitant drug therapy), then PT is monitored more frequently to minimize the risk of complications.

Adverse effects of oral anticoagulants: The major side-effect of oral anticoagulants is bleeding. Bleeding during well-controlled oral anticoagulant therapy is usually due to surgery or other forms of trauma or to local lesions such as peptic ulcer or carcinoma. Spontaneous bleeding may occur if warfarin sodium, given in an excessive dose, results in marked prolongation of the prothrombin time; this bleeding may be severe and even life-threatening.

The nonhemorrhagic side-effects of oral anticoagulants differ according to whether the coumarin derivatives (eg, warfarin sodium) or indanedione are administered. Nonhemorrhagic side-effects of coumarin are uncommon. These include skin necrosis, dermatitis, and a syndrome of painful blue toes. The nonhemorrhagic side-effects occur more frequently with the indanedione derivatives. Hypersensitivity reactions have been reported to occur in 1% to 3% of patients receiving indanedione derivatives; these include rash, fevere, hepatitis, leukopenia, renal failure, and diarrhea and they can be fatal. The indanedione derivatives also produce red discoloration of the urine in many patients which sometimes is confused with hematuria.

Since the nonhemorrhagic side-effects of warfarin are very uncommon, these agents are the oral anticoagulants of choice.

Oral anticoagulants cross the placenta and may cause fetal malformations when used in the first trimester. This complication has been reported with both wartarin and phenindione. Characteristic stippling of the vertebral and tarsal bones associated, on many occasions, with nasal hypoplasia may occur. Microcephaly, blindness, and mental retardation have also been described. Because of these teratogenic effects, oral anticoagulants should not be used in the first trimester, nor should they be used in women who are planning a pregnancy. Furthermore, they should not be used in the latter part of the third trimester because the infant is exposed to the risk of bleeding due to reduced levels of vitamin K–dependent clotting factors.

Heparin does not cross the placenta and is the drug of choice during pregnancy. Heparin therapy, administered in therapeutic doses every 12 hours, results in a prolonged sustained anticoagulant response and can be used in both prophylaxis and treatment of venous thromboembolism.

Oral anticoagulants are also secreted in the milk of nursing mothers, but it is debatable whether the prothrombin time is significantly altered in breast-fed infants, even when mothers receive full therapeutic doses. Thus, the use of these agents in breast-feeding mothers is controversial.

Altered response to oral anticoagulants: A large number of factors influence the response of patients to oral anticoagulants. The most important of these is the interaction of oral anticoagulants with concomitant drug therapy. These interactions may produce either prolongation or reduction in the anticoagulant effect. Drugs that have been reported to interfere or interact with oral anticoagulants are shown in Table 14-4. The most important of these are the barbiturates, phenylbutazone, sulfinpyrazone, large doses of aspirin, anabolic steroids, co-trimoxazol (trimethoprim + sulfamethoxazole), and sulphonamides. Antibiotic drugs only appear to affect oral anticoagulants if dietary sources of vitamin K are reduced, eg, patients on intravenous therapy. The mechanism of drug interactions are numerous and complex and include: (1) reduced absorption of vitamin K (cholestyramine); (2) reduced warfarin absorption (heptabarbital); (3) increased warfarin absorption (nortriptyline hydrochloride); (4) reduced binding of anticoagulants to albumin, which results in increased concentration of a pharmacologically active unbound drug (sulphonamides, phenylbutazone); (5) altered rate of inactivation of warfarin by hepatic microsomal oxidizing systems (barbiturates, glutethimide, rifampin); (6) increased rate of drug inactivation resulting in a more rapid disappearance and thus reduction of the anticoagulant effect (allopurinol, chloramphenicol); (7) increased rate of synthesis of vitamin K–dependent clotting factors producing a relative resistance to the effect of oral anticoagulants (estrogens); (8) increased rate of metabolism of vitamin K–dependent clotting factors and, hence, enchancing of the effect of oral anticoagulants (thyroxine). Drugs may also potentiate the effect of oral anticoagulants on the hemostatic mechanism by impairing platelet function (asprin, carbenicillin, phenylbutazone). Special care should be taken to adjust the dose of oral anticoagulant therapy during the time that other drugs are being taken to minimize the risk of inadequate anticoagulant control.

Increased sensitivity to oral anticoagulants occurs in patients with vitamin K deficiency and in patients with impaired liver function. Increased sensitivity to oral anticoagulants occurs in patients with fever and thyrotoxicosis due to rapid metabolism of vitamin K–dependent clotting factors.

Table 14-4
Drug Interactions with Oral Anticoagulants

Interaction Increasing Anticoagulant Effect	No Significant Interaction	Interaction Decreasing Anticoagulant Effect
Allopurinol	Paracetamol (acetaminophen)	Barbiturates
Anabolic steroids	Chlordiazepoxide	Cholestyramine
Chloramphenicol	Chlorothiazide	Dichloralphenazone
Clofibrate	Diazepam	Phenytoin
Co-trimoxazol (trimethoprim + sulfamethoxazole)	Flurazepam	Diuretics
Dextrothyroxine	Haloperidol	Glutethimide
Disulfiram	Meprobamate	Griseofulvin
Mefenamic acid	Phenothiazines	Heptabarbital
Neomycin	Probenecid	Rifampicin
Nortriptyline		
Oxyphenbutazone		
Phenylbutazone		
Phenyramidol		
Quinidine		
Salicylate		
Sulfaphenazole		
Sulfisoxazole		

Antidote to oral anticoagulants: The antidote to vitamin K antagonists is vitamin K_1. In the situation where excessive prolongation of prothrombin time occurs, management depends on the degree of prolongation and whether the patient is bleeding or not. If the prolongation is mild, ie, less than three times the control value, and the patient is not bleeding, then no specific treatment is necessary, since the PT can be expected to decrease over the next 24 hours if treatment with oral anticoagulants is discontinued. With more marked prolongation in patients who are not bleeding, treatment with small doses of vitamin K_1 given orally or subcutaneously (2.5 to 5 mg) could be considered. With marked prolongation of PT, particularly in patients who either are at risk to bleed or are actively bleeding, vitamin K_1 should be given. If vitamin K_1 is given intravenously, this must be administered with great caution since intravenous injections of this drug may induce, rarely, an anaphylactoid reaction. Other reported side-effects include dizziness, flushing, and sweating. Intravenous vitamin K_1 therefore should be administered at a rate no faster than 1 mg/min. Whenever possible, it is preferable to administer vitamin K_1 subcutaneously to minimize the risk of serious adverse reactions. In most patients, intravenous administration of vitamin K_1 produces a demonstrable effect on the PT within three to four hours and corrects the prolonged PT within six to eight hours. Because the half-life of vitamin K_1 is less than warfarin sodium, a repeat course

296

of vitamin K$_1$ may be necessary. If bleeding is severe and life-threatening, vitamin K$_1$ therapy can be supplemented by using concentrates of factors II, VII, IX, and X.

Thrombolytic Therapy

The frequency of recurrent, clinically suspected venous thromboembolism is low during anticoagulant therapy and this remains the treatment of choice in the majority of patients with venous thromboembolism. Anticoagulant therapy, however, is not ideal because it does not induce thrombolysis. Therefore, in theory it does not eliminate an important potential source of subsequent embolization, nor does it alleviate hemodynamic disturbances associated with major pulmonary embolism, nor prevent damage to the deep venous system which predisposes to postphlebitic syndrome. Thus, although anticoagulant therapy is effective in reducing the important immediate complications of venous thromboembolism, it is relatively ineffective in preventing some of the late sequelae.

For this reason, thrombolytic therapy is advocated as the treatment of choice in selected patients with acute venous thrombosis or massive pulmonary embolism. Advocates of thrombolytic therapy (followed by anticoagulant therapy) point out that thrombolytic therapy can achieve the following objectives of ideal management[36]: (1) thrombi and emboli can be lysed with circulation restored to normal; (2) hemodynamic disturbances can be rapidly reduced; (3) venous valve damage can be prevented or minimized ; (4) postphlebitic syndrome can be minimized or prevented; (5) damage to the pulmonary vascular bed can be prevented or minimized, reducing the likelihood of persistent pulmonary hypertension.

Streptokinase has recently been released for the treatment of established venous thromboembolism. A product of hemolytic streptococci, it is antigenic in man and stimulates the production of neutralizing antibodies.[37] Streptokinase combines with plasminogen to produce a conformational change that exposes an active site. This active site in turn converts the noncomplexed plasminogen to plasmin by proteolytic cleavage. Streptokinase is cleared rapidly from the circulation and has a half-life of approximately 90 minutes.

Urokinase is a β-globulin[37] produced by renal cells. It is present in human urine and is not antigenic in man. This agent acts by directly converting plasminogen to the proteolytic enzyme plasmin with subsequent digestion of fibrin, fibrinogen, and other circulating coagulation factors.

Both streptokinase and urokinase are more effective than heparin in inducing rapid resolution of recent venous thrombi and pulmonary emboli.[38,39] In patients with massive pulmonary embolism, the degree of lysis can be striking. The use of streptokinase for 12 to 24 hours followed by conventional anticoagulant therapy should be considered in patients with massive venous thrombosis of pulmonary embolism.

Thrombolytic therapy is particularly useful in patients with massive pulmonary embolism or in patients with cardiac or pulmonary disease in whom even a small or moderate embolus may be life-threatening. The use of thrombolytic therapy to produce rapid clot lysis in these patient groups may prove life-saving when cardiac and pulmonary function is severely compromised. Thrombolytic therapy with streptokinase has been compared with heparin in randomized trials of patients with acute venous thrombosis.[40,41] The results of these trials indicate that lysis of venous thrombi occurs more frequently with streptokinase than with heparin and that complete lysis of venous thrombi occurs in one third to one half of patients treated with streptokinase within 72 hours of onset of clinical symptoms. Preliminary studies suggest that thrombolytic therapy may reduce postphlebitic complications but this is controversial and awaits the results of more definitive long-term clinical follow-up.

Because streptokinase and urokinase produces lysis of fibrin in hemostatic plugs and wounds, bleeding is a more frequent complication than with heparin. With careful selection of patients, however, the hemorrhagic side-effects of streptokinase or urokinase can be minimized. Review of the published data suggests that the risk of major hemorrhage or intracranial bleeding with streptokinase is approximately twice that associated with heparin therapy. The risk of hemorrhage increases with the length of thrombolytic infusion and often occurs at the site of previous surgery or trauma.

The following guidelines are recommended for patient selection for thrombolytic therapy[36]:

1. The presence of an appropriate clinical indication including documented diagnosis and evidence that the thrombus is of recent origin (less than seven days).

2. Careful evaluation of contraindications. These include:

Absolute contraindications of (a) active internal bleeding and; (b) recent (within two months) cerebrovascular accident or other active intracranial processes.

Relative major contraindications of (a) recent (less than ten days) major surgery or obstetrical delivery, organ biopsy, previous puncture of noncompressible vessels; (b) recent serious gastrointestinal bleeding; (c) recent serious trauma; (d) severe arterial hypertension (> 200 mmHg systolic or greater > 100 mmHg diastolic).

Relative minor contraindications of (a) recent minor trauma including cardiopulmonary resuscitation; (b) high likelihood of left atrial thrombus (ie, mitral disease with atrial fibrillation); (c) bacterial endocarditis; (d) hemostatic defects associated with hepatorenal disease; (e) pregnancy; (f) age over 75 years; (g) diabetic hemorrhagic retinopathy.

Before embarking on thrombolytic therapy, the diagnosis of venous thromboembolism should be established by objective means. If pulmonary angiography is performed to confirm a diagnosis of pulmonary embolism, the angiography catheter should be inserted into the arm vein because hemostasis is easier to achieve than if the femoral vein route is used.

Thrombolytic protocol Prior to commencement of thrombolytic therapy, a base-line PT, PTT, TT, and platelet count should be obtained as well as the base-line hemoglobin level and hematocrit. To minimize the risk of bleeding, invasive arterial procedures should be avoided and venipunctures should be kept to an absolute minimum. If arterial blood samples are required, then blood should be taken from the radial artery and local compression maintained for at least 20 minutes.

Dosage and administration: Streptokinase and urokinase are given intravenously in a priming dose that rapidly induces activation of the fibrinolytic system, which is sustained by continuous effusion for the duration of therapy. Both drugs have a short half-life, so there is a rapid loss of fibrinolytic activity if the treatment is interrupted.

Streptokinase is given in a priming dose sufficiently large to neutralize naturally occurring antibodies resulting from previous streptococcal infections. In the majority of patients, the antibody level can be overcome by a dosage of at least 250,000 units given as a priming dose over 30 minutes. This priming dose neutralizes the antibodies and provides sufficient streptokinase to complex with plasminogen to produce activated plasminogen, which in turn activates uncomplexed plasminogen to plasmin. In patients suspected of having unusually high antibody levels, ie, those recently treated with streptokinase or who have had a recent streptococcal infection, the priming dose can be calculated by performing a streptokinase-resistant test using a commercially available kit. Once priming has been accomplished, the fibrinolytic state is sustained with an effusion of 100,000 to 150,000 units/h. The sustaining dose is designed to maintain the plasminogen/streptokinase complex at levels that produce optimum plasminogen activator activity. If the dose given is excessive, most of the plasminogen is complex with streptokinase and little plasmin can be formed. If the dose of streptokinase is too low, there is a risk of inducing excessively high levels of circulating plasmin.

Urokinase treatment is accomplished by using a priming dose over 15 to 30 minutes to achieve desired levels of activator activity, and this is followed by a sustaining dose. Rapid activation of the fibrinolytic system can be achieved in more than 90% of patients with a priming dose of 4000 units/kg body weight and the activity sustained by an infusion of 4000 units/kg body weight/h for the desired length of time. This thrombolytic state can be maintained indefinitely since resistance does not occur as is the case with streptokinase therapy in which resistance occurs in four to ten days due to a rapid rise in antibody titers.

Monitoring of thrombolytic therapy The effects of thrombolytic therapy can be monitored by a test such as the TT or euglobin lysis time to establish the presence of systemic thrombolytic state, but there is no evidence that these tests predict clinical efficacy or reduce bleeding complications. Monitoring streptokinase is relatively complicated because of the mechanism by which streptokinase works. A TT should be performed approximately two hours after onset of the loading-dose infusion, at which time it should be expected to be prolonged four to five times the control value. A lesser degree of prolongation suggests that the patient's streptokinase antibodies have not been adequately neutralized and it is also an indication for performing streptokinse resistance tests and adjusting the dose accordingly. Once a fibrinolytic state is established, thrombin time should be repeated at four-hour intervals. If the thrombin time remains two to five times the control value, no change in dosage is required. A thrombin time that is less than twice the control value, however, indicates that there is an excess of plasminogen/streptokinase complex relative to the uncomplex plasminogen and that the dose should be decreased by 25% to 50%. A thrombin time that is in excess of five times the control value, on the other hand, suggests that there is too little streptokinase/plasminogen complex relative to uncomplex plasminogen, which is therefore being converted to plasmin and creating an excessive plasma fibrinolytic state. Under these circumstances, the sustaining dose of streptokinase should be increased to approximately 200,000/units/h to increase the rate of complex to free plasminogen. Thus, the average hourly rate of infusion varies from 100,000 to 200,000 units/h following the initial loading dose.

With urokinase infusions, the dose of the drug is decreased by approximately 25% if the TT exceeds four to five times the control value. Tests of fibrinolytic activity such as the euglobulin lysis time can be performed if available, but are not necessary. It is very important to monitor clinically for evidence of bleeding; this is achieved by performing serial hemoglobin determinations and hematocrits at least twice daily and by observing urine and stools for evidence of bleeding. A short course of therapy, less than 24 hours, lessens the risk of bleeding, and for this reason is preferred in patients with pulmonary embolism. However, in patients with venous thrombosis, treatment may be continued for up to 72 hours to achieve complete lysis. After thrombolytic therapy has been discontinued, it should be followed by intravenous after two to four hours, and continued for five to seven days to prevent re-thrombosis. This is particularly important in streptokinase therapy because recurring thrombi are likely to contain very low levels of plasminogen and therefore may be much more resistant to lysis. Then, after five to seven days of intravenous heparin therapy, the usual course of long-term anticoagulant therapy should begin. Plasminogen activator derived from tissue sources is currently under evaluation. This has a more specific fibrinolytic action than urokinase or streptokinase and therefore may be more clinically effective.

Complications of thrombolytic therapy   The major complication of thrombolytic therapy is hemorrhage. Other complications include allergic reactions and fever. Allergic reactions occur in 10% of patients treated with streptokinase. These reactions usually take the form of pruritis or urticaria but approximately 1% to 2% of patients develop anaphylactic reactions. These allergic reactions can be promptly reversed by standard therapy including epinephrine, intravenous corticosteroids, and antihistamines. Fever occurs in about 25% of patients receiving streptokinase and about 10% of patients receiving urokinase.

Hemorrhage is seen in 30% to 50% of patients treated with streptokinase or urokinase for more than 12 hours. The risk of hemorrhage increases with the length of infusion and occurs most often from sites of vascular invasion such as needle puncture wounds, cut-down sites for catheterizations, or from surgical wounds. In about one third of cases, bleeding commences during thrombolytic therapy; in other patients it is first noted after completion of thrombolytic therapy and during anticoagulant therapy. Bleeding may also occur from the genitourinary or gastrointestinal tracts and, occasionally, cerebral bleeding occurs.

Bleeding complications can be reduced by carefully selecting patients and not treating those with contraindications.

Antidote to streptokinase   If bleeding is life-threatening, the fibrinolytic process can be rapidly reversed by an infusion of 5 g of EACA (epsilonaminocapoic acid) given over 30 minutes followed by 1 g/h until hemostasis has been secured. This may be supplemented with transfusions of fresh plasma or cyroprecipitate.

Clinical results of thrombolytic therapy   Complete lysis of venous thrombi occurred in less than 10% of patients treated with heparin but occurred within seven days of onset of symptoms in 35% of patients treated with streptokinase. Significant lysis is seldom evident before 48 hours of treatment and four or more days may be required to achieve complete lysis. This treatment is indicated in younger patients with femoral or ileofemoral vein thrombosis where the long-term benefits of achieving lysis are particularly desirable. Treatment should be started as soon as possible after presentation and should not be administered to patients who have symptoms for more than seven days since it is unlikely to be successful. Treatment is required for 48 to 96 hours; after discontinuation of thrombolytic therapy, the patient should be treated with heparin for five to seven days and with oral anticoagulants to prevent recurrent thrombosis.

Management of Massive Pulmonary Embolism

Most patients who die from pulmonary embolism do so within two hours and in patients who survive more than two hours, the prognosis with standard anticoagulant therapy is excellent and invasive procedures such as embolectomy have little or no place. Rarely, pulmonary embolectomy may be carried out in specialized centers on patients with massive embolism who remain hemodynamically unstable. Cardiopulmonary bypass has been advocated to support the severely decompensated patient while immediate thrombolytic therapy or embolectomy is instituted. Theoretically, life-support systems may provide a breathing space in which to stabilize the patient before embarking upon definitive therapy. Thrombolytic therapy produces rapid lysis and may be helpful in patients with cardiopulmonary decompensation and pulmonary embolism by promoting more rapid resolution of the pulmonary emboli.

Inferior Vena Cava Interruption

The use of inferior vena cava interruption should be considered in the following patients: (1) the patient with acute venous thromboembolism and an absolute contraindication to anticoagulant therapy, (2) the rare patient with massive embolism who survives but in whom recurrent emboli may be disastrous, (3) the rare patient who suffers from objectively documented recurrent embolism while on adequate anticoagulant therapy. Inferior vena cava interruption has the potential of increasing the risk of long-term sequelae (eg, a more severe postphlebitic syndrome). It may be ineffective in preventing late embolic recurrence due to collaterals which develop and bypass the site of the inferior vena cava obstruction. The frequency of these late complications can be reduced by using intracaval devices. These can be introduced into the venous system at a remote site such as the femoral or jugular veins. Such procedures can be performed under local anesthesia and are better tolerated by the gravely ill patient than direct surgical interruption of the vena cava which requires general anesthesia and substantial operative dissection. A recent development in intracaval devices is the Greenfield filter. It has the advantage that it can be inserted under local anesthesia transvenously and, because of its design, has a high rate of patency. The Greenfield filter compares favorably with earlier devices such as the Mobin-Uddin umbrella for protection against pulmonary embolism and has a far superior patency rate. It does not require concomitant anticoagulant therapy and, because the hemodynamic disturbances are less, the sequelae of venous outflow obstruction are minimized.

PREVENTION OF DEEP VEIN THROMBOSIS
AND PULMONARY EMBOLISM

Pulmonary embolism has long been recognized as one of the most important complications of both medical and surgical patients and it has been estimated to be responsible for 100,000 deaths per year in the United States. Many of these deaths occur in terminally ill patients but a significant proportion occur in patients who would otherwise lead a normal life.[42,43] Most of these pulmonary emboli could be prevented by the use of established prophylactic procedures in high-risk patients. It has been estimated, for example, that the routine use of effective prophylaxis in patients undergoing elective general surgery could prevent 4000 to 8000 postoperative deaths annually.[44] Risk factors for deep venous thrombosis have been identified. These include advanced age, a history of previous thromboembolism, the presence of malignancy, cardiac failure, prolonged immobility or paralysis, obesity, and varicose veins. In addition, certain surgical procedures including orthopedic surgery to the lower limbs, and operations involving extensive pelvic surgery or associated direct operative trauma to veins, carry a particularly high risk of postoperative venous thromboembolism. The frequency of fatal pulmonary embolism ranges from 0.1% to 0.8% in patients undergoing general elective surgery,[45-47] 0.3% to 1.7% in patients undergoing elective hip surgery,[48-50] 4% to 7% in patients undergoing emergency hip surgery,[51,52] and 8% in patients following major amputations of the lower extremity.

Although anticoagulant therapy for venous thromboembolism is highly effective, its use in patients with established pulmonary embolism cannot be relied upon to save the maximum number of lives. This is because two thirds or more of patients who die from pulmonary embolism do so within one to two hours of the acute event, too soon for anticoagulant therapy to have an effect on mortality. For this reason, attention has turned to administering prophylactic measures in patients at high risk of venous thromboembolism. Two approaches can be taken to prevent fatal pulmonary embolism. These are the early detection of subclinical deep vein thrombosis by screening of high-risk individuals (eg, screening of postoperative high-risk patients with fibrinogen I 125 leg scanning) and primary prophylaxis using drugs or physical methods that are effective against deep vein thrombosis. Primary prophylaxis is likely to be more effective and less expensive. The ideal primary prophylactic method should be safe, effective, accepted by patients, nurses, and medical staff, and easily administered. It should also be inexpensive and require minimal monitoring.

The mechanisms which are recognized to be important in the pathogenesis of venous thromboembolism are venous stasis, activation of blood coagulation, and endothelial damage. Venous thrombi usually develop at sites of slow or disturbed flow and begin as small deposits of platelet, fibrin, and red cells in valve cusp or in the intramuscular sinuses of leg veins.[48,53] As the thrombus grows, it occludes the lumen of the vein producing stasis and then extends both proximally and distally as a coagulation thrombus composed of red cells with interspersed fibrin. The prophylactic methods which have been evaluated clinically have been directed at one or more of these pathogenic factor mechanisms and include mechanical devices which prevent stasis; anticoagulants which counteract the activation of blood coagulation; and drugs which suppress function of platelets and their interaction with damaged endothelial vessel wall. Results of adequately designed randomized clinical trials provide the basis for the current understanding of prophylaxis against venus thromboembolism.

Oral Anticoagulants

Oral anticoagulants are highly effective for preventing fatal pulmonary embolism in patients undergoing hip surgery, but clinically significant bleeding occurs more frequently than with other measures. Because of the bleeding risk, oral anticoagulants are not widely used for primary prophylaxis. To minimize the risk of bleeding, careful laboratory control is required to maintain the prothrombin time at 1½ to two times the control value.

Oral anticoagulant prophylaxis is likely to be effective for preventing fatal pulmonary embolism in other high-risk groups; eg, patients with fractures of the shaft of the femur.

Subcutaneous Heparin Prophylaxis

Low doses of subcutaneous heparin are effective for preventing venus thrombosis and fatal and nonfatal pulmonary embolism in patients undergoing general surgery, and the administration of low-dose heparin has become an accepted technic of antithrombotic prophylaxis in this patient group.[45,54-64] The effectiveness of the minidose heparin regimen (5000 IU every eight or 12 hours) is based on the observation that concentrations of heparin, although inadequate for preventing the progression of established thrombi, can block the action of activated clotting factors higher in the intrinsic clotting cascade, and thus preventing thrombus formation. Except for the increased frequency of would hematomas, clinically significant bleeding occurs very infrequently. For reasons of both effectiveness and safety, low-dose heparin is the prophylaxis of choice in general surgical patients. Subcutaneous heparin prophylaxis should be continued until the patient is fully ambulant because protection is lost if heparin prophylaxis is discontinued while the patient remains immobilized. Low-dose heparin has not proved to be equally effective in all groups studied. Results of studies evaluating heparin prophylaxis,[64-70] in patients undergoing prostatic surgery,[70-72] or hip surgery are conflicting; thus, at best, heparin prophylaxis is only partially effective in these groups. Low-dose subcutaneous heparin is effective for reducing the frequency of venous thrombosis in patients recovering from myocardial infarction[64] but this approach may not be the prophylactic method of choice in this group because, when used in low doses, heparin may be ineffective for preventing mural thrombosis embolizing systemically.

304

Intravenous Dextran

Dextran is a glucose polymer which was introduced as a volume expander and was then subsequently evaluated as an antithrombotic agent.[73-75] Two sizes of dextran polymer have been used clinically; dextran 70 and dextran 40. The antithrombotic properties of dextran have been attributed to a number of actions[76-79] including: (1) decreased blood viscosity, (2) reduced platelet reactivity with the damaged vessel wall, (3) decreased platelet aggregation, and (4) increased susceptibility to fibrinolysis of the fibrin clot formed in the presence of dextran. Dextran is relatively effective in patients undergoing hip surgery[80-83] and significantly reduces the frequency of postoperative venous thrombosis. Dextran is an effective alternative to low-dose heparin for preventing fatal pulmonary embolism in general surgical patients.[59,84-88]

Dextran use may produce volume overload which can result in cardiac failure, particularly in the elderly patient with reduced cardiac reserve. Hypersensitivity reactions have also been noted which are lower with dextran 40 than dextran 70. Excessive bruising has been noted with the use of dextran but clinically important bleeding has not been a serious problem in general surgical patients.

Because dextran is a highly effective prophylaxis in high-risk patients, with a lower risk of bleeding than oral anticoagulant prophylaxis, it is an acceptable alternative to oral anticoagulants. In patients at less severe risk, it has no advantage over minidose heparin or external pneumatic compression, and is more expensive and requires intravenous infusion.

Intermittent Pneumatic Compression and Other Devices that Enhance Venous Blood Flow in the Legs

It is well established that stasis occurs in leg veins perioperatively and postoperatively in patients who are immobilized. Technics designed to increase blood flow are elastic stockings, leg elevation and intensive physiotherapy, graduated pressure stockings, electric calf muscle stimulation, and intermittent calf compression. The most effective of these is intermittent calf compression and it is of interest that this method enhances not only venous blood flow in the legs but also fibrinolysis. Simple measures[89-93] such as early ambulation and the use of leg elevation are relatively ineffective and should be accompanied by one of the more active prophylactic approaches.

Intermittent external compression of the legs with inflatable boots[66,94-98] or cuffs reduces the pooling of blood in the peripheral veins and increases the rate of velocity of venous flow in the lower extremities. Systemic fibrinolytic activity is also enhanced.

The major advantage to intermittent calf compression is the lack of side-effects. It is an effective method for preventing postoperative deep vein thrombosis in patients undergoing general surgery, urologic surgery, neurosurgery, or major elective knee surgery. Because there are no bleeding complications with external pneumatic compression, the technic is particularly attractive in patients at a potentially high risk of hemorrhagic complications, eg, neurosurgery patients and patients undergoing urologic procedures or major knee surgery.

Antiplatelet Therapy

The use of the antiplatelet drugs sulfinpyrazone, dipyridamole, or aspirin has little place in the prevention of venous thromboembolism. The exception is the observation that aspirin reduces the frequency of postoperative venous thrombosis in men only who have undergone elective total hip replacements.

**Recommended Practical Approaches for
Prevention of Venous Thromboembolism in
Patient Subgroups**

General surgical patients   Subcutaneous low-dose heparin and dextran are both effective agents for preventing fatal and nonfatal postoperative venous thromboembolism in patients undergoing general surgical procedures. Low-dose heparin is more convenient than dextran and therefore the prophylaxis of choice. Low-dose heparin is administered as a 5000-IU dose, two hours preoperatively and then every eight or 12 hours postoperatively.

Intermittent pneumatic compression offers an alternative approach in patients who are at risk from bleeding complications (eg, those undergoing spinal anesthesia). Oral anticoagulant prophylaxis is associated with an increased risk of bleeding and, for this reason, should be reserved for those patients who are at very high risk, such as those with both malignancy and a past history of venous thromboembolism.

The risk of venous thromboembolism in patients undergoing elective abdominal thoracic surgical procedures can be divided into three categories depending on the patient's age, nature and extent of the operative procedure, and on whether or not there is a history of previous thromboembolism (see Table 14-5a). Low-risk patients are those under the age of 40 without previous venous thromboembolism who have uncomplicated operative procedures, and those over the age of 40 with minor surgical procedures lasting less than 30 minutes and which do not result in immobilization. Moderate-risk patients are defined as those over the age of 40 who have abdominal or thoracic procedures performed under general anesthesia and which last for at least 30 minutes. The degree of risk increases with age and risk factors such as malignant disease, extensive surgical dissection, large bowel surgery, varicose veins, and obesity. Finally, a very high-risk group exists who have a history of previous venous thromboembolism or who have extensive pelvic or abdominal surgery for advanced malignant disease.

**Table 14-5a
Categories of Risk and Suggested Prophylaxis in Elective
Abdominal or Thoracic Surgical Patients**

Nature of Thromboembolic Event	Low Risk*	Moderate Risk†	High Risk
Calf vein thrombosis	< 3%	10%–40%	30%–60%
Proximal vein thrombosis	< 1%	2%–8%	6%–12%
Fatal pulmonary embolism	< 0.01%	0.1%–0.7%	1%–2%
Prophylaxis of choice	Early ambulation Graduated compression	Low-dose heparin or intermittent pneumatic compression	Continuous low-to-moderate-dose heparin or intermittent pneumatic compression plus low-dose heparin or oral anticoagulants

*See text for description of low-, moderate-, and high-risk patients.
†Risk increased by obesity, age, malignancy, varicose veins, or prolonged bed rest.

Patients in the low-risk category have less than a 3% chance of developing a thrombosis and it would be reasonable to use physical methods such as graduated compression stockings and early ambulation as the only form of prophylaxis, unless complications develop requiring continued bed rest.

Patients in the moderate-risk category have an increased risk with fatal pulmonary embolism occurring in 0.5% to 0.8% and should be treated prophylactically with lose-dose heparin or, if there is a contraindication to heparin prophylaxis, with intermittent pneumatic compression. Low-dose heparin (5000 IU two hours preoperatively and then every eight or 12 hours postoperatively) has been shown to be effective in reducing venous thrombosis and pulmonary embolism with a minimal risk of bleeding, and this represents the prophylactic method of choice in this group. External pneumatic compression, commenced either at the time of surgery or in the immediate postoperative period and continued until the patient is fully ambulant, appears equally effective in preventing venous thrombosis, but has not been extensively evaluated for the prevention of pulmonary embolism. This represents an acceptable alternative to low-dose heparin and is the method of choice in moderate-risk patients who have increased risk of developing operative or postoperative hemorrhage. Although dextran is also effective, it is less convenient to administer and its use is associated with a greater frequency of side-effects than low-dose heparin or external pneumatic compression and, thus, is not the prophylactic method of choice for moderate-risk patients.

Patients in the very high-risk group are a difficult problem because, if unprotected, they suffer a 1% to 2% frequency of fatal pulmonary emboli. The relative effectiveness of different forms of prophylaxis has not been studied in these patients but, on the basis of current evidence, it is reasonable to suggest one of the following regimens: (1) Continuous intravenous heparin administered by the infusion pump commencing preoperatively and adjusted to maintain the heparin level at 1¼ to 1½ times controlled aPTT. This approach is unlikely to lead to serious bleeding and the dose of heparin can be gradually increased as the risk of bleeding lessens in the postoperative period. (2) A combination of external pneumatic compression with low-dose subcutaneous heparin commencing in the early postoperative period and continued until the patient is fully ambulant. Although not formally tested, it is likely to be effective in preventing major thromboembolic events in this patient group. (3) Oral anticoagulants commencing preoperatively at a dose to maintain the prothrombin time at approximately 1½ times control.

Gynecologic surgery Patients having undergone gynecologic surgery could be divided into low-, moderate-, and high-risk groups in a similar way to those having elective abdominal or thoracic surgery. In the low-risk group, the frequency of venous thromboembolism in patients

Table 14-5b
Risk and Prophylactic Methods in Other Patient Groups

	Risk of Thromboembolic Event (%)	Recommended Prophylaxis
Orthopedic		
Elective hip	40%–60%	Oral anticoagulants commencing postoperatively, or dextran*
Fractured hip	40%–60%	Oral anticoagulants commencing postoperatively
Major knee surgery	60%–70%	External pneumatic compression*
Genitourinary Surgery		
Transurethral	7%–10%	External pneumatic compression*
Abdominal	25%–50%	
Neurosurgery	20%–25%	External pneumatic compression*
Major trauma to lower limbs	50%	External pneumatic compression or dextran or oral anticoagulants after patient has stablized
Myocardial infarction	20%–40%	Low-dose heparin* or full-dose heparin, or oral anticoagulants
Stroke	60%	Intermittent pneumatic compression or low-dose heparin
Other high-risk medical groups		Low-dose heparin

*Efficacy demonstrated by clinical trial.

under 40 having a simple hysterectomy or similar operation is extremely low. These patients do not need specific prophylactic measures although early mobilization should be encouraged. Patients in the moderate-risk group are those above the age of 40 who have a surgical procedure performed that lasts more than 30 minutes. These patients can be treated in the same way as the moderate-risk group in general surgery. Patients in the high-risk group are those over the age of 50 who have an additional risk factor, such as obesity, would infection, varicose veins, malignant disease, heart disease, or previous thromboembolic disease. This group should be treated prophylactically along the lines recommended for high-risk groups in elective general surgery.

Genitourinary surgery External pneumatic compression is the method of choice in patients undergoing prostatic surgery. Patients who have extensive pelvic surgery for invasive carcinoma are at very high risk and can be treated with a combination of pneumatic compression and anticoagulants. Pneumatic compression should be commenced at the time of surgery and continued for the period of immobilization. Heparin or oral anticoagulants can be started postoperatively when the risk of bleeding has diminished.

Neurosurgery Anticoagulants are potentially dangerous in this group because even minimal intracranial bleeding can be catastrophic. External pneumatic compression is effective and is the prophylactic method of choice in neurosurgical patients.

Elective hip surgery Between 1% and 2% of unprotected patients who do have elective hip surgery suffer fatal pulmonary embolism. Oral anticoagulant prophylaxis is effective in this group but it is associated with an increased risk of clinically significant bleeding. Bleeding may be less if oral anticoagulants are started immediately postoperatively. Dextran, using 500 ml twice the day of surgery and 500 ml daily for three to four days, is effective but its widespread acceptance has been slow because of doubt about its safety (mainly the risk of bleeding) and the inconvenience of intravenous administration. On the basis of current evidence, this is the treatment of choice. Results with low-dose heparin and aspirin have been inconsistent and the protection afforded is incomplete. Screening with combined fibrinogen I 125 leg scanning and impedance plethysmography is an alternative which, by early detection and treatment of subclinical deep vein thrombosis, reduces the frequency of fatal pulmonary embolism. However, this approach is considerably more expensive than primary prophylaxis.

Fractured hips The application of effective prophylaxis in patients who have sustained a fractured hip is more difficult than in patients undergoing elective hip surgery.

The risk of fatal pulmonary embolism after surgery for a fractured hip is about 5%. Many of these patients are elderly and therefore are at particularly high risk of bleeding with anticoagulant therapy. Also, there is considerable risk of volume overload if treated prophylactically with dextran. We have used oral anticoagulant prophylaxis in selected patients with fractured hips and begin the oral anticoagulant therapy the day after emergency surgery. If, however, surgery is delayed, treatment is begun but then withheld for 48 hours prior to surgery. The other forms of prophylaxis such as low-dose heparin are, at best, only partially effective in this group. Intermittent pneumatic compression is also not recommended as the sole method of prophylaxis in this group as it may also be only partially effective.

Although effective oral anticoagulant prophylaxis has not been accepted because of the potential risk of major bleeding and the need for laboratory control, no safe, acceptable, proven method of primary prophylaxis is available in this group at present. Therefore, in this group, screening with impedance plethysmography and fibrogen I 125 leg scanning to allow early detection of deep vein thrombosis is a practical alternative.

Major knee surgery Patients undergoing major knee surgery are at potentially high risk of postoperative venous thrombosis, depending on the age of the patient and the extent and nature of the surgery. In young patients undergoing menisectomy, the risk of postoperative thrombosis is relatively low, while in the elderly patient undergoing total knee replacement it is as high as 60%. Intermittent pneumatic compression is a highly effective form of prophylaxis in patients undergoing elective knee surgery and is the method of choice in this patient group.

Major trauma of legs or pelvis Approximately 50% of patients with fractured pelvis or lower limbs develop venous thrombosis. Information on effective prophylactic approaches in these patients is extremely limited. External pneumatic compression could be effective, but if a complete plaster cast is applied to the lower limb or if there is extensive tissue trauma, external compression cannot be used. Alternative forms of prophylaxis are oral anticoagulants commenced 48 to 72 hours after trauma (when it has been clearly established that there is no serious internal injury) and dextran, although the latter could be dangerous in patients with oliguria.

Burns Patients with major burns are at high risk for developing venous thromboembolism. It is likely that low-dose heparin would be effective in these patients and, if practical, is the prophylactic method of choice. Oral anticoagulant therapy, commenced at the time of admission or soon thereafter would be a reasonable alternative.

Myocardial infarction Low-dose heparin is effective in reducing the frequency of venous thrombosis in these patients, but there is no evidence that this approach is effective in preventing systemic embolism. Patients with extensive acute myocardial infarction are at high risk of developing systemic embolism and they should be started on a combination of full-dose heparin and oral anticoagulants when admitted to hospital. Heparin therapy can be stopped after three to five days and oral anticoagulants continued for three to four weeks. Alternative approaches which are likely to be effective include subcutaneous heparin in doses of 7000 to 10,000 IU three times daily while the patient remains hospitalized, or subcutaneous heparin for the first three to four days in combination with oral anticoagulants, the latter to be continued until the patient is discharged. A moderate-dose subcutaneous heparin regimen is particularly useful if facilities for laboratory monitoring are not available. Patients with subendocardial myocardial infarction have a lower risk of systemic embolism, and in these patients it would be reasonable to limit prophylaxis to low-dose heparin while in hospital.

Stroke patients Patients who sustain paralytic stroke are at high risk of developing venous thromboembolism. It is likely that either external pneumatic compression or low-dose heparin would be effective in preventing serious venous thromboembolism in this group. External pneumatic compression has the advantage of not exposing the patient to the risk of intracerebral bleeding.

Other high-risk groups Venous thromboembolism is a common complication of other medical groups. These include patients with chronic obstructive lung disease and patients with other chronic disorders. The use of prophylaxis has not been extensively evaluated in these patients, but it would be reasonable to use either low-dose heparin, pneumatic compression, or oral anticoagulants as prophylaxis in these patients.

Secondary prevention of pulmonary embolism by early detection of venous thrombosis An alternative approach for preventing massive pulmonary embolism is the early detection (and treatment) of subclinical venous thrombosis by the use of currently available screening tests. In the majority of hospitalized patients, venous thrombosis, occurring as a complication of surgery or severe medical illness, is subclinical and cannot be detected by clinical examination. The use of currently available screening tests, in particular, fibrinogen I 125 leg scanning, provides the clinician with the means of early detection and treatment.

Because mass screening of high-risk patients is cost-effective by comparison with primary prophylaxis, the use of screening should be confined to selected patients for whom primary prophylaxis is either not applicable or is ineffective. In medical patients and most surgical patients, fibrinogen I 125 leg scanning of the lower extremities is the screening procedure of choice, being sensitive to thrombi in the calf, distal thigh, and mid-thigh where 95% of thrombi occur in such patients. When the nature of the operation or illness increases the prevalence of iliofemoral thrombi without accompanying calf thrombi, as in total hip replacement or pelvic lymph node dissection, an additional technic sensitive to proximal thrombi should be added, eg, impedance plethysmography. The use of impedance plethysmography alone for screening high-risk patients is of limited value because it fails to detect the majority of calf vein thrombi. Furthermore, it is less sensitive for detecting asymptomatic proximal vein thrombosis since many asymptomatic thrombi are nonobstructive.

Cost effectiveness of prophylaxis Many North American hospitals lack an organized strategy for preventing venous thromboembolism. The reasons for this are complex and range from doubts as to the safety of anticoagulant therapy to lack of awareness that the problem is of significant proportions. The latter situation has arisen because massive or fatal pulmonary embolism is a relatively rare event. It is compounded by the fact that any side-effects attributable to the prophylactic approach are highly visible, whereas the benefits pass unnoticed.

Although there is an extensive body of literature on the safety and efficacy of various prophylactic measures, little attention has been addressed to the economic implications of prophylaxis. Cost-effectiveness analysis allows an objective comparison to be made of the cost of different prophylactic strategies expressed in terms of death due to pulmonary embolism averted. We have performed a cost-effectiveness analysis of strategies for preventing fatal pulmonary embolism based on over 1000 high-risk patients undergoing abdominothoracic surgery. Effectiveness was measured in terms of the number of deaths from pulmonary embolism averted. The total cost incurred by applying an approach against venous thromboembolism can be categorized as follows: (1) the cost of the prophylactic agent or measure, (2) the diagnostic cost of confirming the presence of venous thromboembolism in patients who suffer clinically suspected venous thrombosis or pulmonary embolism, (3) the cost of treating patients with deep-vein thrombosis and nonfatal pulmonary embolism, (4) the cost of excess in-hospital stay for patients requiring treatment of deep-vein thrombosis or pulmonary embolism, (5) the cost of side-effects of the prophylactic measures, and (6) the cost of side-effects of treatment of patients who develop venous thrombosis or pulmonary embolism.

The costs outlined in Table 14-6 are based on those that would be incurred in a hospital in North America (Hamilton, Ontario, Canada).[99] No prophylaxis other than early ambulation and physiotherapy in 1000 general surgical patients would result in eight deaths from massive pulmonary embolism at a cost of approximately $79,927, which represents the costs of treatment incurred by patients developing deep-vein thrombosis and pulmonary embolism. By comparison, low-dose subcutaneous heparin prophylaxis would result in a saving of seven lives per 1000 surgical patients at a cost of approximately $39,722 per 1000 surgical patients. The use of dextran prophylaxis is considerably more

312

Table 14-6
Total Cost of Each Prophylactic Strategy

Strategy	Cost $ (1982)
Traditional (no program) approach	
Venography in 40 patients	3,520
Lung scanning in 30 patients	3,510
Treatment of venous thromboembolism in 32 patients	72,897
Total cost per 1000 patients	79,927
Leg scanning with fibrinogen I 125	
Scanning for 7 days in 1000 patients	85,000
Venography in 135 patients	11,880
Lung scanning in 15 patients	1,755
Treatment of venous thromboembolism in 114 patients	251,826
Total cost per 1000 patients	350,461
Subcutaneous administration of heparin in low doses	
Administration for 7 days to 1000 patients	20,000
Ascending venography in 10 patients	880
Lung scanning in 10 patients	1,170
Treatment of venous thromboembolism in 8 patients	17,672
Total cost per 1000 patients	39,722
Intermittent pneumatic compression of the legs	
Use for 7 days in 1000 patients	33,000
Venography in 10 patients	880
Lung scanning in 10 patients	1,170
Treatment of venous thromboembolism in 8 patients	17,672
Total cost per 1000 patients	52,722
Intravenous administration of dextran	
Administration for 4 days to 1000 patients	103,000
Venography in 20 patients	1,760
Lung scanning in 10 patients	1,170
Treatment of venous thromboembolism in 13 patients	28,717
Total cost per 1000 patients	$ 134,647

expensive and the cost of saving seven lives per 1000 surgical patients is approximately $134,647. Surveillance using early detection with fibrinogen I 125 leg scanning is the most costly. The cost of screening 1000 general surgical patients for seven lives saved by averting massive pulmonary embolism is approximately $333,243. It is clearly evident that the no prophylaxis is cost ineffective. Moreover, the figures do not take into account the economic loss to society of those patients dying from massive pulmonary embolism. If this is taken into account, the burden on society becomes even greater. In the final balance, the decision to use prophylaxis should be based on the observation that it is now possible to avoid much of the tragic and unnecessary loss of life due to massive pulmonary embolism.

REFERENCES

1. Haeger K: Problems of acute deep venous thrombosis. 1. The interpretation of signs and symptoms. *Angiology* 1969;20:219–223.
2. Nicolaides AN, Kakkar VV, Field ES, et al: The origin of deep vein thrombosis: a venographic study. *Br J Radiol* 1971;44:653–663.
3. Gallus AS, Hirsh J, Hull R, et al: Diagnosis of venous thromboembolism. *Semin Thromb Hemostas* 1976;2:203–231.
4. Kakkar VV, Howe CT, Flanc C, et al: National history of postoperative deep vein thrombosis. *Lancet* 1969;2:230–232.
5. McLachlin J, Richards T, Paterson JC: An evaluation of clinical signs in the diagnosis of venous thrombosis. *Arch Surg* 1962;85:738–744.
6. Lea TM: Phlebography. *Arch Surg* 1972;104:145–151.
7. Rabinov K, Paulin S: Roentgen diagnosis of venous thrombosis in the leg. *Arch Surg* 1972;104:135–144.
8. Bettman MA, Paulin S: Leg phlebography: the incidence, nature and modification of undesirable side effects. *Radiology* 1977;122:101–104.
9. Flanc C, Kakkar VV, Clarke MB: The detection of venous thrombosis of the legs using ^{125}I-labelled fibrinogen. *Br J Surg* 1968;55:742–747.
10. Kakkar VV, Nicolaides AN, Renney JTG, et al: ^{125}I-labelled fibrinogen test adapted for routine screening for deep vein thrombosis. *Lancet* 1970;1: 540–542.
11. Wheeler HB, Pearson D, O'Connell D, et al: Impedance phlebography. Technique, interpretation and results. *Arch Surg* 1972;104:164–169.
12. Wheeler HB, O'Connell JA, Anderson FA, et al: Bedside screening for venous thrombosis using occlusive impedance phlebography. *Angiology* 1975;26:199–210.
13. Hull R, Van Aken WG, Hirsh J, et al: Impedance plethysmography using the occlusive cuff technique in the diagnosis of venous thrombosis. *Circulation* 1976;53:696–700.
14. Johnston KW, Kakkar VV, Spindler JJ, et al: A simple method for detecting deep vein thrombosis. An improved electrical impedance technique. *Am J Surg* 1974;127:349–352.
15. Evans DS: The early diagnosis of thromboembolism by ultrasound. *Ann R Coll Surg Engl* 1971;49:225–249.
16. Homes MCG: Deep venous thrombosis of the lower limbs diagnosed by ultrasound. *Med J Aust* 1973;1:427–430.
17. Sigel B, Felix WR, Popky GL, et al: Diagnosis of lower limb venous thrombosis by Doppler ultrasound technique. *Arch Surg* 1972;104:174–179.
18. Strandness DE, Sumner DS: Ultrasonic velocity detector in the diagnosis of thrombophlebitis. *Arch Surg* 1972;104:180–183.
19. Barnes RW, Collicott PE, Mozersky DJ, et al: Non-invasive quantitation of maximum venous outflow in acute thrombophlebitis. *Surgery* 1972;72: 971–979.
20. Cooke ED, Pilcher MF: Deep vein thrombosis: a preclinical diagnosis by thermography. *Br J Surg* 1974;61:971–978.
21. Highman JH, O'Sullivan E, Thomas E: Isotope venography. *Br J Surg* 1973; 60:58–60.
22. Johnson WC, Patten DH, Widrich WC, et al: Technetium 99^{m} isotope venography. *Am J Surg* 1974;127:424–428.
23. Kakkar V: The diagnosis of deep vein thrombosis using the ^{125}I-fibrinogen test. *Arch Surg* 1972;104:152–159.
24. Browse NL: The ^{125}I-fibrinogen uptake test. *Arch Surg* 1972;104:160–163.

25. Kakkar VV: Fibrinogen uptake test for detection of deep vein thrombosis. A review of current practice. *Semin Nucl Med* 1977;7:229–244.

26. Hull R, Hirsh J, Powers P: Impedance plethysmography: The relationship between venous filling and sensitivity and specificity for proximal vein thrombosis. *Circulation* 1978;58:898–902.

27. Biland L, Hull R, Hirsh J, et al: The use of electromyography to detect muscle contraction responsible for falsely positive impedance plethysmographic results. *Thromb Res* 1979;14:811–816.

28. Cranley JJ, Gay AY, Grass AM, et al: A plethysmographic technique for the diagnosis of deep vein thrombosis of the lower extremities. *Surg Gynecol Obstet* 1973;136:385–394.

29. Hull R, Hirsh J: Replacement of venography in suspected venous thrombosis by impedance plethysmography and 125 I-fibrinogen leg scanning. *Ann Intern Med* 1981;94:12–15.

30. Harris WH, Salzman EW, Athanasoulis C, et al: Comparison of 125 I-fibrinogen count scanning with phlebography for detection of venous thrombi after elective hip surgery. *N Engl J Med* 1975;292:665–667.

31. Hull R, Hirsh J, Sackett D, et al: Combined use of leg scanning and impedance plethysmography in suspected venous thrombosis. An alternative to venography. *N Engl J Med* 1977;296:1497–1500.

32. Hull R, Hirsh J, Sackett D, et al: Cost-effectiveness of clinical diagnosis, venography and non-invasive testing in patients with symptomatic deep-vein thrombosis. *N Engl J Med* 1981;304:1561–1567.

33. Hull R, Delmore T, Carter C, et al: Adjusted subcutaneous heparin versus warfarin sodium in the long-term treatment of venous thrombosis. *N Engl J Med* 1982;306:189–194.

34. Hull R, Delmore T, Genton E, et al: Warfarin sodium versus low dose heparin in the long-term treatment of venous thrombosis. *N Engl J Med* 1979;301:855–858.

35. Hull R, Hirsh J, Jay R, et al: A randomized trial of two different intensities of oral anticoagulant therapy in the long-term treatment of patients with proximal vein thrombosis: less intense oral anticoagulant therapy. *N Engl J Med* 1982;307:1676–1681.

36. Thrombolytic therapy in thrombosis: A National Intitute of Health Consensus Development Conference. *Ann Intern Med* 1980;93:141–144.

37. Gallus AS, Hirsh J: Treatment of venous thromboembolic disease. *Semin Thromb Hemostas* 1976;2:291–331.

38. Urokinase pulmonary embolism trials: A national co-operative study. Chapter 11, morbidity and mortality. *Circulation* 1973;47–48 (suppl 2):66–72.

39. Urokinase streptokinase embolism trial. Phase 2 results. A co-operative study. *JAMA* 1974;229:1606–1613.

40. Kakkar VV, Flanc C, Howe CT, et al: Treatment of deep vein thrombosis. A trial of heparin, streptokinase and Arvin. *Br Med J* 1969;1:806–810.

41. Marder VJ, Soulen RL. Atichartakarn V, et al: Quantitative venographic assessment of deep vein thrombosis in the evaluation of streptokinase and heparin therapy. *J Lab Clin Med* 1977;89:1018–1029.

42. Morrell MT, Dunnill MS: The post-mortem incidence of pulmonary embolism in a hospital population. *Br J Surg* 1968;55:347–352.

43. Coon WW, Coller FA: Clinicopathologic correlation in thromboembolism. *Surg Gynecol Obstet* 1959;109:259–269.

44. Fratatoni J, Wessler S: Prophylactic therapy of deep vein thrombosis and pulmonary embolism. US Dept of Health, Education, and Welfare, 1975, pp 76–866.

45. International multicentre trial prevention of fatal postoperative pulmonary embolism by low doses of heparin. *Lancet* 1975;2:45–51.

46. Shepard RM, White HA, Shirkey AL: Anticoagulant prophylaxis of thromboembolism in postsurgical patients. *Am J Surg* 1966;112:698–702.

47. Skinner DB, Salzman EW: Anticoagulant prophylaxis in surgical patients. *Surg Gynecol Obstet* 1967;125:741–746.

48. Harris WH, Salzman EW, DeSanctis RW: The prevention of thromboembolic disease by prophylactic anticoagulants. A controlled study in elective hip surgery. *J Bone Joint Surg Am* 1967;49:81–89.

49. Johnston TC: Clinical follow up of total hip replacement. *Clin Orthop* 1973; 95:118–126.

50. Todd RC, Lightowler CDR, Harris J: Total hip replacement in osteoarthrosis using the Charnley prosthesis. *Br Med J* 1972;2:752–755.

51. Eskeland G, Solheim K, Skjorten F: Anticoagulant prophylaxis, thromboembolism and mortality in elderly patients with hip fractures. A controlled clinical trial. *Acta Chir Scand* 1966;131:16–29.

52. Sevitt S, Gallagher NG: Prevention of venous thrombosis and pulmonary embolism in injured patients. Trial of anticoagulant prophylaxis with phenidione in middle-aged and elderly patients with fractured necks of femur. *Lancet* 1959;2:981–989.

53. Sevitt S: Organization of valve pocket thrombi and the anomalies of double thrombi and valve cusp involvement. *Br J Surg* 1974;61:641–649.

54. Gordon-Smith IC, LeQuesne LP, Grundy DJ, et al: Controlled trial of two regimens of subcutaneous heparin in prevention of postoperative deep vein thrombosis. *Lancet* 1972;1:1133–1135.

55. Kakkar VV, Corrigan T, Spindler J, et al: Efficacy of low doses of heparin in prevention of deep-vein thrombosis after major surgery; a double blind randomized trial. *Lancet* 1972;2:101–106.

56. Nicolaides AN, Dupont PA, Desais S, et al: Small doses of subcutaneous sodium heparin in preventing deep venous thrombosis after major surgery. *Lancet* 1972;2:890–893.

57. Ballard RM, Bradley-Watson PJ, Johnstone FD, et al: Low doses of subcutaneous heparin in the prevention of deep vein thrombosis after gynaecological surgery. *J Obstet Gynecol Br Commonw* 1973;80:469–472.

58. Lahnborg G, Bergstrom K, Friman L, et al: Effect of low-dose heparin on incidence of postoperative pulmonary embolism detected by photoscanning. *Lancet* 1974;1:329–331.

59. Heparin versus dextran in the prevention of deep vein thrombosis. A multiunit controlled trial. *Lancet* 1974;2:118–120.

60. Abernethy EE, Hartsuck JM: Postoperative pulmonary embolism. A prospective study utilizing low-dose heparin. *Am J Surg* 1974;128:739–742.

61. Covey TH, Sherman L, Baue E: Low dose heparin in postoperative patients, a prospective, coded study. *Arch Surg* 1975;110:1021–1025.

62. Rosenberg IL, Evans M, Pollock AV: Prophylaxis of postoperative leg vein thrombosis by low-dose subcutaneous heparin of perioperative calf muscle stimulation: A controlled clinical trial. *Br Med J* 1975;1:649–651.

63. Gruber UF, Duckert F, Fridrick R, et al: Prevention of postoperative thromboembolism by dextran 40, low doses of heparin, or xantinol nicotinate. *Lancet* 1977;1:207–210.

64. Gallus AS, Hirsh J, Tuttle RJ, et al: Small subcutaneous doses of heparin in prevention of venous thrombosis. *N Engl J Med* 1973;288:545–551.

65. Hume M, Kuriakose T, Zuck L, et al: 125 I-fibrinogen and the prevention of venous thrombosis. *Arch Surg* 1973;107:803–806.

66. Hampson WGJ, Harris FC, Lucas HK, et al: Failure of low-dose heparin to

prevent deep vein thrombosis after hip replacement arthroplasty. *Lancet* 1974;2:795–797.

67. Morris GK, Henry APJ, Preston BJ: Prevention of deep vein thrombosis by low-dose heparin in patients undergoing total hip replacement. *Lancet* 1974;2: 797–800.

68. Dechavanne M, Soudin F, Viala JJ, et al: Prevention des thromboses veineuses. Succes de l'heparine a fortes doses lors des coxarthroses. *Nouv Presse Med* 1974;3:1317–1319.

69. Venous thrombosis clinical study group. Small doses of subcutaneous sodium heparin in the prevention of deep vein thrombosis after elective hip operations. *Br J Surg* 1975;62:348–350.

70. Becker J, Borgstrom S, Salzman GF: Incidence of thrombosis associated with epsilon aminocaproic acid administration and with combined epsilon aminocaproic acid and subcutaneous heparin therapy. II: A clinical study with the aid of intravenous phlebography. *Acta Chir Scand* 1970;136:167–171.

71. Coe N, Collins RE, Klein LA, et al: Prevention of deep vein thrombosis in urological patients: a controlled randomized trial of low-dose heparin and external pneumatic compression boots. *Surgery* 1978;83:230–234.

72. Kutnowske M, Vandendris M, Steinberger R, et al: Prevention of postoperative deep vein thrombosis by low-dose heparin in urological surgery. A double-blind randomized study. *Urol Res* 1977;5:123–125.

73. Atik M: Dextran 40 and dextran 70: A review. *Arch Surg* 1967;94:664–672.

74. Data JL, Nies AS: Dextran 40. *Ann Intern Med* 1974;81:500–504.

75. Gruber UF: *Dextran in Blood Replacement*. Berlin-Heidelberg-New York, Springer Verlag 1969, pp 55–104.

76. Ponder E, Ponder RV: Age and molecular weight of dextrans, their coating effects and their interaction with serum albumin. *Nature* 1961;190:277–278.

77. Weiss H: The effect of clinical dextran on platelet aggregation, adhesion, and ADP release in man: in vivo and in vitro studies. *J Lab Clin Med* 1967;69: 37–46.

78. Wallenbeck IAM, Tangen O: On the lysis of fibrin formed in the presence of dextran and other macromolecules. *Thromb Res* 1975;6:75–86.

79. Aberg M, Bergentz SE, Hedner U: The effect of dextran on the lysability of ex vivo thrombi. *Ann Surg* 1975;181:342–345.

80. Ahlberg A, Nylander G, Robertson B, et al: Dextran in prophylaxis of thrombosis in fractures of the hip. *Acta Chir Scand* 1968;387 (suppl):83–85.

81. Johnsson SR, Bygdeman S, Eliasson R: Effect of dextran on postoperative thrombosis. *Acta Chir Scand* 1968;387 (suppl):80–82.

82. Myhe HO, Holen A: Tromboseprofylakse. Dextran eller warfarinnatrium? *Nord Med* 1969;82:1534–1538.

83. Evarts CM, Feil EJ: Prevention of thromboembolic disease after elective surgery of the hip. *J Bone Joint Surg Am* 1971;53:1271–1280.

84. Becker J, Schampi B: The incidence of postoperative venous thrombosis of the legs. A comparative study on the prophylactic effect of dextran 70 and electrical calf-muscle stimulation. *Acta Chir Scand* 1973;139:357–367.

85. Bonnar J, Walsh J: Prevention of thrombosis after pelvic surgery by British dextran 70. *Lancet* 1972;1:614–616.

86. Carter AE, Eban R: The prevention of postoperative deep venous thrombosis with Dextran 70. *Br J Surg* 1973;60:681–683.

87. Bonnar J, Walsh JJ, Haddon M: Thromboembolism following radical surgery for carcinoma-prevention by dextran 70 infusion during and immediately after operation. IVth International Congress on Thrombosis and Haemostasis. Vienna, 1973;278:A.

88. Kline A, Hughes LE, Campbell H: Dextran 70 in prophylaxis of thromboembolic disease after surgery: A clinically oriented randomized double-blind trial. *Br Med J* 1975;2:109–112.

89. Rosengarten DS, Laird J: The effect of leg elevation on the incidence of deep-vein thrombosis after operation. *Br J Surg* 1971;58:182–184.

90. Tsapogas MJ, Goussous H, Peabody RA, et al: Postoperative venous thrombosis and the effectiveness of prophylactic measures. *Arch Surg* 1971;103:561–567.

91. Browse NL, Jackson BT, Mayo ME, et al: The value of mechanical methods of preventing postoperative calf vein thrombosis. *Br J Surg* 1974;61:219–223.

92. Rosengarten DS, Laird J, Jeyasingh K, et al: The failure of compression stockings (Tubigrip) to prevent deep venous thrombosis after operation. *Br J Surg* 1970;57:296–299.

93. Scurr JH, Ibrahim SZ, Faber RG, et al: The efficacy of graduate compression stockings in the prevention of deep vein thrombosis. *Br J Surg* 1977;64:371–373.

94. Sabri S, Roberts VC, Cotton LT: Prevention of early postoperative deep vein thrombosis by intermittent compression of the leg during surgery. *Br Med J* 1971;4:394–396.

95. Roberts VC, Cotton LT: Prevention of postoperative deep vein thrombosis in patients with malignant disease. *Br Med J* 1974;1:358–360.

96. Turpie AGG, Gallus A, Beattie WS, Hirsh J: Prevention of venous thrombosis in patients with intracranial disease by intermittent pneumatic compression of the calf. *Neurology* 1977;27:435–438.

97. Skillman JJ, Collins RE, Coe NP, et al: Prevention of deep vein thrombosis in neurosurgical patients: A controlled, randomized trial of external pneumatic compression boots. *Surgery* 1978;83:354–358.

98. Hills NG, Pflugg JJ, Jeyasingh K, et al: Prevention of deep vein thrombosis by intermittent pneumatic compression of the calf. *Br Med J* 1972;1:131–135.

99. Hull R, Hirsh J, Sackett D, Stoddart G: Cost effectiveness of primary and secondary prevention of fatal pulmonary embolism in high risk surgical patients. *Can Med Assoc J* 1982;127:990–995.

15 *The Management of the Postphlebitic Syndrome and Its Differentiation from Recurrent Deep Vein Thrombosis*

J.R. Leclerc
R.D. Hull
J. Hirsh

Chronic venous insufficiency of the lower extremity refers to a group of venous disorders in which there is dysfunction of venous valves secondary to congenital or acquired disease. Chronic venous insufficiency is caused by primary varicose veins (including perforator incompetence) and the postphlebitic syndrome. The cause of primary varicose veins is uncertain and by definition the disease is limited to the superficial venous system. The postphlebitic syndrome is caused by deep venous incompetence and/or persistent obstruction following deep vein thrombosis. This results in symptoms of dependent leg edema, ache, stasis dermatitis, and in some case ulceration. The symptoms of swelling and pain may be progressive or intermittent. When the latter occurs the clinical presentation may simulate acute recurrent deep vein thrombosis.

In this chapter we propose to discuss the postphlebitic syndrome and its differentiation from acute recurrent deep vein thrombosis.

POSTPHLEBITIC SYNDROME

The frequency with which venous thrombosis is followed by the postphlebitic syndrome is uncertain. This is because no careful prospective study has ever been performed using uniform objective criteria to diagnose the postphlebitic syndrome and the preceding deep vein thrombosis. Clinical studies are made difficult by the fact that there is a long delay between the initial episode of thrombosis and the onset of the postphlebitic syndrome. Despite this shortcoming, attempts have been made in a number of countries to estimate the frequency of the postphlebitic syndrome in the general population. Symptoms of postphlebitic syndrome are reported in approximately 2% of the population in Sweden,[1] and in Switzerland[2] a study carried out in over 4000 chemical workers reported an incidence of severe venous insufficiency with venous ulceration in over 1% of this population. In a Michigan[3] study of more than

"

9000 adults aged over 20, the prevalence of active or healed venous ulcers was 5/1000 population. Extrapolation of this figure to the general population in the United States suggests that approximately 500,000 Americans have, or have had, venous ulceration.

Understanding the pathophysiology of the postphlebitic syndrome requires a knowledge of the normal anatomy and function of the venous system of the lower extremity.

NORMAL ANATOMY OF THE VENOUS SYSTEM

The venous system in the leg consists of three subsystems: the superficial veins, the deep veins, and the communicating branches (Figure 15-1). The superficial venous system consists of two major veins, the long and short saphenous veins which drain into the common femoral and popliteal veins respectively. The deep venous system of the calf consists of two pairs of veins (posterior tibial and peroneal veins) and the anterior tibial vein. All the deep calf veins converge to form the popliteal vein. The popliteal vein becomes the superficial femoral vein at the junction of the proximal part of the politeal fossa and the adductor canal in the thigh. The superficial femoral vein is joined by the deep femoral vein in the upper thigh to form the common femoral vein which becomes the external iliac vein at the level of the inguinal ligament. The external iliac vein is joined by the internal iliac vein in the pelvis to form the common iliac vein and the two common iliac veins converge to form the inferior vena cava. The deep muscular branches of the calf converge to form the soleal and gastrocnemius plexuses. The soleal plexus drains into the posterior tibial vein and the gastrocnemius plexus drains into the popliteal vein. The superficial system is connected with the deep venous system by communicating veins which contain valves directing blood flow from the superficial to the deep system. The communicating branches are more abundant in the calf and their anatomic location is remarkably constant.[4] Numerous bicuspid valves located throughout the entire venous system maintain the upward flow of blood by preventing reflux. They are most abundant in the calf vessels.[4]

NORMAL FUNCTION OF VENOUS SYSTEM

The venous system of the leg and the surrounding muscles are integrated into a functional unit that maintains venous return[5] (Figure 15-2). In the motionless upright position, the hydrostatic pressure in the dorsal vein of the foot is a function of the vertical column of blood extending from the ankle to the heart and approximates 90 mmHg.[6] This high venous pressure is prevented from being transmitted to the superficial

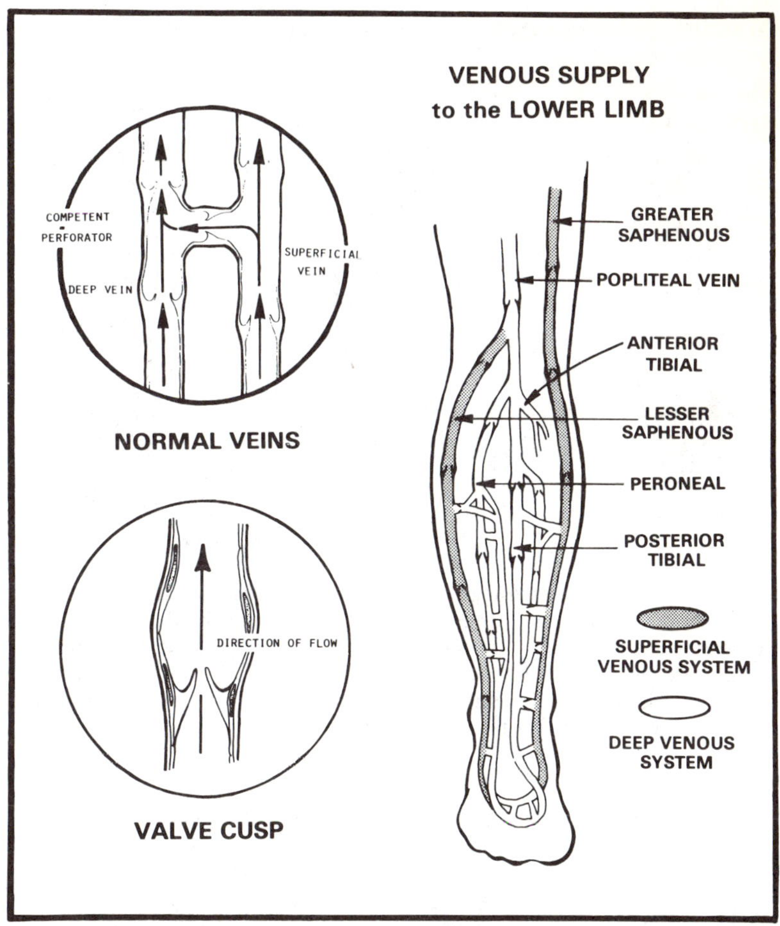

Figure 15-1 Diagram of deep and superficial veins in the leg showing long saphenous (greater saphenous) vein, short saphenous (lesser saphenous) vein, peroneal and posterior tibial veins, and popliteal vein. Circled insets show communicating vein between the superficial and the deep venous system and a valve cusp pocket of a deep vein.

veins by competent valves in the perforating veins. During exercise the deep venous reservoir of the calf empties as a result of muscle contraction. Distal reflux and reflux into the superficial venous system is prevented by competent valves in the deep veins and perforators respectively. During calf contraction the standing venous pressure at the ankle is reduced to 20 mmHg.[6,7] Postexercise, the peripheral venous pressure returns to the preexercise level as the arteriolar inflow refills the deep venous reservoir (Figure 15-3). The recovery time for the distal venous pressure to return to the preexercise baseline level is greater than 20 seconds in normal subjects.[8]

CALF MUSCLE PUMP

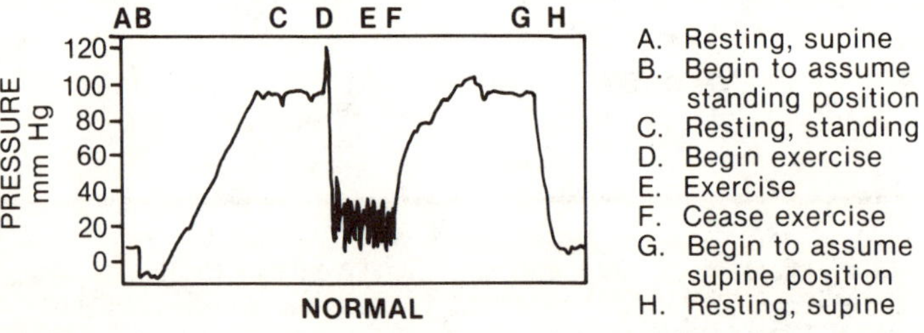

Figure 15-2   Calf muscle pump: During calf muscle relaxation, blood in the deep and superficial veins of the lower limb flows slowly toward the heart from the superficial to the deep venous system (left panel). During the calf muscle contraction, blood in the deep venous system is rapidly propelled toward the heart and if the valves in the connecting veins between the superficial and the deep system are competent, there is no reflux into the superficial system (middle and right panels).

Figure 15-3   Pressure tracing recording from the long saphenous vein at ankle in a normal person. Note rapid decrease in pressure during exercise and return to base-line level with cessation of exercise. (Reproduced from Nicolaides[12] with permission of CV Mosby Co.)

PATHOPHYSIOLOGY OF POSTPHLEBITIC SYNDROME

The postphlebitic syndrome occurs as a consequence of the generation of abnormally high pressure in the deep and superficial veins of the leg.[7] This chronic venous hypertension occurs as a consequence of valvular incompetence with or without outflow obstruction, secondary to venous thrombosis (Figure 15-4). In the motionless erect position, the

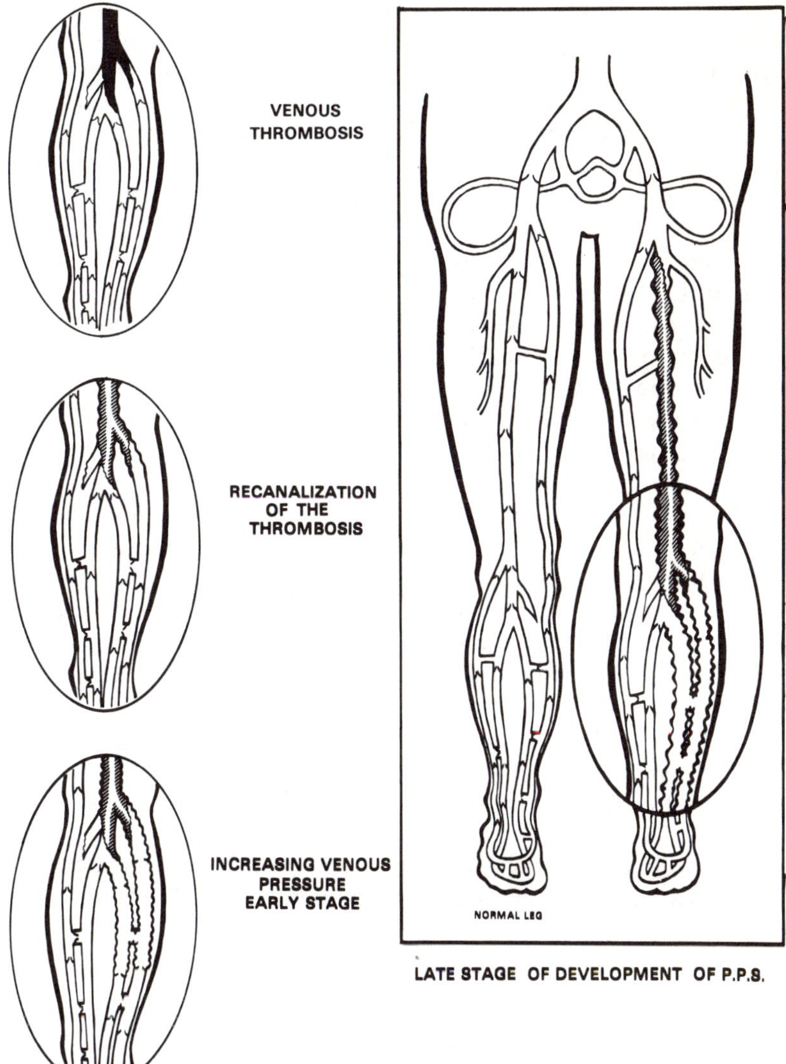

Figure 15-4 Development of the postphlebitic syndrome (PPS). Following acute venous thrombosis (upper panel, left) the thrombus recanalizes (middle panel) leading to valvular destruction and an increase in venous pressure; this in turn results in distention of veins distal to the recanalized segment (lower panel). The resulting venous distention produces further venous dilatation which in turn leads to more extensive valvular incompetence and the development of the postphlebitic syndrome with pain, swelling, pigmentation and, it its most severe form, ulceration. (Reproduced from Johnson[7] with permission of Year Book Medical Publishers.)

hydrostatic pressure in the deep venous system is transmitted to the superficial veins if the valves of the perforators are incompetent. Incompetence of these valves may be caused by their direct involvement by the thrombotic process or by dilatation of the distal veins as a consequence of proximal obstruction. During exercise, venous emptying is impaired due to reflux[9-12] and there is an increase in pressure in the superficial veins if the perforators are incompetent[13] (Figure 15-5). The postphlebitic syndrome can occur without perforator vein incompetence; under these circumstances the symptoms are due to chronic venous hypertension alone.[14]

Chronic venous hypertension may also lead to secondary valvular incompetence and varicosities in the superficial and saphenous veins. Saphenofemoral incompetence increases the inefficiency of the peripheral venous pump since up to 25% of the blood flow will participate in a "circus" movement, ie, a reflux through the saphenofemoral junction.[7] It has been suggested that the competence of the popliteal valves is an important factor in determining the ambulatory venous pressure in postthrombotic limbs.[15]

Venous ulceration is the most serious complication of the postphlebitic syndrome. It is associated with perforator incompetence and abnormal reflux into the superficial veins but its precise pathogenesis remains to be determined.[16-18] Venous ulceration is associated with a thickening of the skin and subcutaneous tissue (called lipodermatosclerosis) and with skin pigmentation. The latter is caused by repeated bleeding from dermal capillaries which results in the deposition of hemosiderin.[19]

SYMPTOMS AND SIGNS OF POSTPHLEBITIC SYNDROME

The clinical manifestations are caused by chronic venous hypertension, perforator incompetence, and incompetence of the superficial veins (Table 15-1).

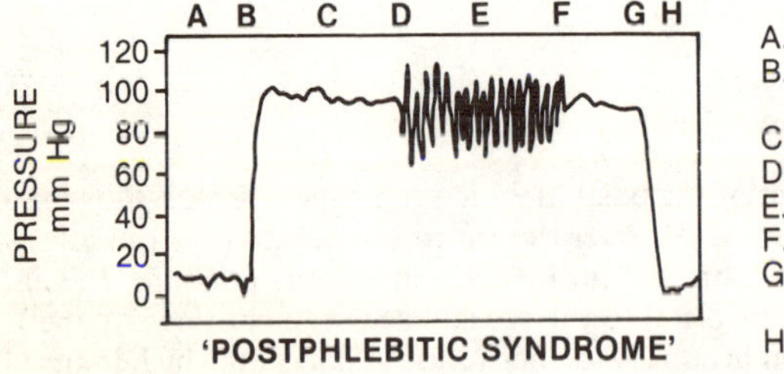

Figure 15-5 Pressure tracing recording from the long saphenous vein at ankle in a patient with the postphlebitic syndrome. Note the lack of pressure reduction in response to exercise. (Reproduced from Nicolaides[12] with permission of CV Mosby Co.)

Table 15-1
Clinical Features of the Postphlebitic Syndrome

Dependent edema
Heavy, aching sensation in leg
Prominent venules around ankle
Pigmentation and induration around lower leg and ankle
Ulceration in the region of medial malleolus
Venous claudication

Swelling

The initial symptoms of the postphlebitic syndrome are swelling and dependent edema of the ankle and the calf which are most marked after the patient has been standing or walking.[20] The swelling may be intermittent and is usually relieved by rest and leg elevation. Marked swelling of the thigh may occur after proximal vein thrombosis.

Pain

Heavy, aching pain in the calf and proximal leg is typically present.[21] It is exacerbated by standing up and relieved by rest and leg elevation.

Venous Claudication

This rare symptom may occur after iliofemoral thrombosis. Patients complain of bursting pain in the thigh or calf which is produced by walking and particularly by climbing. It can mimic arterial claudication.[22] It is caused by exacerbation of venous hypertension during exercise which occurs as a consequence of severe outflow obstruction.[22]

Stasis Dermatitis

With time and the development of incompetent perforators, pigmentation, induration, and prominent venules develop around the ankle and lower third of the leg.

Venous Ulcer

Venous ulceration develops in the region of the medial malleolus. Ulceration in the region of the lateral medial malleolus is usually not caused by the postphlebitic syndrome.[23] Ulceration is a late manifestation of the postphlebitic syndrome which may be initiated by trauma but can occur spontaneously. Venous ulceration is usually not painful. It is the most serious manifestation of the postphlebitic syndrome and is responsible for marked disability. Achilles tendon fibrosis may occur when ulcers have developed close to the tendon and are left untreated for a prolonged period.[24] Chronic infection with a variety of infecting bacteria and fungi is often present at the site of ulceration. Venous ulcers usually respond to conservative management but have a tendency to recur.

Varicosities

Varicosities are caused by secondary destruction of the valves of the superficial veins.

RECURRENT DEEP VENOUS THROMBOSIS AND ITS DIFFERENTIATION FROM THE POSTPHLEBITIC SYNDROME

The clinical manifestations of the postphlebitic syndrome, especially if intermittent, may be difficult to differentiate from deep vein thrombosis.[25] In patients with established postphlebitic syndrome who develop an exacerbation of pain and swelling, superimposed recurrent deep vein thrombosis should always be ruled out. The importance of differentiation between these two conditions cannot be made on clinical grounds.[26] We have recently demonstrated the value of the combination of impedance plethysmography and leg scanning in either ruling in or ruling our recurrent deep vein thrombosis in this setting.[27] Venography alone is of limited value because the diagnostic hallmark of acute thrombosis, a constant intraluminal defect, may be masked due to obliteration and recanalization of the involved veins.[26]

In this prospective study, we evaluated impedance plethysmography and leg scanning plus venography for the diagnosis of recurrent deep vein thrombosis in 270 patients considered by their physician to be experiencing symptoms and signs of acute recurrent deep vein thrombosis.[28] The results demonstrated that these patients could be separated into two groups, a negative cohort (patients in whom both noninvasive tests are negative and in whom it is safe to withhold anticoagulant therapy) and a positive cohort (patients in whom one and/or the other noninvasive test is positive requiring anticoagulant therapy). One hundred and eight-one of 270 patients (67%) had negative impedance plethysmograph and leg scanning results; only three of these 181 patients (1.7%) returned with recurrent venous thromboembolism during long-term follow-up, and no patient died from pulmonary embolism. In contrast, patients with positive impedance plethysmography or leg scan results had a high frequency of acute recurrent deep venous thrombosis on long-term follow-up; 18 of 89 (20.2%) developed new episodes of documented venous thromboembolism including four deaths from pulmonary embolism, a highly statistically significant difference. In the majority of positive patients, recurrent venous thromboembolism occurred after anticoagulant therapy had been terminated either inadvertently or following three months of therapy.

This diagnostic approach has a high clinical utility since it was possible to establish definitive management in 257 of 270 patients (95%). It is also highly cost effective, since 181 of 270 patients (67%) were spared the need for in-hospital care and long-term anticoagulant therapy.

The diagnostic algorithm shown in Figure 15-6 is of considerable clinical relevance because for the first time it provides the clinician with a practical approach to the patient with clinically suspected recurrent deep vein thrombosis.

DIAGNOSIS OF POSTPHLEBITIC SYNDROME

There is no definitive diagnostic test for the postphlebitic syndrome but objective evidence of the prior episode of deep vein thrombosis plus one or more of the following abnormalities, deep valve incompetence, ambulatory venous hypertension, persistent outflow obstruction in a patient with appropriate symptoms, constitute sufficient evidence to make this diagnosis.

Direct Visualization of Previous Deep Venous Thrombosis

When a patient with suspected chronic venous insufficiency is first seen, ascending venography is useful to confirm previous deep vein thrombosis. Most patients after a deep venous thrombosis show persistent

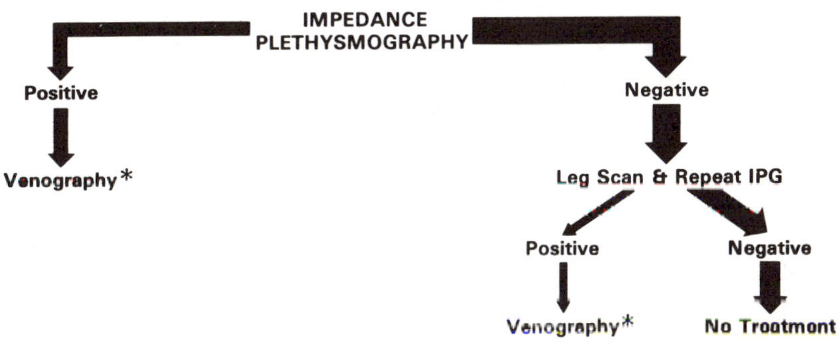

Figure 15-6 Recommended approach for patients with clinically suspected acute recurrent deep vein thrombosis.

abnormalities on venography such as recanalized postphlebitic veins, collateral channels, and varicose superficial veins.[29] However, the hemodynamic consequences and patency of the valves cannot be evaluated with ascending venography. Descending venography is more effective in demonstrating valvular incompetence.[30] However, it is more invasive than ascending venography since it requires a femoral puncture and detects mainly valvular incompetence of the saphenofemoral system.

Assessment of Outflow Obstruction

Persistent outflow obstruction is uncommonly seen in patients with the postphlebitic syndrome. Two tests can be used to measure outflow obstruction: impedance plethysmography[29] and strain-gauge plethysmography.[12,31-33] Most quantitative experience on outflow obstruction has been obtained by strain-gauge plethysmography.

Strain-gauge plethysmography   This technic is performed with a mercury-in-Silastic strain-gauge plethysmograph connected to a pen recorder. The strain-gauge is placed around the thickest part of the calf and detects volume change. This technic provides quantitative information on the output of the calf pump at rest and during exercise. The maximum venous outflow can be determined with the patient supine and legs elevated 10 degrees to the horizontal. A cuff around the thigh is inflated at 60 mmHg for two minutes and then released suddenly. The maximum venous outflow is derived from the recording of the slope of the emptying curve during the first second after the thigh cuff (Figure 15-7). For the determination of the maximum venous outflow during exercise, the patient is asked to stand up and to repeatedly raise himself/herself on the toes ("tiptoeing") at the rate of one movement per second for a period of 20 seconds. The ambulatory volume change, which is the maximum volume change in the calf during this exercise, is obtained and expressed in milliliters per 100 milliliters of tissue (Figure 15-8). As incompetence of the saphenous and superficial veins can give abnormal results with this test, the exercise test is repeated with the cuff just below the knee inflated at 100 mmHg to occlude the superficial veins. If only the superficial veins are diseased this last step will normalize the test. A decrease in calf volume greater than 1.5 ml/100 ml during exercise means that the calf pump is efficient.[12] In contrast, a decrease in calf volume by less than 0.75 ml/100 ml or an increase in calf volume means that the calf muscle pump is inefficient.

Assessment of Reflux in the Microcirculation of the Skin

Photoplethysmography   uses an infrared light-emitting diode and an adjacent phototransistor to receive back-scattered light reflected from the superficial layer of the skin.[34] The amount of reflected light varies with the number of red blood cells in the cutaneous microcirculation.

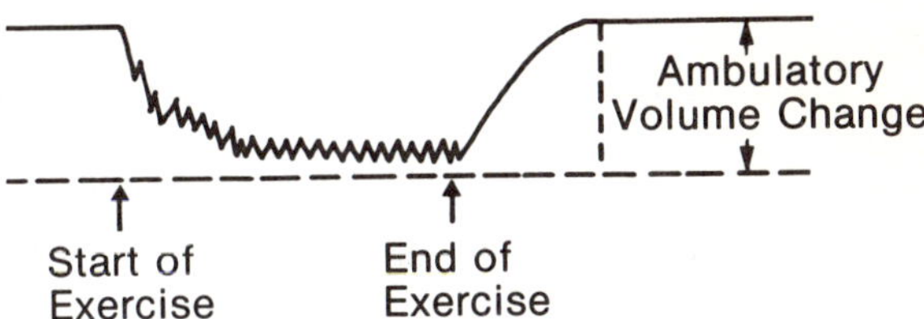

Figure 15-7 Principle of strain-gauge plethysmography. Diagram shows change in calf volume during venous occlusion (cuff on) and after sudden release of the cuff with the leg elevated 10 degrees. The maximum venous outflow is derived from the initial slope of the emptying curve during the first second after release of the cuff.

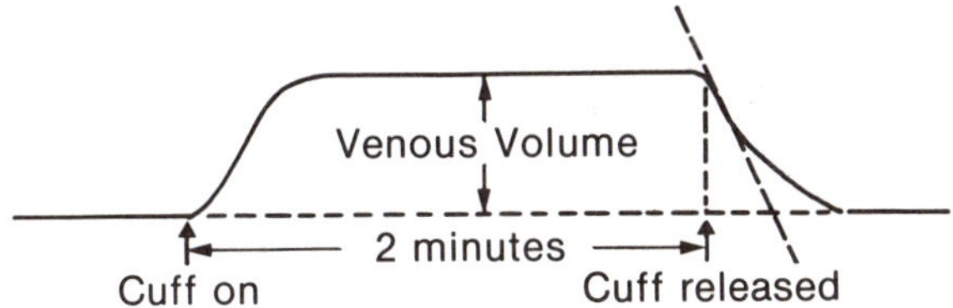

Figure 15-8 Tracing of ambulatory change in calf volume before, during, and immediately after an exercise period of 30 seconds ("tiptoeing").

The transducer is connected to a recorder which shows relative changes in skin blood content over the course of time. In a normal subject, the skin blood content decreases significantly in response to active or passive calf muscle exercise. The recovery time for the recording to return to the pre-exercise base-line level in the normal subject is usually over 20 seconds[8] (Figure 15-9a). In patients with chronic venous insufficiency, the recovery time is markedly shortened (Figure 15-9b). The photoplethysmograph permits unique assessment of altered cutaneous hemodynamics in patients with postphlebitic syndrome. The abnormalities of skin blood response to leg exercise is thought to bear a relationship to the presence and severity of postphlebitic dermatitis and stasis ulceration. This test is abnormal only if there is incompetence of the perforating veins as seen in advanced postphlebitic syndrome. Therefore, patients who have valve incompetence proven by Doppler ultrasound can occasionally have normal photoplethysmographic tracings. It would thus appear that photoplethysmography and strain-gauge plethysmography are potentially complementary.

The two plethysmography technics need to be evaluated by properly designed clinical trials.

Assessment of Valvular Competence in the Deep Venous System

Qualitative evaluation with Doppler ultrasound is the most simple and rapid method to detect venous reflux.[35] With this technic, the patient

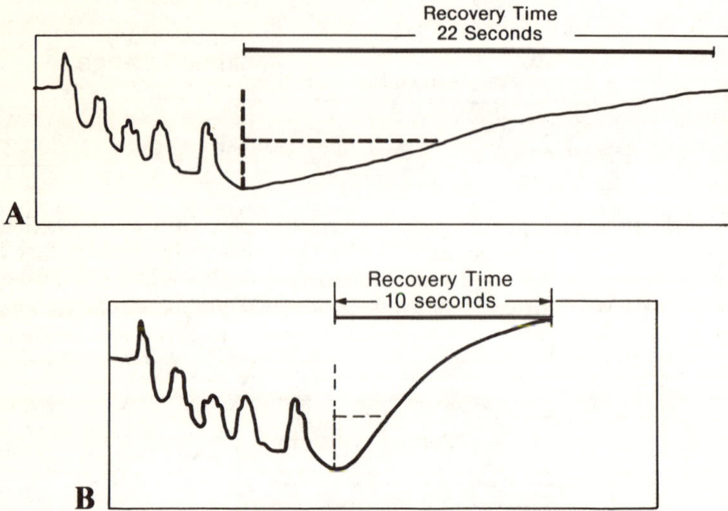

Figure 15-9 Recording from photoplethysmograph transducer in a normal subject (**A**), and a patient with postphlebitic syndrome (**B**). Note the markedly shortened recovery time in the postphlebitic syndrome.

is examined in the recumbent position. The presence of reflux is elicited by compressing the area proximal to the valve being examined and listening distally with the probe. A positive test for venous reflux in the presence of the appropriate signs and symptoms supports a diagnosis of postphlebitic syndrome. This technic is also useful to detect perforator incompetence. Its major limitations are that it is qualitative and requires an experienced user. A tracing of the result can be obtained using a directional Doppler with a recording chart (Figure 15-10).

Summary of Diagnosis of Postphlebitic Syndrome

In patients with progressive symptoms and signs, the diagnosis can be established by demonstrating presence of previous deep vein thrombosis by venography, plus an abnormality in any one of the tests described above. The demonstration of reflux in the deep venous system will correctly identify the majority of patients with the postphlebitic syndrome. In patients with recurrent or episodic symptoms, it is important to exclude an acute recurrence of venous thrombosis by the combination of impedance plethysmography and leg scanning.

PREVENTION OF POSTPHLEBITIC SYNDROME

Early treatment of deep vein thrombosis with anticoagulants limits clot extension. Theoretically this should minimize valvular damage and decrease the incidence of postphlebitic syndrome. It has been suggested that the early use of heparin in the treatment of deep vein thrombosis has decreased the incidence of postphlebitic syndrome in recent year, but this remains to be proved.

Three approaches can be used to prevent the postphlebitic syndrome: primary prophylaxis in high-risk patients, early detection of asymptomatic thrombosis, and rapid dissolution of thrombi in patients with extensive venous thrombosis by thrombolytic therapy. While it is likely that the latter two approaches would reduce the postphlebitic syndrome, definitive proof supporting this contention is lacking.[36] Clinical trials comparing the effects of streptokinase and heparin using serial venography to assess thrombolysis have shown that lysis of venous thrombi occurs much more frequently with thrombolytic agents than with heparin. Thus, a measurable decrease in thrombus size is seen in less than 30% of patients treated with heparin compared with 60% and 75% of patients treated with streptokinase. Complete lysis of venous thrombi occurs in less than 10% of patients treated with heparin, but is seen in 35% of patients treated with streptokinase within seven days of onset of symptoms. Significant lysis is seldom evident before 48 hours of treatment, and four or more days may be required to achieve complete lysis. In a number of studies, follow-up venograms have demonstrated that early patency is usually maintained and, in the small number of cases in which it has been tested, valve function remained intact. Whether the

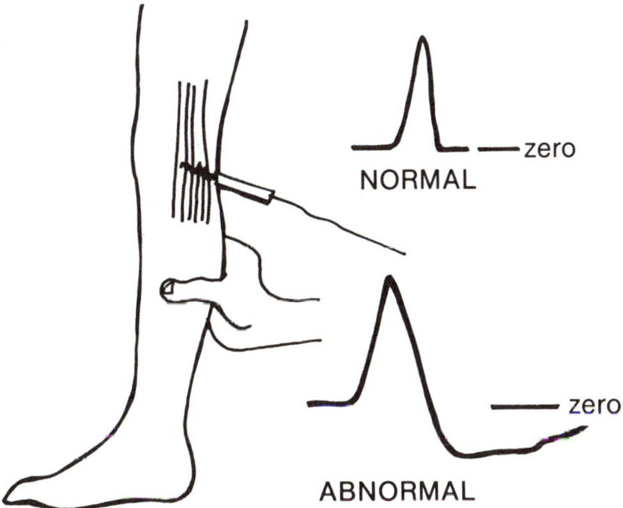

Figure 15-10 Directional Doppler examination of the popliteal valve. Diagram shows position of probe and calf compression. Upper tracing: flow toward the heart on compression without reflux on release. Lower tracing: reversal of flow on release of compression signifies reflux (tracing below zero line).

long-term effects of achieving early lysis of thrombi decreases the incidence of postphlebitic syndrome needs to be investigated by properly designed randomized clinical trials.

TREATMENT OF POSTPHLEBITIC SYNDROME

Treatment of patients with postphlebitic syndrome is based on conservative measures aimed at increasing venous return to the heart and preventing stasis. Most patients respond favorably to a conservative approach and very few patients require corrective surgery.[24]

Leg elevation is effective in improving the venous return by gravity and is helpful in controlling symptoms of dependent edema. Patients should be encouraged to elevate the leg periodically during the day as part of their daily routine.

Pressure gradient elastic stockings compress the superficial veins, force blood flow into the deep veins, and prevent venous stasis.[37] Although graduate pressure stockings do not completely correct the abnormal venous hemodynamics, most patients experience subjective relief. It is important to ensure that the patient wears a correctly fitted stocking. Either knee-high or full-length stockings may be worn.

Patients with venous ulcers also benefit from a conservative approach. Most leg ulcers regress with conservative measures.[24] Compression bandaging, like the Unna boot, is considered to be of value in the treatment of postphlebitic leg ulcers. When cellulitis is not present, an Unna boot can be used for intervals of three weeks until the ulcer is completely healed. Topical application of proteolytic enzymes is used by some in the belief that it facilitates the healing rate of ulcers.[38] Chronic infection with various bacteria and fungi is often present at the site of ulcers. Treatment by means of potassium permanganate soaks of 1:10,000 dilution three times daily for 30-minute periods for three days helps in controlling local infection and keep the would dry. Parenteral antibiotics are not used unless the patient has a widespread cellulitis.

In the minority of patients with ulcers refractory to conservative measures, ulcer resection with skin grafting may be indicated. A variety of corrective surgical procedures have been proposed: ligation of incompetent perforators,[39] reconstruction of femoral valves,[40,41] ligation of popliteal veins,[42] and resection of superficial varicosities and saphenous veins.[43] In patients with leg ulcers secondary to saphenous incompetence and communicating branches, incompetence without disease of the deep system, ligation of incompetent perforators, and resection of saphenous veins may be useful to prevent ulcer recurrence.[43] Finally, foot care is also important. Prophylactic medications such as talcum and fungicidal powder for the moist foot or leg wearing an elastic support are prescribed. Corns, calluses, and thickened toe nails are best managed by a podiatrist.

REFERENCES

1. Gjores JE: The incidence of venous thrombosis and its sequalae in certain districts of Sweden. *Acta Chir Scand* 1956;206(suppl):1–88.
2. Hirsh J, Genton E, Hull R: The post phlebitic syndrome, in Hirch J, Genton E, Hull R (eds): *Venous Thromboembolism*. New York, Grune & Stratton, 1981, pp 63–66.
3. Coon WW, Willis PW, Keller JB: Venous thrombeoembolism and other venous disease in Tecumseh Community Health Study. *Circulation* 1973; 48:839–846.
4. Dodd H, Cockett FB: The surgical anatomy of the veins of the lower limbs, in *The Pathology and Surgery of Veins of the Lower Limb*, Edinburgh, Churchill Livingstone, 1976, pp 18–49.
5. Bauer G: Patho-physiology and treatment of the lower leg stasis syndrome. *Angiology* 1950;1:1–8.
6. Negus D: The post thrombotic syndrome. *Ann R Coll Surg Engl* 1970; 47:92–105.
7. Johnson G: Chronic venous insufficiency of the lower extremity: an overview, in Foley W (ed): *Advances in the Management of Cardiovascular Disease*. Chicago, Year Book Medical Publ, 1980, pp 195–205.
8. Abramowitz HB, Queral LA, Flinn WR, et al: The use of photoplethysmography in the assessment of venous insufficiency: a comparison to venous pressure measurements. *Surgery* 1979;86:434–441.
9. DeCamp PT, Ward JA, Ochsner A: Ambulatory venous pressure studies in post-phlebitic and other disease states. *Surgery* 1951;29:42–52.
10. Hojemsgard IC, Sturp H: Venous pressure in primary and post-thrombotic varicose veins. *Acta Chir Scand* 1950;99:133–153.
11. Pollack AA, Taylor BE, Myers DD, et al: The effect of exercise and body position on the venous pressure at the ankle in patients having venous valvular defect. *J Clin Invest* 1949;28:559–563.
12. Nicolaides AN: Noninvasive assessment of primary and secondary varicose veins, in Bernstein EF (ed): *Noninvasive Diagnostic Techniques in Vascular Disease*. St. Louis, CV Mosby Co, 1982, pp 575–586.
13. Burnand KG, O'Donnell TF, Thomas ML, et al: The relative importance of incompetent communicating veins in the production of varicose veins and venous ulcers. *Surgery* 1977;82:9–14.
14. Browse NL: Venous insufficiency: non operative management, in Bang N, Glover J, Holden R, Triplett D (eds): *Thrombosis and Atherosclerosis*. Chicago, Year Book Medical Publ, 1982, pp 275–281.
15. Shull KC, Nicolaides AN, Miles C, et al: Significance of popliteal reflux in relation to ambulatory venous pressure and ulceration. *Arch Surg* 1970; 114:1304–1306.
16. Burnand KG, Whimster I, Clemenson G, et al: The relationship between the number of capillaries in the skin of the venous ulcer-bearing area of the lower leg and the fall in foot vein pressure during exercise. *Br J Surg* 1979;68:297–300.
17. Wolf JHN, Morland M, Browse NL: The fibrinolytic therapy of varicose veins. *Br J Surg* 1979;66:185–187.
18. Browse NL, Gray L, Jarett PEM, et al: Blood and vein-wall fibrinolytic activity in health and vascular disease. *Br Med J* 1977;1:478–481.
19. Browse NL, Burnand KG: The post phlebitic syndrome: a new look, in Bergan JJ, Yao JST (eds): *Venous Problems*. Chicago, Year Book Medical Publ, pp 395–404.

20. Hirsh J: Natural history of venous thromboembolism in Bang N, Glover J, Holden R, Triplett D (eds): *Thrombosis and Atherosclerosis*. Chicago, Year Book Medical Publ, 1982, pp 27–35.

21. Negus D: Calf pain in the post thrombotic-syndrome. *Br Med J* 1968; 2:156–158.

22. Tripolitis AJ, Milligan EB, Bodily KC, et al: The physiology of venous claudication. *Am J Surg* 1980;139:447–448.

23. Barker WS: The post phlebitic syndrome: management by surgical means, in Bergan JJ, Yao JST (eds): *Venous Problems*. Chicago, Year Book Medical Publ, 1978, pp 383–393.

24. Owens JC: The post phlebitic syndrome: management by conservative means, in Bergan JJ, Yao JST (eds): *Venous Problems*. Chicago, Year Book Medical Publ, 1978, pp 369–383.

25. Hirsh J, Hull RD: Natural history and clinical features of venous thrombosis, in Colman RW, Hirsh J, Marder VJ, Salzman EW (eds): *Hemostasis and Thrombosis*, Philadelphia, Lippincott, 1982, pp 831–843.

26. Hirsh J, Genton E, Hull R: Differential diagnosis of clinical features of venous thrombosis, in Hirsh J, Genton E, Hull R (eds): *Venous Thromboembolism*, New York, Grune & Stratton, 1981, pp 82–89.

27. Hull R, Carter C, Ockelford P, et al: The use of noninvasive testing and venography for the diagnosis of acute recurrent deep vein thrombosis, abstracted. *Thromb Haemost* 1981;46:168.

28. Hull RD, Carter C, Jay R, et al: The diagnosis of acute recurrent deep vein thrombosis: a diagnostic challenge. *Circulation* 1983;67:901–906.

29. Hirsh J, Genton E, Hull R: Diagnosis of venous thrombosis, in Hirsh J, Genton E, Hull R (eds): *Venous Thromboembolism*. New York, Grune & Stratton, 1981, pp 234–318.

30. Herman RJ, Neiman HL, Yao JST, et al: Descending venography a method of evaluating lower extremity venous valvular function. *Radiology* 1980; 137:63–69.

31. Barnes RW, Collicott PE, Mozersky DJ, et al: Noninvasive quantitation of venous reflux in the post phlebitic syndrome. *Surg Gynecol Obstet* 1973; 136:769–773.

32. Mason R, Giron S: Noninvasive evaluation of venous function in chronic venous disease. *Surgery* 1982;91:312–317.

33. Barnes RW, Collicott PE, Sumner DS: Noninvasive quantitation of venous hemodynamics in the post phlebitic syndrome. *Arch Surg* 1973;107:807–814.

34. Barnes RW, Yao JST: Photoplethysmography in chronic venous insufficiency in noninvasive diagnostic techniques, in Bernstein EF (ed): *Noninvasive Diagnostic Techniques in Vascular Disease*. St. Louis, CV Mosby Co, 1982, pp 514–521.

35. Barnes RW: Doppler ultrasonic diagnosis of venous disease in Bernstein EF (ed): *Noninvasive Diagnostic Techniques in Vascular Disease*. St. Louis, CV Mosby Co, 1982, pp 452–458.

36. Hirsh J, Genton E, Hull R: Thrombolytic Drugs, in Hirsh J, Genton E, Hull R (eds): *Venous Thromboembolism*. New York, Grune & Stratton, 1981, pp 198–208.

37. Jones MAG, Webb R, Rees I, et al: A physiological study of elastic compression stockings in venous disorders of the leg. *Br J Surg* 1980;67:569–572.

38. Gordon B: The use of topical proteolytic enzymes in the treatment of post-thrombotic leg ulcers. *Br J Clin Pract* 1975;29:143–146.

39. Schanzer H, Converse Peirce E: A rational approach to surgery of the chronic venous stasis syndrome. *Ann Surg* 1982;195:25–29.

40. Kistner RL: Post-phlebitic syndrome: cure by surgical repair of the incompetent femoral valve. *J Cardiovasc Surg (Torino)* 1976;17:85–86.
41. Johnson ND, Queral LA, Flinn WR, et al: Late objective assessment of venous valve surgery. *Arch Surg* 1981;116:1461–1466.
42. Bauer G: The aetiology of leg ulcers and their treatment by resection of the popliteal vein. *J Intern de Chir* 1948;8:937–967.
43. Antal SC, Reiss R: Post-thrombotic leg ulcer and its surgical treatment. *Am J Surg* 1976;131:710–713.
44. Burnand K, O'Donnell T, Thomas L, et al: Relation between post-phlebitic changes in the deep veins and results of surgical treatment of venous ulcers. *Lancet* 1976;1:936–938.

16 *Mesenteric, Portal, and Hepatic Vein Thrombosis*

John A. Payne

Thrombosis of the splanchnic veins, the portal vein and its radicals, and the hepatic vein produces a spectrum of bowel dysfunction, portal hypertension, and hepatic injury. Depending upon location, rate of development, and coexistent disease, these lesions may be asymptomatic or rapidly lethal. Acutely symptomatic lesions generally produce infarction of the affected tissue. Survivors of bowel infarction may be incapacitated by the short-bowel syndrome. Patients with chronic hepatic vein thrombosis (Budd-Chiari syndrome) often have major problems with gastrointestinal (GI) hemorrhage, ascites, and malnutrition.

ANATOMY

The venous drainage from the stomach is carried by the short gastric veins to the splenic and the coronary veins, which join the portal vein. The pancreatic and splenic venous flow is carried by the splenic vein along the superior margin of the pancreas and unites near the head of the pancreas with the venous drainage from the colon, carried by the inferior mesenteric vein. The splenic vein then joins the superior mesenteric vein to form the portal vein. After receiving the coronary vein, the portal vein branches at the hilum into the right and left portal veins. The left portal vein connects with the vestigial umbilical vein, lying within the ligamentum teres.

Within the liver, an extraordinary perfusion system is found, wherein the major portion of blood is supplied by the portal system, and the driving pressure necessary to perfuse the liver is supplied by the hepatic artery. Blood traverses the hepatic sinusoids to be collected in terminal hepatic venules that subsequently combine to create the several hepatic veins. Drainage into the inferior vena cava occurs just below the diaphragm with channels draining the right, left, and caudate lobes arranged in two groups. The upper veins drain the left lobe and most of the right lobe. The lower group drains the caudate, quadrate, and remainder of the right lobes.

MESENTERIC VEIN THROMBOSIS

Venous thrombosis produces hemodynamic stasis, ischemia, and lymphedema. The involved segment of bowel ceases its absorptive function and motility, becoming swollen from a combination of local edema and reactive hyperemia. The altered segment is subject to become the leading edge for intersusception, the site of perforation or subsequent stricture. Bacterial overgrowth and invasion occur in the injured segment and may lead to sepsis in the absence of peritonitis. The release of vasoactive agents affects the local arterial supply. Arterial constriction may persist despite thrombectomy and require chemotherapy or surgical extirpation for correction.

Systemic hypotension and hemoconcentration from splanchnic pooling and hemorrhage may cause renal tubular necrosis and shock.

Diagnosis

Patients with mesenteric vein thrombosis develop abdominal pain which may be crampy and intermittent or steady and diffuse, depending on the extent of involvement and the degree of bowel decompensation. Infarction, peritonitis, and death may develop within six to 12 hours. Relatively minor insults may resolve without apparent sequelae. A lack of impressive physical findings in a patient with severe pain is highly characteristic.

Biochemical tests are of little value in confirming the diagnosis. Preliminary data suggest that elevated serum phosphate may be helpful in identifying mesenteric vascular compromise, but this correlation has not been established, nor has a mechanism been proposed. Massive bowel infarction may elevate serum amylase, but in general amylase levels remain normal. Ascites may be present, usually in modest amount, and will typically be exudative and bloody. Frank or occult blood in the stool is an important clue, indicative of the loss of mucosal integrity.

Plain films of the abdomen are frequently abnormal, but the finding of focal ileus or small amounts of ascites is not specific enough to establish a diagnosis. Occasionally, mucosal edema (thumbprinting) can be seen when intraluminal air is present. Barium studies may reveal typical changes of mucosal edema, impaired motility, and ulcerations, but the extent of bowel involvement may be underestimated (see Figure 10-4).

Both abdominal ultrasound and computed tomography (CT) have been useful in demonstrating thrombosis of the superior mesenteric vein (Figure 16-1). Failure to demonstrate thrombi does not eliminate the possibility of involvement of segmental veins, however, and additional studies with technetium 99 or abdominal angiography may provide useful supporting information. The technetium 99 scan may show prolonged stasis in the splanchnic circulation. Arteriography, which should only be done in a well-hydrated patient, may disclose focal arteriolar spasm, prolonged arterial phase, opacification of the bowel wall, and delayed venous drainage.

At laparotomy, the characteristic dusky red, devitalized bowel, with thrombi demonstrable upon transection of the mesenteric venules, is

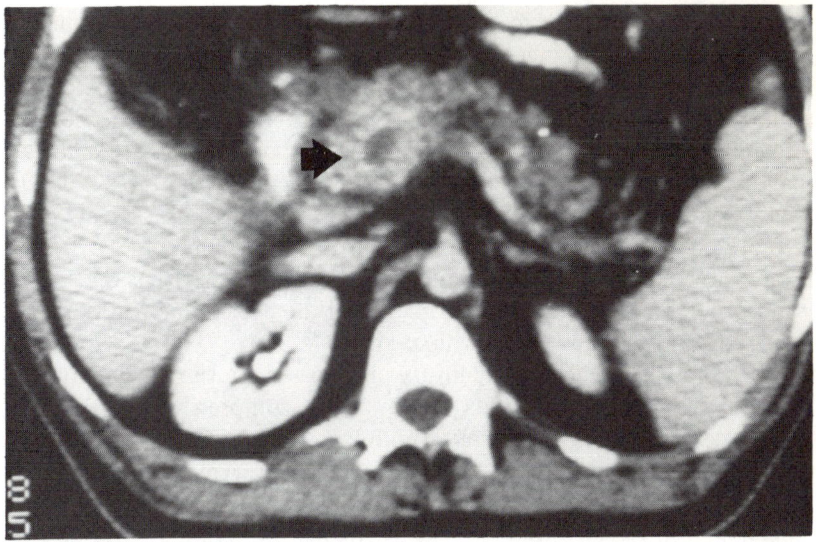

Figure 16-1   Computed tomogram of the upper abdomen, demonstrating a central thrombus in the dilated superior mesenteric vein (as indicated by the arrow). Patient developed fever, abdominal pain, and ileus. Subsequent laparotomy disclosed a periappendiceal abscess and mesenteric venous thrombosis.

often clearly demarcated from adjacent viable bowel. Commonly, the proximal extent of the thrombosis includes the superior mesenteric vein or the portal vein, with retrograde involvement of the tributaries. The extent of reactive arterial spasm is poorly evaluated by inspection and palpation and repeat exploration or intra-arterial infusion of vasodilators is frequently advisable.

Etiology and Pathophysiology

Most instances of mesenteric venous thrombosis may be ascribed to portal stasis due to portal hypertension in cirrhosis, inflammation due to intra-abdominal trauma, infections, or operations, or altered hemostasis due to coagulopathies from local or distant malignant processes. Rarely, primary coagulopathies will be identified to account for localized thrombi. Fully 25% of cases of mesenteric thrombosis occur without recognized antecedent cause.

Relatively little is known about the characteristics of the coagulation system within the splanchnic circulation of man, but several intriguing features have emerged from studies in dogs. Prostaglandins, thromboxane, and prostacyclin are derived from unsaturated fatty acids, primarily arachidonic acid (eicosatetraenoic acid). Release of arachidonic acid from tissue stores, or possibly from assimilation from the gut, is influenced by triglyceride lipase, phosphatase A_2, the kinins, and angiotensin.

After metabolism by cyclooxygenase, thromboxane, prostacyclin, or prostaglandin are produced in response to local tissue needs. Thromboxane A_2 constricts vessels and induces platelet aggregation. Prostacyclin dilates vessels and prevents platelet aggregation. The balance between thromboxane and prostaglandin synthesis may potentially have substantial effects upon the modulation of mesenteric thrombosis. Clearly, dietary effects must be investigated as well. The role of this system in syndromes of idiopathic mesenteric vein thrombosis, pulmonary hypertension following portocaval shunting, primary portal hypertension (Banti's syndrome), and nodular transformation of the liver (noncirrhotic portal hypertension) remains to be evaluated.

Cirrhosis When hepatic injury produces cirrhosis, the hepatic vascular bed is scarred with a loss of sinusoids, compression of sinusoids, and portal venules by regenerative nodules, and loss of the presinusoidal sphincter control mechanism which normally prevents transmission of hepatic arterial pressure to the portal bed. These changes may be augmented in the alcoholic patient by the accumulation of fat and protein within hepatocytes causing additional sinusoidal compression and portal hypertension. Initially, the tendency for stagnation of mesenteric blood flow is countered by hemoconcentration and increased lymph production, until the drainage capacity of the thoracic duct and other abdominal lymphatics is overcome and ascites develops. There is congestion of the splanchnic bed with redistribution of the circulating blood volume. With time, collaterals develop that partially relieve the portal hypertension and congestion. In addition to the relative venous stasis inherent in this situation there are changes in blood flow patterns which reduce the clearance of metabolites by the liver. Introduction of a surgical portal-systemic shunt, while reducing stasis, augments the bypass of the liver and has been associated with chronic embolization to the lungs and pulmonary hypertension on occasion. Thrombosis of surgically created shunts is generally attributed to technic of local turbulence. In neither of these situations have the role of prostaglandins or coagulation factors been systemically studied.

Inflammation Mesenteric vein thrombosis may complicate an intra-abdominal abscess or phlegmon. In such instances, the cause for the sudden deterioration of the patient's condition may be suggested by finding hemorrhagic ascitic fluid or a characteristic lesion by abdominal ultrasound or CT scans. Aggressive intervention and improved diagnostic technics have reduced mortality from superior mesenteric vein thrombosis from 80% to 20%. A high index of suspicion must be maintained in following patients with intra-abdominal inflammation, for changes in clinical state may be subtle and easily attributed to the primary process. Even if successful drainage of an abscess and embolectomy of affected veins is accomplished, careful attention must be paid to regional arterial spasm which may lead to postoperative ischemia and disruption of anastamoses. The use of intra-arterial papaverine may prove to be helpful in this setting as well as in the treatment of nonocclusive arterial ischemia (see Chapter 12).

Primary and secondary coagulopathies   Mesenteric venous thrombosis, pulmonary emboli, and superficial or deep venous thrombosis occur in patients with hypercoagulable states. A systematic evaluation for such a condition should be undertaken in any patient without portal hypertension or abdominal abscess who presents with sudden onset of melena, abdominal pain, and bloody ascites. Several carcinomas, notably carcinoma of the pancreas, may produce a hypercoagulable state with incidental involvement of the mesenteric vessels. Polycythemia rubra vera, paroxysmal nocturnal hemoglobinuria, and sickle cell disease may also involve the mesenteric vessels when they produce a hypercoaguable state. Splenectomy often is followed by thrombocytosis when performed to alleviate hypersplenism. Propagation of a thrombus from the oversewn splenic vein has been documented on occasion.

Treatment

Treatment of mesenteric venous thrombosis is supportive with thrombectomy and/or resection of ischemic or infarcted bowel. Postoperative anticoagulation and vasodilator therapy seem to be appropriate. A "second look" operation with 48 hours of resection is often needed before one can be assured that all involved bowel has been removed.

In those cases where a treatable predisposing condition can be identified, appropriate therapy should prevent a recurrence. When extensive bowel resection leads to choleric enteropathy or short bowel syndrome, management can be quite complex. Details regarding these difficult situations should be sought in the surgical and gastrointestinal literature devoted to these problems.

PORTAL VEIN THROMBOSIS

Thrombosis of the portal vein is surprisingly well tolerated in the absence of sepsis, undoubtedly because of the ability of the hepatic artery to sustain blood flow until collateralization (cavernous transformation) occurs (Figure 16-2). In addition to the processes that induce mesenteric thrombi, several conditions particularly predispose a patient to extrahepatic portal vein thrombosis. These include schistosomiasis, cirrhosis, neonatal omphalitis, or invasion of the portal vein by hepatoma. Idiopathic hepatoportal sclerosis appears to be an unusual condition produced by multiple emboli in the portal system with obliteration of small intrahepatic portal venules and fibrosis of portal tracts.

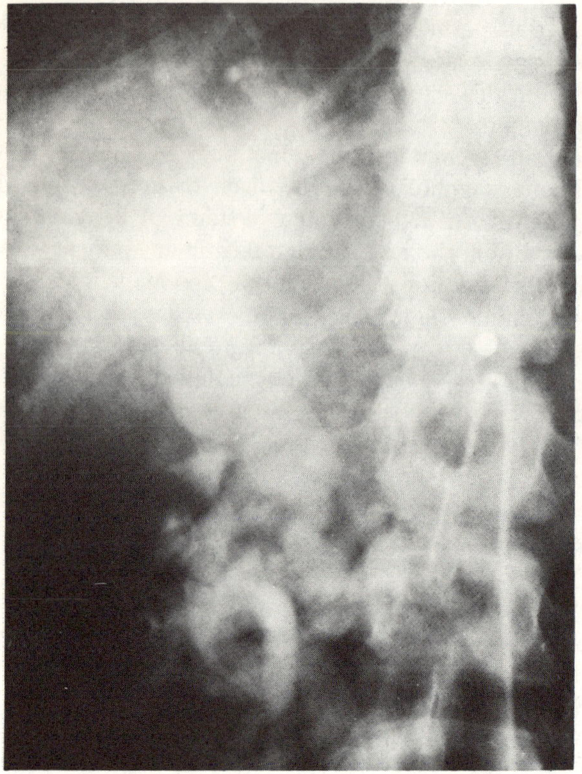

Figure 16-2 Venous phase of splanchnic arteriogram revealing cavernous transformation of the portal vein. Patient was a 14-year-old girl with recurrent hemorrhage from variceal hemorrhage. No predisposing cause for portal vein thrombosis identified.

The physiologic consequences of portal vein thrombosis are splanchnic stasis, altered bowel motility, and increased splanchnic lymph production. Collateral vessels develop rapidly to restore portal flow to the liver and to alleviate portal hypertension through extrahepatic channels. These latter vessels develop in the retroperitoneum, the anterior abdominal wall, the splenic fossa, and the submucosa of the rectum and esophagus. Splenomegaly in produced because of passive congestion and immune stimulation by gut and diet-derived antigens which bypass the Kupffer cell clearing mechanism. Ascites may develop from portal vein thrombosis without associated cirrhosis, but generally is mild and tends to resolve with time. When portal vein thrombosis occurs with cirrhosis, formerly manageable ascites may become intractable.

Specific therapy, ie, portal venous embolectomy, is not warranted. Most of the manifestations of portal vein thrombosis are well tolerated unless hemorrhage from esophageal varices develops. Vascular shunts are generally contraindicated for lack of a suitable vessel. Surgical transection of the esophagus with splenectomy (Sigura procedure) will usually afford relief from severe hemorrhage despite a high recurrence rate of varix formation. Subsequent variceal hemorrhage can usually be managed conservatively. The recent interest in endoscopic sclerosis of esophageal varices has a strong appeal in this setting, and may well prove to be the optimal approach, but postsclerotic complications of esophageal ulceration, perforation, infection, disseminated intravascular coagulation, and potential pulmonary hypertension are reason for caution.

HEPATIC VEIN THROMBOSIS

Thrombosis of the hepatic vein, the Budd-Chiari syndrome, is manifested by a decline in hepatic synthetic function and evidence of portal hypertension. Generally the onset is acute, the deterioration of clinical status occurring over several weeks to months, and the patient dies from hepatic failure or the complications of portal hypertension. With the widespread use of radionuclide scans and angiograms has come the realization that a fortunate minority of patients with Budd-Chiari syndrome develop the condition over a span of months to years. In these patients collateral vessels and recanalization of thrombosed hepatic veins mitigate an otherwise bleak prognosis.

Pathogenesis

The cause(s) of the Budd-Chiari syndrome, which generally occurs without evidence of systemic thrombosis, are mechanical or idiopathic. Mechanical obstruction from hepatomas, adrenal cell carcinoma, leimyosarcoma, or renal cell carcinoma occluding the hepatic venous system is well documented; such uncontrolled tumor growth presages death. A second condition, inferior vena caval webs (congenital), is also associated with the syndrome, particularly in Orientals. A final mechanical factor is based on the observation that polycystic liver disease and perihilar liver abscesses may impinge on the venous outflow and produce thrombosis.

The familiar list of conditions which produce systemic thromboses can all cause hepatic vein thrombosis. These conditions include polycythemia rubra vera, paroxysmal nocturnal hemoglobinuria, use of oral contraceptives, sickle cell hemoglobinopathy and myeloproliferative disorders.

Clinical Manifestations

Whatever the process which initiates hepatic venous thrombosis, there is prompt centrolobular (zone 3) congestion in the affected hepatic acini. Redistribution of blood flow away from the block occurs through intra-hepatic vessels; ischemic necrosis of the centrolobular hepatocytes with diapedesis of erythrocytes into the space of Disse is evident. If the process is focal and self-limited, recovery will be uneventful without sequelae (Figure 16-3). Serial hepatic scintigrams demonstrate a progressive diminution of tracer uptake in the right lobe of the liver, with enlargement and a dramatic shift of tracer uptake to the caudate lobe (Figure 16-4). This characteristic pattern may precede the development of clinical symptoms by years and should be sought in the routine follow-up of patients with polycythemia vera and paroxysmal nocturnal hemoglobinuria (Figure 16-5).

When the onset of hepatic vein occlusion is abrupt, the patient's condition deteriorates rapidly with hepatocellular failure, massive ascites, and painful hepatomegaly. Bilirubin clearance is usually well maintained so that jaundice is minimal or nonexistent.

Liver biopsy is often difficult to obtain because of the critical state of the patient. It may indicate veno-occlusive disease, an unusual condition produced by the ingestion of *Senecio* alkaloid plants, or follow therapy with hepatic irradiation, 6-thioguanine, arsphenamine, and urethane. Liver biopsy is also helpful in assessing chronicity (Figure 16-6). A biopsy cannot distinguish whether the initiating lesion is intrahepatic, caval, or pericardial, although the more homogeneous the status of venous thrombi

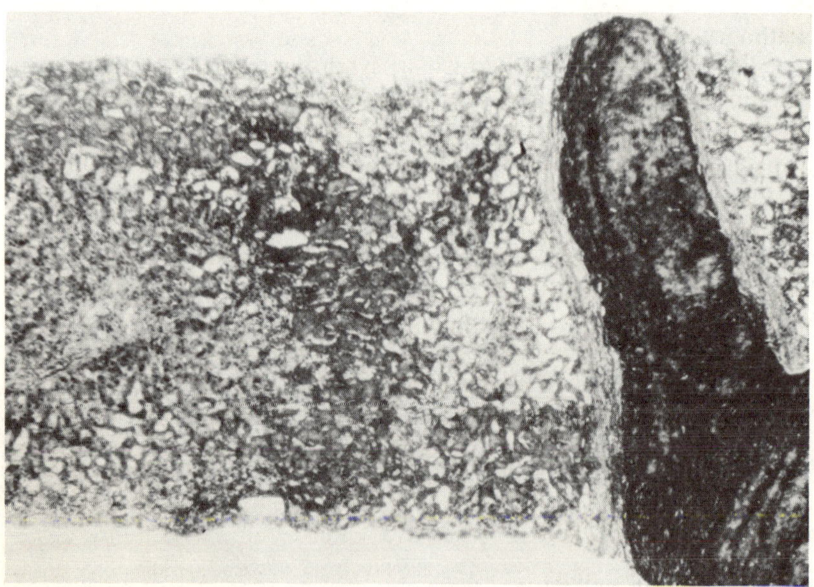

Figure 16-3 Photomicrograph demonstrating acute thrombosis of a terminal hepatic venule with sinusoidal congestion, and hepatocyte atrophy. Acute Budd-Chiari syndrome in patient with lymphoma.

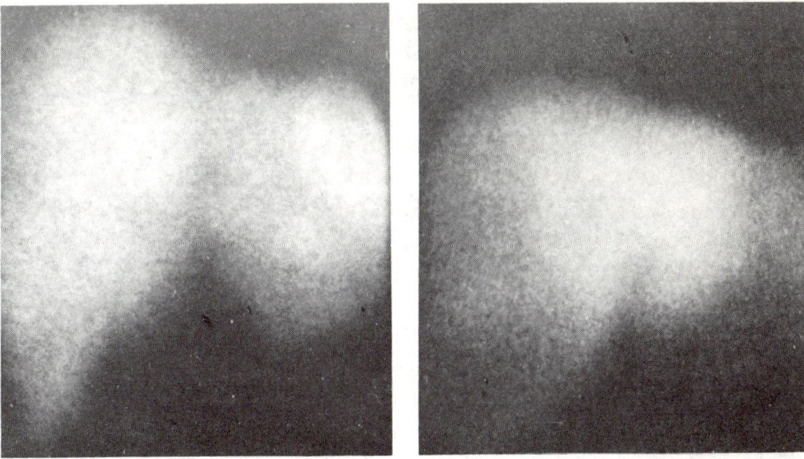

Figure 16-4 Serial hepatic scintiscans, with a four-month interval demonstrating an enlargement and intensification of technetium 99 uptake by the caudate lobe, with marked reduction in uptake over lateral right lobe. Same patient as in Figure 16-3.

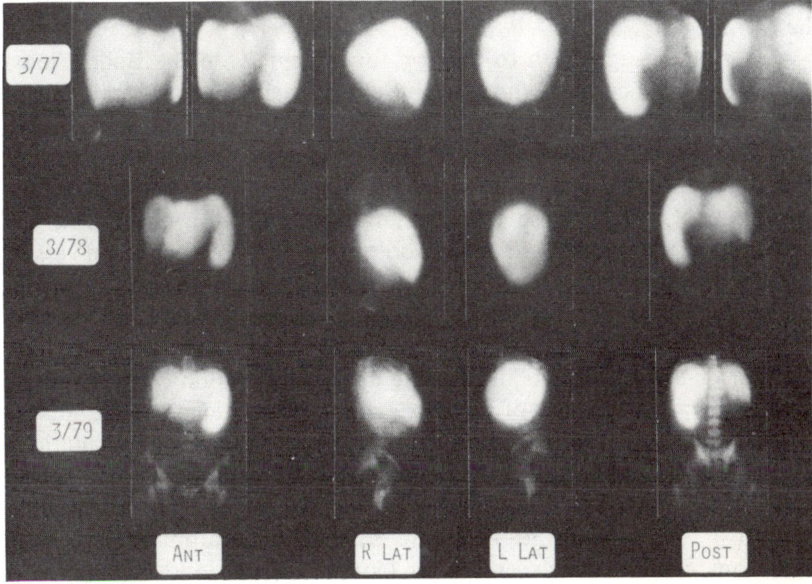

Figure 16-5 Serial hepatic scintiscans from a patient with polycythemia rubra vera, demonstrating evolution of typical findings over a period of several years. Patient died from variceal hemorrhage and hepatic failure.

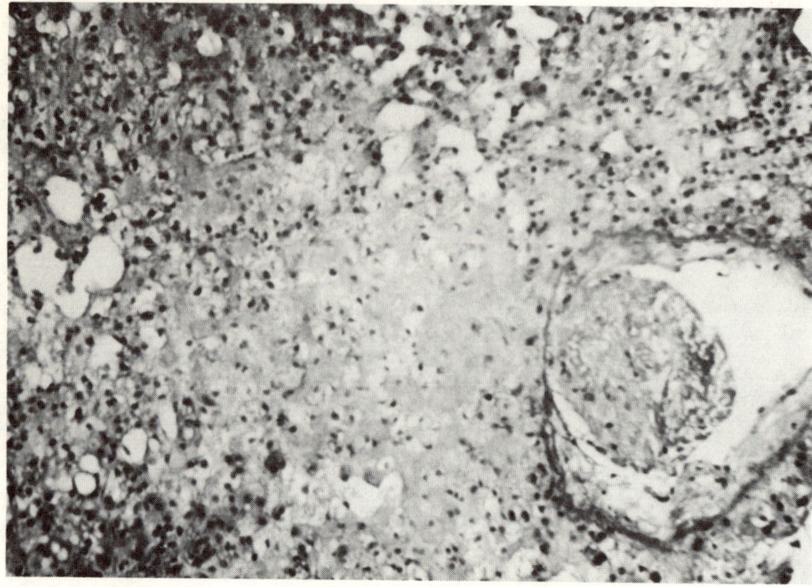

Figure 16-6 Photomicrography of organized thrombus in terminal hepatic venule, indicative of chronic Budd-Chiari syndrome.

throughout the specimen, the more likely the obstructing lesion is apt to be extrahepatic.

A rational approach to therapy for patients with the Budd-Chiari syndrome is difficult, for the available clinical data are anecdotal and experimental data are derived from an acute model. For the most part, one can rarely distinguish between cases of abrupt onset and those of a chronic nature that come to clinical attention because of sudden decompensation. Clearly, those tactics that reverse a fresh thrombus, eg, thrombolytic therapy or surgical embolectomy, cannot be used on vessels occluded by organized thrombi. In fact, surgical decompression of the portal system, preserving the portal vein as an outflow tract by use of a side-to-side portocaval shunt or a mesocaval H-graft, may produce beneficial or deleterious effects, depending upon the duration of the process, the regenerative capacity of the liver, and the dependence of the surviving parenchyma upon the hepatotropic factors of the portal circulation.

The initial step in therapy is to establish the location of the vascular obstruction and the duration of the process. Angiographic studies, while the most specific for this task, are somewhat hazardous because of splanchnic pooling which renders the kidneys oligemic and susceptible to dye-induced acute tubular necrosis. Abdominal ultrasound, CT scans, and nuclide angiographs may disclose inferior vena caval obstruction. The relative propensity of Orientals to develop Budd-Chiari syndrome due to web or diaphragm near the hepatic vein ostia is an important consideration for prompt surgical thrombectomy; web resection may be curative.

Detection of constrictive pericarditis may be surprisingly difficult. This condition may mimic the Budd-Chiari syndrome in nearly every respect and may require pressure measurements by placement of a Swan-Ganz catheter or formal right-sided cardiac catheterization for clear definition. Chest roentgenography, cardiac ultrasound, and clinical examination are not sufficiently accurate to eliminate the possibility of constrictive pericarditis.

As previously indicated, a liver biopsy might disclose an active, recent thombosing process susceptible to fibrinolytic therapy. Hemorrhage from the biopsy site would be expected with the use of fibrinolytic agents, so ironically, if their use is contemplated, the best evidence to support their use cannot be obtained. A radioactive fibrinogen scan may be the

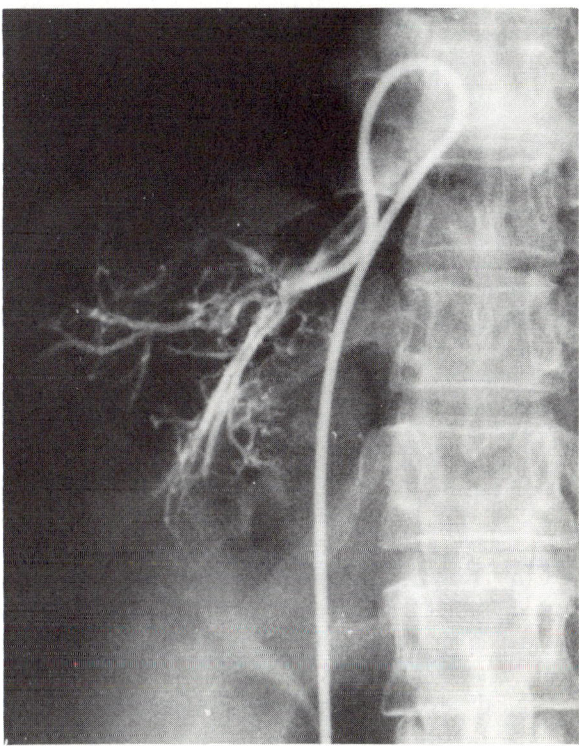

Figure 16-7 Hepatic venogram from a patient with polycythemia rubra vera demonstrating alteration of venous pattern (spider-web change) and probable thrombus in the hepatic vein proximal to the catheter tip. Patient has survived five years following placement of a LeVeen shunt on low-dose aspirin therapy.

most appropriate investigative tool to establish an active process but experience with its use in this setting is meager.

The best established, least invasive tool to make the diagnosis of Budd-Chiari syndrome is the hepatic scintiscan. When intense caudate lobe uptake and enlargement is demonstrable in the appropriate clinical setting, the diagnosis can be firmly established.

Approximately half of the patients with Budd-Chiari syndrome will have less specific "maldistribution" of nuclide uptake, which does assist the diagnostician.

Characteristic changes may be found on hepatic venogram (Figure 16-7), which shows a ragged, irregular, and focally occluded venous system. Inability to cannulate the hepatic veins is suggestive, but may reflect inexperience or unusual anatomy rather than occlusion. The added benefits of demonstrating inferior vena cava patency and obtaining hepatic wedge pressure measurements may assist considerably in ascribing ascites to presinusoidal, sinusoidal, or postsinusoidal portal hypertension.

A recent report demonstrated hepatic vein occlusion by CT and abdominal ultrasound. If these findings are extended, these noninvasive methods may be the safest, most reliable technics in the future.

Treatment

Aggressive therapy with fibrinolytic agents is most clearly indicated when the onset of the syndrome is abrupt and the clinical setting, eg, early postpartum state, suggests an active process rather than decompensation of a chronic process. A rapidly enlarging liver and increasing ascites, high serum enzyme levels, and lack of compensatory hypertrophy of the caudate lobe on scintiscan support an acute process. When the use of fibrinolytic agents is intended, invasive procedures such as arteriotomy, liver biopsy, and exploratory laparotomy will create sites of potentially hazardous hemorrhage at therapeutic levels of fibrinolysis and should be avoided. One often cannot wait for ten days, the recommended interval between surgery and fibrinolytic therapy, when surgery or biopsy is required to establish an irrefutable diagnosis. Such delay will also impair the effectiveness of fibrinolytic therapy because of the increased degree of thrombus organization developing during the interval.

A second therapeutic intervention, which seems to be more appropriate when treating a subacute or chronic Budd-Chiari syndrome, is the construction of a side-to-side portocaval shunt or a mesocaval H-graft shunt. Both procedures enhance the role of the portal vein as an outflow conduit and make hepatic survival dependent upon hepatic arterial blood flow. Acute experiments in dogs and anecdotal success in man indicate that a skilled surgeon can successfully perform these operations in critically ill subjects, with a reasonable chance for survival. Such a diversion must make the liver relatively oligemic, and whether improved liver function postoperatively is due to relief of congestion or interruption of the clotting process is unknown. Long-term survival seems to be best in patients with a protracted course prior to abrupt decompensation and it may be that survival in this group is dependent upon recanalization of old thrombi as much as the portal diversion. To be sure, portal diversion is likely to ameliorate the complications of this Budd-Chiari syndrome, bleeding gastritis, varices, ascites, mesenteric venous stasis, mesenteric thrombosis and malnutrition, even though the stage may be set for eventual liver atrophy and liver failure.

Once an initial intervention has been carried out, chronic anticoagulation should be instituted. If warfarin sodium is chosen, liver synthetic capacity may be monitored by factor V levels. Should the coagulopathy not be controlled, however, falling levels of factor V may be attributed inappropriately to hepatic decompensation. Furthermore, the often tenuous liver reserve may make the use of warfarin excessively dangerous. For these reasons, there is strong appeal for the use of platelet function inhibitors such as aspirin and dipyramidole. One to two ASA daily will likely impair platelet aggregation sufficiently to prevent recurrence of the coagulopathy. Long-term studies are not available to support this contention, but in the author's experience this approach seems to have merit. When chronic aspirin therapy is used in patients with unrelieved portal hypertension, careful monitoring for GI bleeding is prudent because of the known tendency for such patients to have hemorrhagic gastritis.

Ascites may respond to diuresis with an aldosterone antagonist and a loop diuretic. Dietary salt restriction may minimize the need for natriuresis in the exceptional patient. Dehydration is of particular concern because of the possible induction of fatal vena caval, mesenteric, portal, or renal vein thromboses in patients with coagulopathies, so that careful monitoring of weight, serum BUN, creatinine electrolytes, and urine osomolality is indicated. The goal of diuretic therapy is to enhance mobility and nutrition rather than elimination of demonstrable ascites.

In patients whose coagulopathy is controlled and in whom ascites is refractory, placement of a LeVeen shunt may be helpful. The enhanced renal function, nutrition, and abdominal silhouette must be weighed against the possibility of life-threatening intravascular coagulopathy, sepsis, or shunt and suprior vena caval thrombosis. An occasional patient will also develop bleeding varices or congestive heart failure early in the postoperative period. Despite these risks, some patients do remarkably well after shunt placement.

Adequate nutrition may be difficult to supply to patients with chronic Budd-Chiari syndrome. Gut edema can impair absorption, chronic massive ascites can compress the stomach and reduce intake, and the frequent evolution of chronic Budd-Chiari syndrome to cirrhosis can add problems of hepatic encephalopathy and amino acid imbalance to ill patients with minimal nutritional reserve. Dietary salt restriction, ingestion of proteins relatively low in aromatic amino acids, and provision of calories through the use of medium-chain triglyceride oils can be of benefit in selected cases. Supplemental vitamins are advisable.

Finally, the role of liver transplantation remains to be evaluated. Provided the anatomical alterations of the inferior vena cava and the portal vein are not great, and the underlying process which induced the syndrome can be controlled or eliminated, there is hope that some of these patients can be salvaged.

ACKNOWLEDGMENT

Drs. Jerry Petasnick, Claire Smith, and David Turner provided illustrative radiographs and scintiscans. Charlene Schwar provided secretarial assistance.

REFERENCES

1. Grendell JH, Ockner RK: Mesenteric venous thrombosis. *Gastroenterology* 1982;82:358–372.
2. Marder VJ: The use of thrombolytic agents: choice of patient, drug administration, laboratory monitoring. *Ann Intern Med* 1979;90:802–808.
3. Mitchell MC, Boitnott JK, Kaufman S, et al: Budd-Chiari syndrome: etiology, diagnosis and management. *Medicine* 1982;61:199–218.
4. Orloff MJ, Stipa S, Ziparo V (eds): *Medical and Surgical Problems of Portal Hypertension*. New York, Academic Press, 1980.

17 *Pulmonary Embolism*

James W. West

Pulmonary thromboembolism is a clinical condition which deserves the careful attention of physicians and students. It is a common disorder, with an estimated 500,000 persons annually suffering a pulmonary embolism.[1] It is a serious disorder, with at least 50,000 deaths per years in the United States alone.[2] Effective therapy for embolism exists, which yields a 90% survival rate once therapy has been given.[3] Approximately 90% of patients will survive more than one hour after the embolic event, and should be candidates to receive this therapy. However, patients die unnecessarily since the diagnosis is established and therapy instituted in only one third of these patients.[3] In addition to underdiagnosing pulmonary thromboembolism, many experts believe that our common diagnostic approach to patients with suspected embolism leads to a serious incidence of false-positive results, or overdiagnosis, exposing patients unnecessarily to the hazards of anticoagulation therapy.[4] The final frustration in this sequence is that the careful attention that physicians give to pulmonary thromboembolism is partly misdirected. Although pulmonary embolism may be the most common acute pulmonary problem in hospitalized patients, it is not primarily a pulmonary disease.[5] It is a complication of deep venous thrombosis, which is a disease that is, to a great degree, preventable. Several excellent reviews of the topic of pulmonary embolism are available.[5-9] The reader is referred to these for a more detailed discussion of pulmonary embolism.

PATHOGENESIS

Origin of Deep Venous Thrombosis

The etiology and pathogenesis of deep venous thrombosis have been described in detail in a previous chapter. For the purpose of this discussion, it will be sufficient to emphasize only two points. First, almost all pulmonary thromboemboli arise from a deep vein thrombosis. Second, the risk factors which predispose to the development of deep venous thrombosis are necessarily the same risk factors which predispose to the occurrence of pulmonary emboli. The major risk factors are: prior history of deep venous thrombosis, venous valvular insufficiency in the legs, prolonged bed rest or immobility, congestive heart failure, obesity, trauma to pelvis and lower extremities, the postoperative and postpartum period, extensive body burns, and systemic malignancy.

It should be apparent from the causal relationship between deep venous thrombosis and pulmonary emboli that the only hope for decreasing the frequency of emboli lies with the prevention or earlier detection of deep venous thrombosis.

Origin of Emboli

Pulmonary thromboemboli arise in the deep venous system. Current estimates state that about 95% of pulmonary emboli originate in the deep veins of the legs.[5] The remaining few emboli arise as mural thrombi in the right ventricle, thrombi in pelvic veins, such as the prostatic veins or uterine veins, or in renal or hepatic veins. Although thrombophlebitis in the veins of the upper extremity is quite common in hospitalized patients, it apparently does not give rise to pulmonary emboli. This may be due to the intense local inflammatory response, which may rapidly produce attachment and organization of the thrombi. Alternatively, since these veins are relatively quite small compared to the deep veins of the leg, emboli could arise which are too small to produce clinical manifestations.

Although emboli originating in the right ventricle, hepatic veins, and renal veins are rare, they are nonetheless important since caval interruption procedures will not prevent recurrence from these sites. The physician's index of suspicion should, therefore, be high in patients with underlying rheumatic valvular disease, cor pulmonale, Budd-Chiari syndrome, and chronic renal disease with marked proteinuria which could be due to renal vein thrombosis.

Within the deep venous system of the legs, the vast majority of emboli probably arise from the veins above the knee.[10,11] Certainly many deep vein thrombi are extensions of thrombi that have started in veins below the knee. The greater frequency of emboli complicating thigh vein thrombosis could be related to the larger caliber of these veins. Emboli from these large thrombi would result in more significant pulmonary arterial obstruction and more clinically apparent symptoms and signs. Thrombi may, of course, arise primarily in the veins of the thigh, especially following hip trauma or surgery. The relative frequency of these two events, primary thrombosis of thigh veins or calf vein thrombosis extending into thigh veins, is important since the physical signs of deep venous thrombosis in the thigh are even less reliable and more variably present than those in calf vein thrombosis.

It should be mentioned that thrombi of the superficial veins of the lower leg rarely result in emboli. Should an embolus occur, it probably represents extension of the thrombus into the deep venous system. As mentioned in the context of upper extremity thrombophlebitis, emboli could be occurring which are too small to be clinically apparent.

PATHOPHYSIOLOGY

Once a thrombus, or a part of a thrombus, detaches from its site of origin in the deep venous system, normal venous return will carry it through the right-sided chambers of the heart, where it may be held up or fragmented, to the pulmonary arterial system. After the embolus lodges in a pulmonary artery, it will produce partial or complete interruption of the arterial flow to a portion of the lung. The amount of the pulmonary arterial circulation that is compromised will vary according to the size of the embolus. A massive embolus will occlude 50% or more of the pulmonary vascular bed.[12] Examples of a massive embolus would be a "saddle" embolus to the pulmonary artery trunk, or an embolus to the left or right main pulmonary artery. A submassive embolism is one that results in occlusion of less than 50% of the pulmonary vascular bed, such as a lobar or segmented artery embolus. Categorization of the size of an embolus should be based on quantification of the defect visualized with the perfusion lung scan or the pulmonary arteriogram.

The pathophysiologic consequences of a pulmonary embolism are of two types: respiratory and hemodynamic.[5]

Respiratory Pathophysiology

There are three major respiratory consequences of pulmonary embolism: the production of alveolar dead space, reduction in volume of the embolized portion of lung, and loss of surfactant.[5]

Alveolar dead space is that volume of lung which has absent or significantly reduced arterial perfusion but with persistent ventilation. Such a nonperfused but ventilated zone is the obvious immediate result of an embolus. The ventilation to this area cannot partake in gas exchange and is therefore wasted. Since the ventilatory requirement of a patient after an embolism is at least unchanged and commonly is increased, the total ventilation will have to be increased significantly to compensate for the added dead space. As a minimum effect, the increased demand for total ventilation may contribute to the patient's sense of dyspnea. If a large-enough volume of lung has been so affected, then the patient may not be able to compensate adequately for the additional dead space, and acute ventilatory failure may supervene. This is especially true of patients with underlying severe obstructive lung disease who may have markedly increased dead space as a base line, as well as minimal reserve ventilatory capacity.

The second major respiratory consequence of an embolism is a reduction in the volume of the embolized portion of lung. The reduction in lung volume cannot be explained only by the loss of the perfusing volume of blood, nor is it due to bronchoconstriction alone. Rather constriction of the smooth muscle in the terminal bronchioles and alveolar ducts occurs. These smooth muscle fibers are arranged longitudinally as well as circumferentially.[13] Contraction of the longitudinal fibers will have the effect of reducing the volume of the distal alveoli.[14] This will result in a decrease in the alveolar dead space produced by the embolus. The postulated mechanism for this "pneumoconstriction" is of interest.[5] The alveolar partial pressure of carbon dioxide will be markedly reduced in the embolized zone since it is ventilated with inspired gas which is almost carbon dioxide–free. Hypocapnic areas of the lung have been demonstrated to undergo pneumoconstriction, which can be reversed by inhalation of a carbon dioxide–air mixture.[15] Local hypoxia may also be playing a role since supplemental oxygen can also reverse the pneumoconstriction in experimental models.[16] The role played by humoral agents such as serotonin, histamine, and bradykinin is controversial.[17] Although these agents have been demonstrated to produce bronchoconstriction following microembolization in some animal species, extrapolating the results to macroembolization in humans is risky.

Loss of surfactant, the third major respiratory consequence of pulmonary emoblism, is also the last to develop. By about 24 hours after cessation of blood flow to a segment of lung, the surfactant activity will have declined markedly.[18] The deficiency in surfactant will predispose to the development of atelectasis of this segment. In addition, interstitial fluid will be more likely to transude into the alveolar space, producing pulmonary edema in the segment, since surfactant normally plays a role in maintaining the impermeability of the alveolar capillary membrane.[5]

The processes of pneumoconstriction and loss of surfactant will have the effect of producing in the embolized segment significant volume loss and fluid-filling of air spaces. This will have the histologic appearance of "congestive atelectasis." It is this pathologic process which produces the majority of pulmonary parenchymal radiographic densities associated with emboli, rather than true tissue infarction, which is uncommon.

Hypoxemia is a result of the respiratory, and possibly hemodynamic, consequences of pulmonary embolism. The exact mechanism of its production, however, is not known definitely. It should be remembered that alveolar dead space, with its high ventilation-perfusion ratio will not by itself produce hypoxemia. It is likely that a low ventilation-perfusion mismatch, specifically with ventilation decreased relative to perfusion, is the explanation for hypoxemia. Certainly low ventilation-perfusion ratio defects have been documented in experimental pulmonary embolism using the multiple inert gas technic.[19] Such a defect could be produced by bronchoconstriction/pneumoconstriction around, or at the edge of, the emoblized segment where there remains relatively intact arterial perfusion. Alternatively, nonembolized segments of lung could be exposed to severe overperfusion with blood shunted away from the embolized vascular bed, which will also result in ventilation being reduced in relation to relatively increased perfusion. Other explanations for the hypoxemia have been advanced,[6] ranging from anatomic shunting of venous blood through a patent foramen ovale, pleural vessels, or other channels, to a widened arterial-venous oxygen gradient due to a diminished cardiac output, which would magnify the effects of normal venous admixture. There are probably different mechanisms for the production of hypoxemia at different stages in the evolution of the embolus. An excellent example of this would be at the time the embolus is starting to resolve, since perfusion will then be restored to a congested, atelectatic segment.[5]

Hemodynamic Pathophysiology

The initial, and main, hemodynamic result of pulmonary embolism is acute reduction in the pulmonary vascular cross-sectional area.[5] The subsequent hemodynamic consequence will be secondary to this, although other mechanisms may play a role.

The reduction in patent vascular bed will result in an immediate increase in the pulmonary vascular resistance. If the resistance is increased significantly, and if the cardiac output is to be maintained, the pulmonary artery pressure must rise and the right ventricular work will be increased. Therefore, the net hemodynamic consequences of pulmonary embolism are increases in the pulmonary vascular resistance, pulmonary artery pressure, and right ventricular work.[5]

As mentioned above, the pulmonary vascular resistance must be increased significantly to produce an elevation of the pulmonary artery pressure. The normal pulmonary vascular reserve capacity is such that about 50% of the cross-sectional area must be lost before sustained pulmonary hypertension will be seen at normal levels of cardiac output.[5,20] If more than 50% of the vascular bed is occluded, then pulmonary hypertension will result, with its attendant increased right ventricular work, if the cardiac output is maintained. The greater the degree of occlusion, the higher will be the pulmonary artery pressure.[21] There are limits to the right ventricle's ability to compensate for embolic occlusion and to develop pressure. Several studies have shown that, in patients without prior history of cardiopulmonary disease, the maximum mean pulmonary artery pressure that can be developed is 40 mmHg.[21-23] The right ventricle is thin-walled and is not prepared to develop high pressures and perform a significantly increased amount of work. A previously normal right ventricle will dilate significantly at a mean pulmonary artery pressure of 40 mmHg, which may result in acute tricuspid regurgitation.[24] If this pressure load is sustained, then the cardiac output may fall, and acute cor pulmonale and shock may follow.

The extent of embolic occlusion is, then, one of the three major determinants of the severity of the hemodynamic consequences of pulmonary embolism. The other two are the cardiovascular status of the patient before the embolism, and the action of reflex and humoral factors.[5]

If a disease of the heart or lungs exists in a patient which has already impaired the pulmonary vascular reserve capacity, then a relatively smaller degree of vascular occlusion due to pulmonary embolism will result in greater pulmonary arterial hypertension and right ventricular strain.[5,6,21] Examples of such cardiovascular and pulmonary diseases are: congestive heart failure, aortic or mitral valve disease, previous pulmonary embolism, and chronic obstructive pulmonary disease. Detailed hemodynamic evaluations of pulmonary embolism patients with and without preexisting cardiopulmonary disease have documented these relationships.[21] It is also a common clinical observation that a moderate-sized embolus can prove fatal in a patient with obstructive lung disease or heart failure, whereas an otherwise normal patient will usually survive even a massive embolism.[5]

The role played by reflex and humoral factors in determining the severity of the hemodynamic responses to embolism is controversial. Reflex pulmonary artery vasoconstriction has been found in response to emboli in dogs.[25] Also, in experimental animals, pulmonary vasoconstriction in response to the release of serotonin from platelets has been documented.[26-28] If these reflex and humoral mechanisms are operative in humans, it is easy to see how they would increase the burden on the right ventricle, over and above that produced by mechanical occlusion. To what extent they contribute to determining the hemodynamic response to embolism in humans remains uncertain.[5]

Pulmonary Infarction

True pulmonary infarction, ischemic death of lung tissue, is a rare consequence of embolism. It has been estimated that fewer than 10% of emboli result in death of lung parenchyma.[5] This may be due, in part, to the fact that there is commonly some blood flow past an embolus. More important, however, are the other two sources of oxygen supply to lung tissue besides the pulmonary artery, namely the bronchial arteries and the airways. Loss of one of these sources, if the others are intact, probably does not result in infarction. Rather, it appears that two of the sources must be compromised to lead to infarction. Therefore, pulmonary infarction is more likely to occur in patients with underlying left ventricular failure or obstructive lung diesease, which is an accepted clinical observation.[5,29] The availability of two alternate sources of oxygen supply to the lung tissue probably also explains why infarctions are more likely to occur after small, peripheral emboli than following large, central ones. In a small, peripheral lung segment there may be less bronchial arterial anastomotic flow available to support tissue viability, and a much more minor airway abnormality could significantly impair the penetration of ventilation.

NATURAL HISTORY

Even as the above pathophysiologic sequence is occurring, the pulmonary thromboembolism itself is starting the process of resolution. The most frequent course of thromboembolic obstruction beyond the acute event is restoration of vascular patency.[5,30] As is the case with venous thromboses, the two processes which lead to this resolution are fibrinolysis and organization. Since these processes have been described already in chapter 4, the discussion here will be brief.

There are two sources of the fibrinolytic process: circulating fibrinolytic activity, and activity released from the pulmonary vascular endothelium at the site of the embolism. Fibrinolytic dissolution can occur quite rapidly, in as short a time as a few hours in dogs,[30] and, interestingly, can progress postmortem. The rate of resolution is not well-known in humans, but, based on angiographic and scintigraphic data, can occur in as little as two days.[5] There is probably marked patient-to-patient variability in the rate of fibrinolytic activity. The speed of fibrinolytic resolution can also be affected by the embolus itself. Older thrombi, especially if there has been some organization prior to embolization, will be relatively resistant to fibrinolysis.[31]

Organization is the second process for restoring vascular patency, and occurs more slowly, requiring days to weeks for maximum effect.[5] In this process, the embolus becomes invested with an endothelial covering and gradually becomes attached to, and incorporated into, the vessel wall. The endothelial cells extend into the embolus, eventually forming new channels through it. This recanalization can lead to no discernible residua, or it can lead to varying degrees of endothelial scarring or "web" formation. The frequency of permanent residual defects is not known, but is apparently not common since fewer than 10% of patients have perfusion scar defects beyond six weeks following the embolus.

DIAGNOSIS

Clinical Manifestations

The symptoms and signs of pulmonary thromboembolism are nonspecific. The abnormalities which can be seen on routine laboratory tests, chest films, or the electrocardiogram cannot be considered pathognomonic. It is then necessary for the physician to consider the possibility of pulmonary embolism in any patient who has significant risk and has a compatible presentation. The Urokinase-Streptokinase Pulmonary Embolus Trial (USPET)[12,32] was a multicenter controlled study of 327 patients with angiographically documented pulmonary emboli performed between 1968 and 1973. Although it was designed to evaluate the effect of fibrinolytic therapy on emboli, it also carefully documented the clinical manifestations displayed by these patients. It is these data that will form the basis for the subsequent description.

Symptoms and signs　Dyspnea is the most common symptom, occurring in 88% of patients. It occurs with only slightly increased frequency in patients with massive as opposed to submassive emboli,[6] and in patients with pre-existing cardiopulmonary disease as opposed to those without.[33] The dyspnea is usually of sudden onset and can be transient, clearing in minutes to hours, and clearing in two days in 50% of the USPET patients.

Pleuritic chest pain occurred in 73% of patients and is significantly more common in submassive emboli, which are more likely to produce infarction or congestive atelectasis.[5] Nonpleuritic substernal pain or tightness occurs much less commonly than pleuritic pain and is present more commonly in massive emboli.[34]

Apprehension and cough occur in a little more than half the patients. Hemoptysis was present in 34% of patients, and, like pleuritic chest pain, is more common in submassive emboli. Syncope, palpitations, and angina are found in less than 15% of patients.[35] The commonly taught combination of dyspnea, pleuritic chest pain, and hemoptysis was seen in only 28% of all patients and less frequently in patients with massive emboli.[36]

Tachypnea is the most consistent physical finding and is seen in 88% of patients. Tachycardia was seen in only 43% of patients. These findings can be of short duration. Localized rales and an increased pulmonic component of the second heart sound ($\uparrow S_2 P$) are present in about one half the cases. Fever (temperature $> 37.8\,°C$) is found in approximately 40% of patients. Evidence of thrombophlebitis is present in about one third of patients. Cyanosis and a pleural friction rub are seen in less than 20% of cases.

Although all the above symptoms and signs are nonspecific, and would serve poorly to differentiate a patient with an embolus from one with pneumonia or a myocardial infarction, they tend to occur together in more recognizable syndromes.[33] The circulatory collapse syndrome, characterized by shock or syncope, is correlated with more extensive emboli, and occurs in about 20% of patients. The pulmonary infarction syndrome, presenting with pleuritic chest pain and/or hemoptysis, occurs in approximately 66% of patients. (It should be remembered that a true pulmonary infarction is occurring in only a fraction of these patients.) The uncomplicated pulmonary embolism syndrome, characterized by dyspnea, nonpleuritic chest pain, and tachypnea, is seen in about 15% of patients.

Routine blood tests   There are no routine blood tests that can help to establish the diagnosis of pulmonary embolism. It had been suggested that the finding of an elevated serum lactic dehydrogenase, an elevated serum bilirubin, and a normal serum glutamic oxaloacetic transaminase, all occurring simultaneously, is evidence for pulmonary infarction.[37] However, these findings are not specific for pulmonary infarction, and occur only infrequently.[38] The white blood cell count can be normal or elevated, but is usually less than $15,000/\mu l$. Breakdown products of fibrinogen and fibrin have not proved to be helpful, nor have technics using plasma DNA levels or the nitroblue tetrazolium assay.[6]

Arterial blood gases   Arterial blood gases drawn while the patient is breathing room air, although a valuable test, cannot be considered to have diagnostic significance. Hypoxemia is found in most patients with a pulmonary embolus. A PO_2 greater than 80 mmHg was found in only 10% of patients in phases I and II of the USPET.[12,32,36] Use of the alveolar arterial gradient of oxygen is more sensitive than just the arterial PO_2. This calculation takes into account that hyperventilation, and a resultant reduced arterial PCO_2, is commonly present. This can cause an elevation in the arterial PO_2 and can mask the oxygenation defect due to an embolus. But even the alveolar-arterial gradient is normal in rare cases of pulmonary embolus.

Chest radiography   Although there are many chest radiograph abnormalities that can be produced by pulmonary embolism, the chest film is commonly considered normal and is rarely diagnostic.[13] The high incidence of radiographic abnormalities quoted in the literature[12,39] is misleading and is probably due to the fact that the presence of an embolus was already established. The chest radiograph is usually one of the first pieces of laboratory information available, however, and careful evaluation can yield helpful information.

Pulmonary parenchymal infiltrations can be produced by emboli and represent congestive atelectasis or, less commonly, pulmonary infarction. The densities are pleura-based, and are almost always seen in the lower and mid-lung fields. If seen in profile, the density is usually rounded, with the convexity directed toward the hilum ("Hampton's hump"). If seen frontally, however, the density is irregular and inhomogeneous. More than 90% of the densities will resolve within weeks, with no residual scar.[13] On rare occasions a pulmonary infarct will cavitate, and in these instances a complicating infectious process should be considered. Smaller, nonsegmental densities, usually horizontal in orientation, representing "platelike" atelectasis are sometimes present.

Elevation of a hemidiaphragm is a subtle and not uncommon clue. It represents volume loss of the lung on that side. The diaphragm can be seen fluoroscopically to be freely moveable, so that the elevation should not be attributed to "splinting" due to chest pain.[13]

Changes in the radiographic appearance of the pulmonary vasculature are commonly subtle and are more easily seen in retrospect. If a pre-embolus chest film is available for comparison, the diagnostic value will be improved. Distention of a proximal pulmonary artery due to the presence of a thrombus which has been impacted distally by pulmonary blood flow is the most common vascular abnormality. Sometimes the vessel downstream to the embolus can appear narrowed or cut off. Oligemia of the lung field affected by the embolus ("Westermark's sign") can be focal and limited or can be extensive depending on the size of the embolus. Unilateral oligemia may be overlooked in the presence of more obvious hyperperfusion of the opposite lung (Figure 17-1).

A pleural effusion can be seen in a minority of patients, more frequently accompanying submassive embolism with infarction, and can

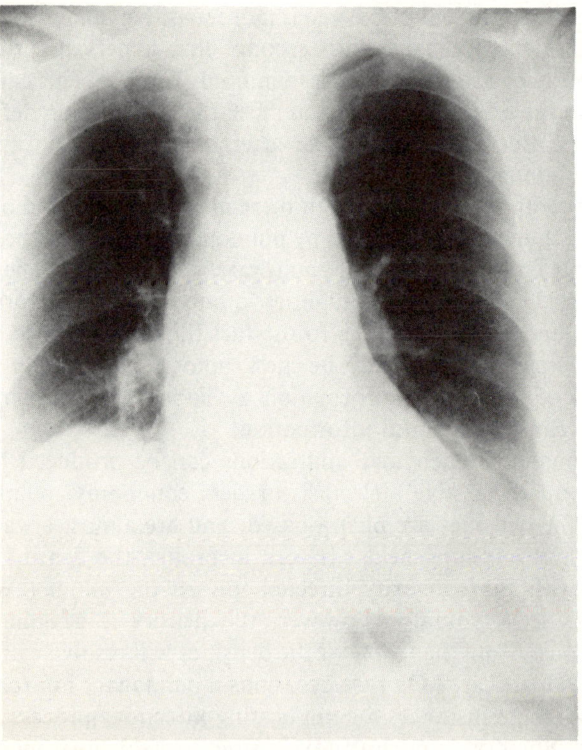

Figure 17-1   An admission posteroanterior chest radiograph of a patient with massive pulmonary embolism reveals a significantly elevated right hemidiaphragm, a distended right lower lobe pulmonary artery, and a paucity of vascular markings in the right lung. A decubitus film also revealed a small right pleural effusion.

occasionally be large enough to obscure the underlying parenchymal density. However, it is much more commonly small, and may not be apparent unless decubitus views are obtained.

Electrocardiogram   Like the other clinical examinations mentioned above, the electrocardiogram can reveal only suggestive information. It frequently is normal or shows only a sinus tachycardia. The most common abnormality found in the USPET patients was T wave inversion.[12] Nonspecific S-T segment elevation or depression were also common. Left axis deviation was more common than right axis deviation. Changes suggestive of acute cor pulmonale ($S_1Q_3T_3$, right bundle branch block, P pulmonale) occurred in less than 20% of patients. Premature ventricular beats were the most common rhythm disturbances. Atrial fibrillation was present in less than 5% of patients.

Lung scanning   If a patient is suspected of having had a pulmonary embolus on the basis of the above clinical manifestations, then testing is usually pursued in order to firmly and objectively establish the patient's diagnosis. Lung scanning is frequently the first step in this process.

The perfusion lung scan is performed by injecting intravenously macroaggregates of albumin which have been labeled with a gamma-emitting isotope, like technetium 99m. These particles will be distributed throughout the pulmonary vasculature, wherever pulmonary arterial perfusion is intact. Because the particles are 10 to 50 μm in diameter, they will be held up in the precapillary arterioles. If there is impairment of vascular perfusion to an area of lung, then the radioactive particles will not be distributed to the lung beyond these abnormalities. Examples of processes which can impair perfusion are: pulmonary embolus, pulmonary vasculitis, pulmonary arterial vasospasm, external compression of a central artery by a neoplasm, or obliteration of the vessel by destructive processes like emphysema, pulmonary fibrosis, pneumonia, or a peripheral neoplasm. A gamma-sensing device outside the chest is then used to detect the pattern of deposition of the particles. Areas of the lung with relatively diminished or absent gamma activity will then be recognized as "perfusion defects." The correspondence of the distribution and extent of perfusion defect to the anatomy of the lung should be considered. If the defect corresponds to a segment of a lobe, or to an entire lobe, this finding would be more significant than if the defect was subsegmental in extent.

The perfusion lung scan must be interpreted with a recent chest radiograph at hand. Even the incomplete list of processes causing perfusion noted above suggests that many of those processes will be visible on the radiograph. If there is a radiographic abnormality which corresponds in position to the perfusion defect, then the differential diagnosis of the scan will be the same as that of the radiograph, which may include pulmonary embolus with infarction or atelectasis, of course. If the area of lung displaying the perfusion defect is radiographically normal, then the differential diagnosis is more limited. Besides pulmonary emboli, this pattern could be explained by a pulmonary arteritis or primary airway or air-space disease, like asthma, emphysema, bronchitis, endobronchial tumor, or foreign body. In order to screen for an airway or air-space abnormality causing a perfusion defect, the ventilation scan has been used.

The ventilation scan is performed by having the patient breathe an inert, radioactive gas, like xenon 133. The scanning device will then demonstrate the pattern of distribution of ventilation. It is best to monitor this pattern during the patient's first breath, as the patient continues to breathe the radioactive gas from a closed-circuit ("wash-in" phase), at equilibrium, and as the patient progressively breathes the gas out ("wash-out" phase). If there is an abnormality of the distribution of ventilation, this will appear as an area of delayed uptake or elimination of the tracer gas, or an inhomogeneity of the pattern at equilibrium.

Combining the ventilation scan with the perfusion scan should permit the differentiation of processes producing abnormalities of both ventilation and perfusion ("matched defects") from those producing only an abnormality of perfusion ("mismatched defect"). The finding of a mismatched defect would then imply the presence of vascular obstruction and would be considered to have a high probability of being due to an embolus. However, to complicate matters still further, if an embolus is associated with pneumoconstriction or developing congestive atelectasis, then there can be a matched ventilation-perfusion defect due to a pulmonary embolus.[4]

There are several advantages of lung scanning as the initial step in screening for a pulmonary embolus after suggestive clinical manifestations have been found. Present technology permits multiple views to be performed in a short time, and, where facilities permit, it can even be performed at the patient's bedside. It is relatively noninvasive and safe, and can be repeated in order to follow the resolution of an embolus or to screen for a recurrent embolus, using previous scans as a base line for comparison. It chief advantage, however, is its sensitivity. A normal perfusion lung scan effectively rules out the possibility of an embolus.[5-7,40] In contrast to this marked sensitivity, there is a very poor specificity to the interpretation of the perfusion defect. This is apparent by reviewing the variety of processes which can produce perfusion defects.

Lung scanning is, then, a useful procedure but cannot be considered to have uniform diagnostic significance independent of the clinical situation. Certainly a normal perfusion scan is sufficient evidence to rule out the possibility of pulmonary embolus.[41] However, an abnormal scan, including the ventilation scan, must be interpreted with the clinical presentation in mind. If the patient is in a high-risk group for pulmonary embolism and has suggestive clinical manifestations, then the finding of multiple segmental or lobar mismatched defects with a normal chest radiograph would be considered adequate for a presumptive diagnosis of pulmonary emboli (Figures 17-2 and 17-3).[42] If the defects have a subsegmental distribution, are multiple but not all mismatched, or if the defects are correlated with radiographic abnormalities, then these ventilation-perfusion scan results can neither establish nor exclude the diagnosis of pulmonary embolism.[43] The work-up should then proceed to the definitive test, pulmonary angiography.

Pulmonary angiography   Pulmonary angiography permits visualization of an embolus as well as definition of its extent, and provides the

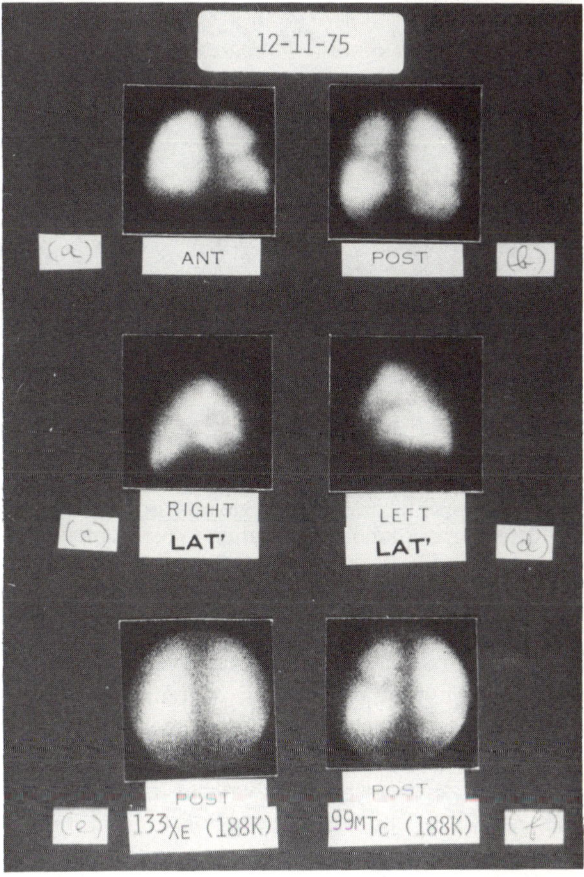

Figure 17-2   Series of lung scans on a patient with suspected pulmonary embolism: (a)–(d): Four-view perfusion lung scan showing segmented perfusion defects in the left, mid-, and upper lung zones. (e) Posterior view of the ventilation scan revealing normal distribution of ventilation. (f) Posterior view of perfusion scan done simultaneously with (e) documenting mismatched perfusion defects on the left. (Lung scans courtesy of David A. Turner, MD, Rush–Presbyterian–St. Luke's Medical Center.)

364

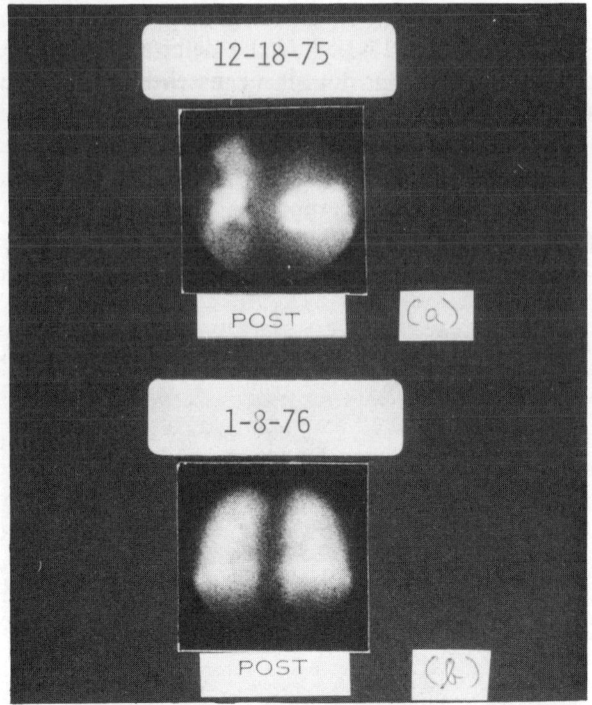

Figure 17-3 (a) Posterior view of perfusion lung scan performed on same patient as in Figure 17-2 immediately after an episode of cardiovascular collapse. There have now been superimposed several new segmental perfusion defects on the left, as well as a new right upper lobar defect. Angiogram documented extensive intravascular filling defects corresponding in location to perfusion defects. (b) Significant resolution of perfusion defects three weeks later. (Lung scans courtesy of David A. Turner, MD, Rush–Presbyterian–St. Luke's Medical Center.)

greatest diagnostic certainty of any test available. Because of its invasiveness, the risk of arrhythmias, the risk of renal, cardiovascular, and allergic complications of the dye-load, and its cost, it should not be considered necessary in every patient suspected of having a pulmonary embolism. If a young patient presents with historical and clinical manifestations suggestive of pulmonary embolism and has mismatched defects on lung scanning in areas of the lung not associated with a radiographic abnormality, then this can be considered an adequate basis for establishing the diagnoses of embolism and instituting anticoagulation. In an older patient whose evaluation still leaves doubt as to the diagnosis, or who has a predictably greater risk from anticoagulation, angiography is indicated. Certainly if surgical intervention (such as caval interruption or embolectomy) or thrombolytic therapy is being considered, then incontrovertible angiographic demonstration of the embolus is necessary.

Ideally, angiography should be performed within 48 hours of the suspected embolic event.[44] Delay beyond this time may occasionally result in loss of angiographic detail as the normal fibrinolytic activity causes the clot to diminish in size, or break up into a shower of smaller clots which may embolize too far distally to be detected reliably. The contrast injection should be made in the main pulmonary artery or more distally in the pulmonary vasculature; injecting into the right ventricle, right atrium, or the central or peripheral venous system will significantly reduce the detection capability of the study. Selective angiography in lobar or segmental arteries, directed by the findings on lung scan or chest radiograph, may enhance diagnostic yield. If available, hemodynamic data, such as pulmonary capillary wedge pressure, pulmonary artery and right ventricular pressures, and cardiac output, should be measured through the central catheter to improve the overall evaluation of the patient's status.

There are two angiographic findings which are considered diagnostic for pulmonary emboli: intraluminal filling defect in a pulmonary artery, or abrupt cut-off of a major artery.[44,45] Delay in flow, regional diminution of perfusion, or a decrease in vessel caliber are nonspecific findings (Figure 17-4).

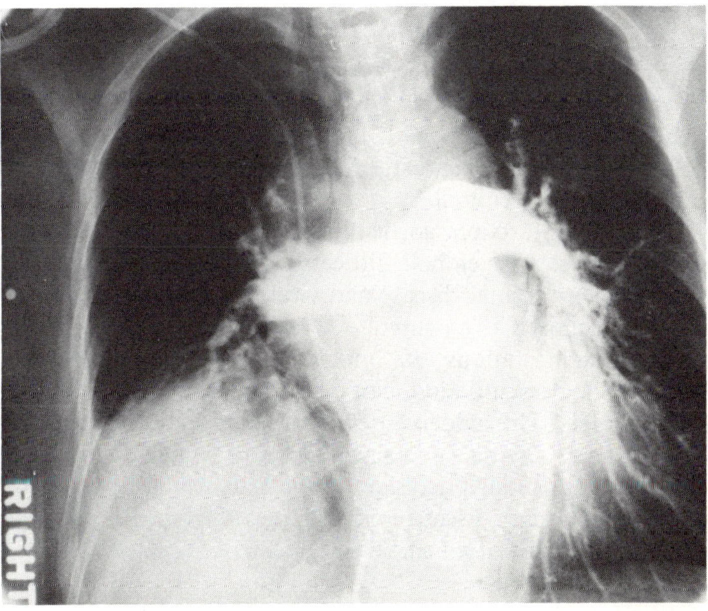

Figure 17-4 Pulmonary angiogram performed on same patient as in Figure 17-1. A filling defect is visible in the right main pulmonary artery at the takeoff of the right upper lobe artery. There is also markedly diminished flow to the entire right lung and the left upper lobe.

The incidence of complications of pulmonary angiography is 4%, while the mortality in large series is less than 0.5%.[4,7] This is considerably greater morbidity and mortality than would be seen with lung scanning. However, the nonspecificity of clinical presentation, routine testing, and lung scanning still leads to many false-positive diagnoses. In these patients, the risk of anticoagulation therapy is unwarranted and is considerably greater than the risk of angiography. Representative studies evaluating the risk of heparin and coumarin-derivative anticoagulation have found significant complications in 25% to 30%, and mortality, related directly to the anticoagulation, of 1% to 2.4%.[46,47] The importance of definitively establishing the diagnosis of pulmonary embolism with angiography whenever the proceeding evaluation leaves significant doubt, is therefore, apparent.[43]

DIFFERENTIAL DIAGNOSIS

Pulmonary embolism is a difficult diagnosis to make on clinical grounds because its common manifestations are the same as those of several other common medical problems. The clinician must have a high index of suspicion of pulmonary embolus even when these other processes seem more likely. Only in this way can the number of emboli not diagnosed be reduced.

Pneumonia, both bacterial and viral, commonly produces dyspnea, pleuritic chest pain, apprehension, cough, tachypnea, tachycardia, fever, and rales just as pulmonary embolism does. Purulent sputum production and marked leukocytosis would, of course, favor pneumonia, but are variably present. In this context, postoperative fever and atelectasis can be manifestations of emboli.[5]

Myocardial infarction, aortic dissection, and pneumothorax can all be easily confused with emboli. Processes producing acute pleuritis, including collagen-vascular disease and viral or tuberculous pleurisy may also be misdiagnosed as an embolus.[5]

Subtle manifestations of emboli, especially syncope, recurrent dyspnea, and hyperventilation, can mimic neurologic, cardiac, and psychiatric disorders. The sudden onset of atrial fibrillation in a patient with pre-existing heart disease, sudden worsening of a patient with congestive heart failure, and sudden deterioration in a patient with severe chronic obstructive pulmonary disease are all settings where a pulmonary embolism is likely to be overlooked.

DIAGNOSTIC WORK-UP

The extent of the diagnostic evaluation which is adequate in the setting of suspected embolism must be tailored to the individual patient.

The factors that must be considered in making this decision are: (1) the severity of the patient's condition, and (2) the risk of the therapeutic intervention being considered.[5,45]

If the patient is hemodynamically or metabolically unstable following the possible embolic event, with manifestations such as acute right ventricular failure, shock, ventilatory insufficiency, or severe hypoxemia, then the diagnosis of pulmonary embolism must be established or excluded with the greatest certainty and as rapidly as possible. Unless there was a very serious contraindication, most clinicians would initiate anticoagulation therapy with a bolus of heparin in a dose of 10,000 to 20,000 IU as they started the evaluation. Certainly an ECG, arterial blood gases, and a chest radiograph would be indispensible. Unless an alternative diagnosis, such as myocardial infarction, pneumothorax, or aortic dissection became apparent, the next step would be angiography. If the patient is less acutely ill, then perfusion lung scanning could be done before planning for angiography. If the perfusion scan is normal, then a diagnosis other than pulmonary embolism should be pursued. If the perfusion scan is abnormal, then a ventilation scan could be added to improve the specificity of the results. If the findings are less extensive than multiple lobar or segmental mismatched defects, then angiography is indicated. This is especially important in the patient with underlying cardiopulmonary disease, in whom the nonspecificity of other than angiographic results is greater, and in whom the prognosis is poorer, requiring consideration of thrombolytic therapy or surgical intervention.[45]

The risk of the therapeutic intervention being weighed must be considered simultaneously with the severity of illness. In the case of a young patient without other medical problems, heparin therapy may be warranted on the basis of compatible clinical manifestations and perfusion scan defects not associated with radiographic abnormalities. If anticoagulation therapy is being considered for an elderly patient with complicating medical illnesses, then the diagnostic certainty of an angiogram may be necessary. Certainly if thrombolytic therapy, caval interruption, or embolectomy is being considered, angiography is absolutely necessary.

Besides these clinical concerns, there are practical considerations to be weighed by the clinician, such as the availability and reliability of lung scanning and pulmonary angiography. The physician should be aware of these situations at his/her hospital.

TREATMENT

The generally accepted management of patients with pulmonary embolism, consisting of anticoagulation therapy, and other therapeutic interventions, such as thrombolytic therapy, caval interruption, and surgical embolectomy, will be discussed below. However, it is important

368

to remind the clinician of some of the uncertainties underlying this therapy.

There has been no prospective, randomized, controlled study of the efficacy of anticoagulation therapy in patients with angiographically documented pulmonary embolism. The study most commonly cited to justify anticoagulant therapy is that of Barritt and Jordan.[48] There were several problems with this study. Entry of patients into this study depended on referral, which may have biased the population. The population was small, with a total of 35 patients. The diagnosis of pulmonary embolism was based on clinical manifestations alone. Three of the five deaths in the untreated group were probably not directly related to embolism.[49]

That anticoagulation is the appropriate form of therapy for deep venous thrombosis, which presumably underlies almost all instances of pulmonary embolism, is accepted (see chapter 6). That heparin therapy has theoretical advantages in managing the biochemical events which accompany emboli is also accepted.[50] Lacking an appropriately controlled study, however, the present "standard of practice" should be considered to be based on the accumulated experience of generations of clinicians as expressed by many thoughtful experts.[5-7,51,52]

Anticoagulant Therapy

Heparin Anticoagulation therapy is started with heparin. Oral anticoagulants have a delayed onset of antithrombotic activity and should not be used as initial therapy. Heparin both inhibits the activation of thrombin and inactivates thrombin which has already been formed. Far more heparin is required to inactivate formed thrombin than to inhibit its formation. For this reason, the dose used to prevent clot formation is much smaller than that used to "treat" an already-formed thrombus.[50] Another action of heparin is to inhibit the aggregation of platelets on the surface of the thrombus.[53] Experimental evidence suggests that humoral mediators contained in platelets can be released as the platelets, newly aggregated on the fresh embolus, undergo degranulation.[26,27] These mediators, including histamine, serotonin, prostaglandin, endoperoxides, and thromboxanes, produce both vasoconstriction and bronchoconstriction. The significance of these processes depends on the magnitude and extent of the embolic event and requires a large amount of heparin for inhibition.[5,6]

An initial dose of 10,000 IU of sodium heparin is administered intravenously as a bolus. This is followed in approximately two hours by a continuous intravenous infusion of 1000 to 1500 IU/h. The presence of adequate anticoagulation is documented with an activated partial thromboplastin time (aPTT). Resistance to the effect of heparin is an unusual occurrence, but if present, is commonly due to a congenital deficiency of antithrombin III, a plasma factor necessary for heparin's action. Antithrombin-III deficiency can also be seen with severe liver disease or a severe ongoing thrombotic process.[8] The continuous infusion dose is adjusted to maintain the aPTT 2 to 2½ times normal, or approximately 60 to 80 seconds.

Sodium heparin may also be administered as an intravenous bolus every 4 hours, usually in a dose of 5000 to 7500 IU. The aPTT is then drawn immediately prior to the next planned dose in order to adjust the heparin dosage. The continuous intravenous infusion is the preferred method of delivering heparin, if a mechanical pump is available to ensure a reliably uniform delivery rate. The incidence of bleeding complications may be less with continuous infusion than with bolus administration, and the aPTT can be obtained at any time during the infusion rather than just before the next dose.[54,55]

If a continuous infusion is not practical, intravenous bolus administration should be chosen. Although subcutaneous administration was the formerly used method, it is no longer recommended.

The aPTT should be determined as frequently as necessary until the appropriate dose is determined. This usually means two or three determinations in the first 24 hours of heparin therapy. Thereafter, it should be determined at least daily. Some clinicians prefer to document adequate anticoagulation with the aPTT on only one occasion, just after initiating therapy.[41] Further observation for adequacy of heparin effect and for possible bleeding complications is then performed on a clinical basis.

It is important to avoid aspirin or other platelet-inhibiting drugs during the course of anticoagulation therapy whether with heparin or coumarin derivatives, in order to minimize the risk of bleeding complications.

Heparin should be started as early in the course of a patient with suspected embolism. The more seriously compromised is the patient's hemodynamic and respiratory condition, and the more likely the diagnosis of embolism, the earlier heparin should be started. It is not uncommon to start anticoagulation before data from lung scan or angiography are available.

Once the diagnosis of pulmonary embolism is accepted, the clinician must determine the duration of heparin therapy, and tentatively plan the duration of anticoagulation therapy. Heparin is usually continued for the first 7 to 10 days after the embolic event. During this interval, it is assumed that adherence and organization, or resolution, of thromboemboli has occurred.[30]

The appropriate duration of oral anticoagulant therapy is controversial. This is especially so in patients who do not have a continuing risk factor for the development of deep venous thrombophlebitis, such as congestive heart failure, immobilization, cancer, or peripheral venous disease. In those patients who were previously healthy, and may have had their embolism complicate trauma, an operation, or childbirth, the suggested duration varies widely. Recommendations extend from seven to ten days,[5] through one month,[8] 30 days to 4 months,[6] to at least 6 months.[26] In most patients 6 months is chosen by many clinicians. In those patients with an ongoing risk of venous thrombosis, anticoagulation should be continued as long as there is a likelihood of embolism.

Coumarin derivatives   If anticoagulation therapy is to be continued longer than two weeks, parenteral heparin therapy becomes impractical. Oral therapy with a coumarin derivative, like warfarin, is the appropriate choice for long-term anticoagulation. Coumarin anticoagulants act by inhibiting hepatic production of active, vitamin K–dependent clotting factors (factors II, VII, IX, X). The resultant anticoagulant effect can be monitored by measuring the prothrombin time (PT). A PT prolonged to about 1½ to 2 times the control value is considered to represent adequate anticoagulation. Approximately 3 to 6 days are required to affect the PT to this degree. For this reason, warfarin is usually started after the first few days of heparin therapy. The PT is monitored daily, and heparin is tapered and stopped once the PT is within the therapeutic range, for two or three days. Once anticoagulation is stable, the frequency of checking the PT decreases, but it is usually determined weekly in outpatients for the duration of therapy. Physicians responsible for prescribing and monitoring long-term anticoagulation with warfarin must be alert for the many possible interactions of this agent with other drugs. Besides the agents which can inhibit platelet function (aspirin, indomethacin, nonsteroidal anti-inflammatory agents), there are many drugs which can potentiate the effect of warfarin (cimetidine, quinidine, trimethoprin-sulfamethoxazole, antibiotics which can alter bowel flora, chloral hydrate). Many other drugs can inhibit warfarin's effect (oral contraceptives, corticosteriods, barbiturates, rifampin). Warfarin can also potentiate the effect of certain drugs (diphenyl hydantoin, tolbutamide). A complete listing of drug interactions has been published by Rosenow.[7]

Supportive Measures

Additional medical care may be necessary for patients with an embolism, and are applied as the clinical condition demands. Oxygen therapy is almost always necessary to reverse hypoxemia. This is usually accomplished with simple oxygen delivery devices. However, on occasion institution of a high-flow system, or even intubation, is necessary to provide 100% oxygen. Rarely, truly massive emboli will impair carbon dioxide elimination, necessitating mechanical ventilatory support. If hypotension accompanies the embolism, a pressor agent, such as dopamine, may be necessary. If the hypotension does not improve in the first few hours of heparin therapy and conservative management, then additional measures such as thrombolytic therapy or surgical embolectomy must be considered.

Thrombolytic therapy Urokinase and streptokinase are enzymes which activate plasminogen. The resulting proteolytic enzyme, plasmin, produces the lysis of clots by breaking down fibrin, fibrinogen, and other clotting factors. The activated fibrinolytic system can then effect more rapid resolution of thromboemboli. This "medical embolectomy" can produce the beneficial effects of hastening the resolution of the detrimental respiratory and hemodynamic consequences of a pulmonary embolus. The USPET, phases 1 and 2, did indeed, demonstrate more rapid resolution of emboli following 12 to 24 hours therapy with these agents compared to heparin therapy alone.[12,32] The resolution was documented using lung scan, angiographic, and hemodynamic data. There was no difference in survival between the groups of patients receiving thrombolytic therapy and those receiving heparin alone. By two weeks, there was no demonstrable difference in extent of resolution between the groups, as judged by lung scan.[8] An increased incidence of bleeding complications was found, however, in the patients receiving thrombolytic therapy. Because of the efficacy of urokinase and streptokinase in stimulating the lysis of any recent clot, multiple relative contraindications must be kept in mind: surgical procedure or childbirth within the preceding ten days; pregnancy, stroke, or CNS trauma or surgery within the preceding two months; kidney or liver biopsies within two weeks; peptic ulcer disease; any active bleeding process; atrial fibrillation; bacterial endocarditis; severe hypertension; renal or hepatic failure. Careful attention should be paid to sites of recent arterial punctures or intravenous catheter placement.[7,8] In view of the multiple contraindications, thrombolytic therapy has not become a part of the routine management of pulmonary embolism.

In the setting of an angiographically documented pulmonary embolism which has produced life-threatening hemodynamic compromise in a patient without contraindications, thrombolytic therapy with urokinase or streptokinase should be considered. The heparin infusion should be stopped and, once the aPTT has returned to within 10 seconds of control, a 12-hour course of continuous infusion thrombolytic therapy can be started. Loading and maintenance dose guidelines are described by the manufacturer. A prolonged thrombin time, an elevated level of fibrin degradation products, or a decreased fibrinogen can be tested for, and compared to base-line results, to document the induction of a "thrombolytic state."[8] Once the infusion of urokinase or streptokinase is completed, heparin infusion may be restarted.

Surgical embolectomy In patients with acute, massive, angiographically demonstrated pulmonary embolism who have refractory hypotension in spite of optimum supportive measures, heparinization, and possibly thrombolytic therapy, surgical embolectomy may be considered. This is especially true of patients free of serious underlying medical illnesses.[9] In the best of hands, using extracorporeal circulation to support the patient, the operative mortality alone is almost 25%,[56] and the ultimate survival is less than 40%. Unless a medical center can offer angiography and a prepared surgical team on an emergency basis, surgical embolectomy may not be a realistic alternative.

Inferior vena caval interruption Interruption of the inferior vena cava, either by surgical ligation or plication, or by transvenous placement of a Mobin-Uddin type "umbrella" filter[57] or a Hunter-Sessions occluding balloon[58] is a procedure being done with decreasing frequency. It was originally postulated that caval interruption would prevent recurrences of emboli. However, since large collateral channels can develop, this has not proved to be uniformly successful.[5] In addition, the procedure has been associated with reports of some frightening complications, such as embolism of the umbrella filter and perforation of the inferior vena cava.[59,60] In the modern era of aggressive application of effective anticoagulation, the applicability of caval interruption procedure has been significantly limited. Accepted indications for an interruption procedure are: (1) demonstrated recurrence of embolism after the first few days of adequate anticoagulation; (2) following a life-threatening embolism in a patient with a serious risk of recurrence; (3) following a pulmonary embolism in a patient who has an absolute contraindication for anticoagulation therapy; and (4) following the rare instance of surgical embolectomy, since anticoagulation will be temporarily contraindicated.[5,7]

If caval interruption is indicated, then the Hunter-Sessions balloon appears to be the procedure of choice. It is placed under local anesthesia with only a small neck incision. It will produce complete occlusion of the inferior vena cava, completely preventing recurrent pulmonary emboli in the short term. It also has not been associated with any complications such as dislodgment or perforation of the vena cava.

REFERENCES

1. Wilson JE III: Pulmonary embolism: Diagnosis and treatment. *Clin Notes Respir Dis* 1981;19(4):3–13.
2. Wessler S: Venous thromboembolism: Scope of the problem, in *Prophylactic Therapy of Deep Vein Thrombosis and Pulmonary Embolism*. US Dept of Health, Education, and Welfare publication No. (NIH)76-866, 1976, pp 1–10.
3. Dalen JE, Alpert JS: Natural history of pulmonary embolism, in Sasahara AA, Sonnenblick EH, Lesch M (eds): *Pulmonary Emboli*. New York, Grune & Stratton, 1975, pp 77–88.
4. Robin ED: Overdiagnosis and overtreatment of pulmonary embolism: the emperor may have no clothes. *Ann Intern Med* 1977;87:775.
5. Moser KM: Pulmonary embolism. *Am Rev Respir Dis* 1977;115:829–852.
6. Stein M: Pulmonary embolism, in Simmons DH (ed): *Current Pulmonology*. Boston, Houghton Mifflin, 1979, vol 1, pp 125–161.

7. Rosenow EC, Osmundson PJ, Brown ML: Pulmonary embolism. *Mayo Clin Proc* 1981;56:161–178.

8. Hyers TM: Massive pulmonary embolism, in Sahn SA (ed): *Pulmonary Emergencies*. New York, Churchill Livingstone, 1982, pp 197–224.

9. Wolfe WG, Sabiston DC: *Pulmonary Embolism*. Philadelphia, WB Saunders Co, 1980, pp 117–146.

10. Sevitt S, Gallagher NG: Venous thrombosis and pulmonary embolism. A clinicopathological study in injured and burned patients. *Br J Surg* 1961;48:475–489.

11. Kakkar VV, Howe CT, Flanc C, et al: Natural history of postoperative deep vein thrombosis. *Lancet* 1969;2:230–232.

12. Urokinase Pulmonary Embolism Trial. A national cooperative study. *Circulation* 1973;(suppl 2).

13. Simon M: Plain film and angiographic aspects of pulmonary embolism, in Moser KM, Stein M (eds): *Pulmonary Thromboembolism*. Chicago, Year Book Medical Publ, 1973, pp 197–215.

14. Nadel JA: Alveolar duct constriction after barium sulfate microembolism, in Sasahara AA, Stein M (eds): *Pulmonary Embolic Disease*. New York, Grune & Stratton, Inc, 1965, pp 153–161.

15. Severinghaus JW, Swenson EW, Finley TN, et al: Unilateral hypoventilation produced by occlusion of one pulmonary artery. *J Appl Physiol* 1961;16:53–60.

16. Tisi GM, Wolfe WG, Fallat RJ, et al: Effects of O_2 and CO_2 on airway smooth muscle following pulmonary vascular occlusion. *J Appl Physiol* 1970;28:570–753.

17. Stein M, Levy SE: Reflex and humoral responses to pulmonary embolism, in Sasahara AA, Sonnenblick EH, Lesch M: *Pulmonary Emboli*. New York, Grune & Stratton, 1975, pp 5–12.

18. Finley TH, Swenson EW, Clement JA, et al: Changes in mechanical properties, appearance, and surface activity of extracts of one lung following occlusion of its pulmonary artery in the dog. *Physiologist* 1960;3:56–66.

19. Dantzker DR, Wagner PD, Tornabene VW, et al: Gas exchange after pulmonary thromboembolization in dogs. *Circ Res* 1978;42:92–103.

20. Brandfonbrener M, Turino GM, Himmelstein A: Effects of occlusion of one pulmonary artery on pulmonary circulation in man. *Fed Proc* 1958;17:19.

21. McIntyre KM, Sasahara AA: Determinants of cardiovascular responses to pulmonary embolism, in Moser KM, Stein M (eds): *Pulmonary Thromboembolism*. Chicago, Year Book Medical Publ, 1973, pp 144–159.

22. Miller GA, Sutton GC: Acute Massive Pulmonary Embolism. Clinical and hemodynamic findings in 23 patients studied by cardiac catheterization and pulmonary arteriography. *Br Heart J* 1970;32:518–523.

23. Dexter L, Smith GT: Quantitative studies of pulmonary embolism. *Am J Med Sci* 1964;247:641–648.

24. Knapp RS, Mullens CB: Progressive tricuspid regurgitation as a limit to right ventricular output in acute pulmonary hypertension. *Clin Res* 1972;20:69.

25. Marshall R, Allison PR: Pulmonary embolism by small blood clots. Physiological responses in the anesthetized dog. *Thorax* 1962;17:289–297.

26. Thomas DP, Stein M, Tanabe G, et al: Mechanism of bronchoconstriction produced by thromboemboli in dogs. *Am J Physiol* 1964;206:1207–1212.

27. Thomas DP, Gurewich V, Ashford TP: Platelet adherence to thromboemboli in relation to the pathogenesis and treatment of pulmonary embolism. *N Engl J Med* 1966;274:953–956.

28. Gurewich V, Cohen JL, Thomas DP: Humoral factors in massive pulmonary embolism: An experimental study. *Am Heart J* 1968;76:784–794.
29. Dalen JE, Haffajee CI, Alpert JS, et al: Pulmonary embolism, pulmonary hemorrhage and pulmonary infarction. *N Engl J Med* 1977;296:1431–1435.
30. Wessler S, Freiman DG, Ballon JD, et al: Experimental pulmonary embolism with serum-induced thrombi. *Am J Pathol* 1961;38:89–101.
31. Freiman DG, Wessler S, Lertzman M: Experimental pulmonary embolism with serum-induced thrombi aged in vivo. *Am J Pathol* 1961;39:95–102.
32. Urokinase Streptokinase Pulmonary Embolism Trial: Phase 2 results. *JAMA* 1973;229:1606–1613.
33. Stein PD, Willis PW, DeMets DL: History and physical exmination in acute pulmonary embolism in patients without preexisting cardiac or pulmonary disease. *Am J Cardiol* 1981;47:218–223.
34. Wenger NK, Stein PD, Willis PW: Massive acute pulmonary embolism. *JAMA* 1972;220:843–844.
35. Clinical Presentation of Pulmonary Embolism, in Wolfe WG, Sabiston DC (eds): *Pulmonary Embolism*. Philadelphia, WB Saunders Co, 1980, pp 63–67.
36. Bell WR, Simon TL, DeMets DL: The clinical features of submassive and massive pulmonary emboli. *Am J Med* 1977;62:355–360.
37. Wacker WEC, Rosenthal M, Snodgrass PJ: A triad for the diagnosis of pulmonary embolism and infarction. *JAMA* 1961;178:8.
38. Cordley EL: Enzyme profiles in the evaluation of pulmonary infarction. *JAMA* 1969;207:1307.
39. Torrance DJ: *The Chest Film in Massive Pulmonary Embolism*. Springfield, Ill, Charles C Thomas, 1963.
40. Ashburn WL, Moser KM: Pulmonary ventilation and perfusion scanning, in Moser KM, Stein M (eds): *Pulmonary Thromboembolism*. Chicago, Year Book Medical Publ, 1973, pp 216–230.
41. Moser KM: Diagnosis and management of pulmonary embolism. *Hosp Prac*, Oct 1980;10:57–68.
42. McNeil BJ: A diagnostic strategy using ventilation-perfusion studies in patients suspect for pulmonary embolism. *J Nucl Med* 1976;17:613–616.
43. Hull RD, Hirsh J, Carter CJ, et al: Pulmonary angiography, ventilation lung scanning, and venography for clinically suspected pulmonary embolism with abnormal perfusion lung scan. *Ann Intern Med* 1983;98:891–899.
44. Morris S: Plain film and angiographic aspects of pulmonary embolism, in Moser KM, Stein M (eds): *Pulmonary Thromboembolism*. Chicago, Year Book Medical Publ, 1973, pp 197–215.
45. Sharma GV, Sasahara AA: Diagnosis and treatment of pulmonary embolism. *Med Clin North Am* 1979;63:239–250.
46. Jick H, Slone D, Borda IT, Shapiro S: Efficacy and toxicity of heparin in relation to age and sex. *N Engl J Med* 1968;279:284–286.
47. Cheely R, McCantney WH, Perry JR, et al: The role of noninvasive tests versus pulmonary angiography in the diagnosis of pulmonary embolism. *Am J Med* 1981;70:17–22.
48. Barritt DW, Jordan SC: Anticoagulant drugs in the treatment of pulmonary embolism. *Lancet* 1960;1:1309–1312.
49. Egermayer P: Value of anticoagulants in the treatment of pulmonary embolism. *J R Soc Med* 1981;74:675–681.
50. Colman RW: Prophylaxis and treatment of thromboembolism based on pathophysiology of clotting mechanisms, in Fishman AD (ed): *Pulmonary Disease and Disorders*. New York, McGraw-Hill Book Co, 1980, pp 827–834.

51. O'Sullivan EF, Hirsh J, McCarthy RA, et al: Heparin in the treatment of venous thromboembolic disease. *Med J Aust* 1968;2:153–159.

52. Kernohan JR, Todd C: Heparin therapy in thromboembolic disease. *Lancet* 1966;1:621–623.

53. Thomas DP: The anticoagulant therapy of venous thromboembolism, in Moser KM, Stein M (eds): *Pulmonary Thromboembolism*. Chicago, Year Book Medical Publ, 1973, pp 271–279.

54. Salzman EW, Deykin D, Shapiro RM, Rosenberg R: Management of heparin therapy. *N Engl J Med* 1975;292:1046–1050.

55. Mant MJ, Thong KL, Birtwhistle RV, et al: Hemorrhagic complications of heparin therapy. *Lancet* 1977;1:1133–1135.

56. Tschirkov A, Krause E, Evert O, et al: Surgical management of massive pulmonary embolism. *J Thorac Cardiovasc Surg* 1978;75:730–733.

57. Mobin-Uddin K, Utley JR, Bryant LR: The inferior vena cava umbrella filter. *Prog Cardiovasc Dis* 1975;17:391–396.

58. Hunter JA, Dye WS, Javid H, et al: Permanent transvenous occlusion of the inferior vena cava: Experience with 60 patients. *Ann Surg* 1977;186:491–498.

59. Adelson J, Steer ML, Glotzer DJ, et al: Thromboembolism after insertion of the Mobin-Uddin caval filter. *Surgery* 1980;87:184–189.

60. Phillips MR, Widrich WC, Johnson WC: Perforation of the inferior vena cava by the Kim-Ray Greenfield filter. *Surgery* 1980;87:233–235.

18 *Blood Surface Interaction During Cardiopulmonary Bypass*

L. Henry Edmunds, Jr

The heart-lung machine exposes blood to synthetic surfaces, temperature gradients, and mechanical and rheologic trauma. As a result, blood elements are damaged and depleted, and some elements are activated. Surface contact activates the coagulation cascade, and unless thrombosis is prevented, extracorporeal perfusion is not possible. Although other anticoagulants such as calcium binding agents (EDTA, citrate) or reptilase may be used in vitro, heparin is required in vivo. Several properties of heparin make this drug indispensable for extracorporeal perfusion. The drug is nontoxic in nearly all patients; it effectively inhibits coagulation at several points in the coagulation cascade; and it is rapidly reversible with protamine sulfate. Thus the study of blood-surface interactions during cardiopulmonary bypass is the study of heparinized blood within extracorporeal perfusion systems.

Extracorporeal perfusion devices injure both formed and unformed blood elements, dilute and deplete blood of certain constituents, add foreign materials to the blood, and cause release of some of the contents of platelets, red cells, and white cells. Moreover, extracorporeal perfusion deranges body homeostasis in many additional ways that are only partially understood.[1] The effects of anesthesia, operation, various drugs, nonpulsatile blood flow,[2] responses of endocrine organs, inhibition of atrial and stretch receptors, cooling and rewarming, the functional reserve of various organ systems, etc, in addition to the changes that occur within circulating, heparinized blood, all contribute to the morbidity and occasional mortality of cardiopulmonary bypass. Although this chapter focuses on the interaction of blood and extracorporeal perfusion systems, the impact of operation and a period of bypass should not be overlooked.

THE HEART-LUNG MACHINE

The major components of cardiopulmonary bypass systems are venous catheters, blood reservoir, pump, oxygenator, heat exchanger, filter, and arterial catheter. Most commercial bubble oxygenators consist

377

of a blood reservoir, oxygenator, and heat exchanger in one unit (Figure 18-1). This unit is placed upstream to the pump. When a membrane oxygenator is used, the pump is placed between a venous reservoir and either the heat exchanger or the oxygenator (Figure 18-2). Both systems include two cardiotomy sucker systems and a venting system for the left ventricle.

A variety of synthetic materials are used to construct the heart-lung machine. Although much effort has been expended to discover thrombo-resistant materials, this property is *not* a requirement in extracorporeal perfusion systems. Polyvinyl chloride, polydimethyl siloxane, pyrolytic carbon, polyurethanes, stainless steel, Dacron, Teflon, nylon, polycarbonate, and methyl methacrylate are some of the materials used in the construction of heart-lung machines. The properties of synthetic materials unpredictably affect reactions with blood which is not anticoagulated, but have little effect on heparinized blood.

Other factors also affect blood trauma and reactivity of blood elements in extracorporeal perfusion systems. Within the heart-lung machine blood flow is not streamlined. Blood itself is a noncompressible, viscous, non-Newtonian suspension of particles. Within the heart-lung machine blood encounters sharp projections and angles, irregular surfaces, narrow areas, and expanded areas. The velocity of flow changes radically within the machine. Blood is subjected to a variety of shear stresses, turbulence, cavitation pressures, secondary flows, and flow

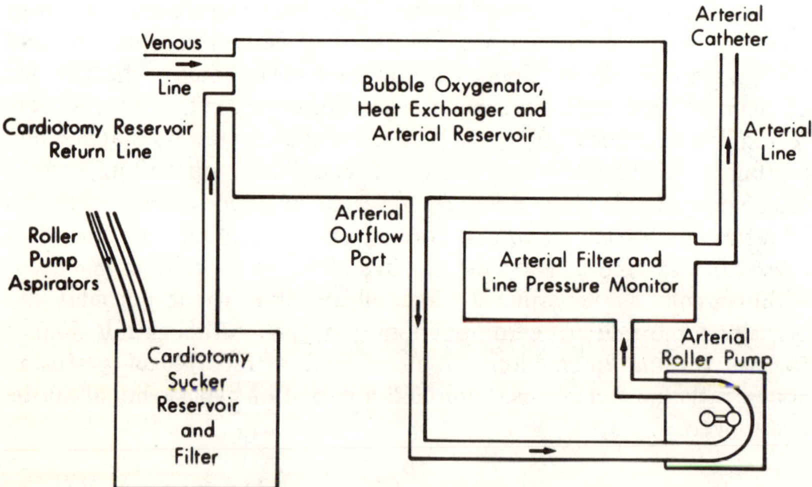

Figure 18-1 Block diagram of a heart-lung machine utilizing a bubble oxygenator. The oxygenator usually contains a heat exchanger for cooling and warming blood and serves as a reservoir for the downstream roller or centrifugal perfusion pump. (Reproduced with permission from Edmunds LH Jr, Stephenson LW.[1])

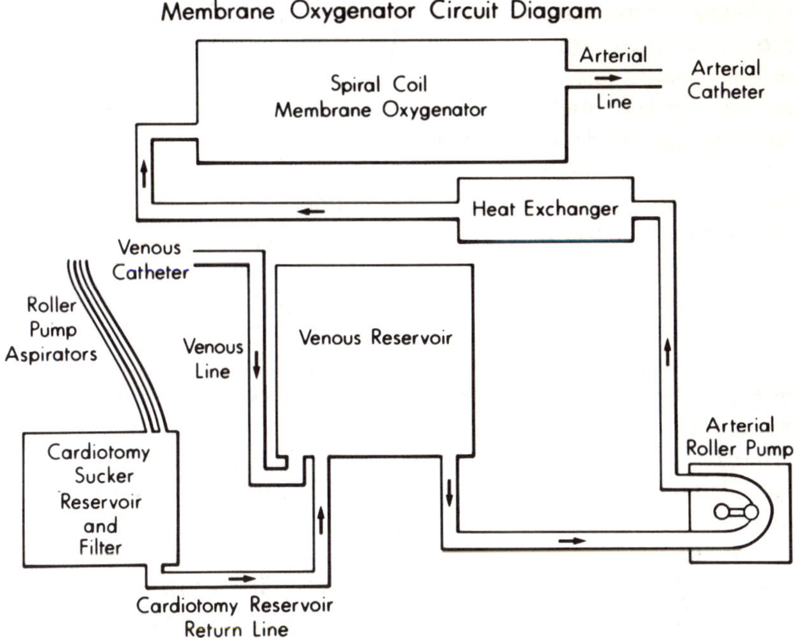

Figure 18-2 Block diagram of a heart-lung machine utilizing a membrane oxygenator. Some commercial oxygenators contain a heat exchanger within the oxygenating unit. The cardiotomy sucker system is used to recover blood shed into the operative field and is identical in both membrane and bubble oxygenator systems. (Reproduced with permission from Edmunds LH Jr, Stephenson LW.[1])

separation phenomena. Many of these physical forces, the admixture of air and foreign materials to the blood, and the necessity of exposing blood to large areas of gas or synthetic material to achieve oxygen and carbon dioxide exchange injure some blood elements and activate others. All tend to increase blood-surface interaction and to increase platelet adhesion and thrombosis.

SURFACE ACTIVATION OF COAGULATION

Blood contact with all known surfaces except endothelial cells binds and activates factor XII, which forms active fragments, XIIa and XIIf by proteolytic transformation.[3] High molecular weight kininogen enhances surface binding of factor XII and also enhances activation of factor XII and the formation of active fragments by kallekrein. Kallekrein is formed from prekallekrein which is activated by both XIIa and XIIf and is enhanced by high molecular weight kininogen. Factor XIIa also activates factor XI and the coagulation cascade via the intrinsic pathway.

When blood contacts a foreign surface plasma proteins are adsorbed onto the surface to form a layer 50 nm thick within five seconds and 125 nm thick within one minute.[4] Plasma proteins are adsorbed selectively and competitively and not in proportion to their bulk concentration. Chemical and physical properties of the synthetic surface affect adsorption[5] but unfortunately physical properties of wetability, surface-free energy, electrocharge, and surface texture do not predictably determine adsorbed protein concentrations. Fibrinogen is preferentially adsorbed as compared to albumin, globulin, lipoproteins, and other proteins including coagulation proteins.[6] Within 30 seconds of blood contact, fibrinogen appears to undergo a conformational change or is partially replaced by high molecular weight kininogen.[7] In any event, adsorbed fibrinogen no longer reacts with fibrinogen antibody,[6] and, furthermore, surface affinity for platelets markedly decreases. Prior to the change in fibrinogen, platelets are strongly attracted to the fibrinogen-covered surface. Prior exposure of the surface to albumin solutions reduces fibrinogen adsorption and platelet adhesion.[8]

Circulating platelets adhere to fibrinogen-covered surfaces and immediately change from discs to spiny spheres.[9] First, individual platelets adhere to the surface; these coalesce to form an irregular monolayer and eventually increase to form rounded mounds[9] (Figure 18-3). Surface-activated platelets, enhanced by release of adenosine diphosphate (ADP) from red cells, also form aggregates within the flowing blood stream.[10] The presence of red cells, areas of high flow, high shear stress, and turbulence increase platelet adhesion. The number of adherent platelets is directly proportional to the surface area in contact with blood.

Further activation of platelets causes release of granule contents which contain coagulation factors, calcium, serotonin, acid hydrolyases, adenine nucleotides, platelet-specific proteins, and factors affecting chemotaxis, vascular permeability, and mitogenesis. In addition, activated platelets can stimulate formation of endoperoxidases and thromboxane A_2, and powerful vasoconstrictor. Release of some of these products in turn activates other platelets.

Activation of platelets releases platelet procoagulant activity which can stimulate the *intrinsic* pathway of the coagulation cascade.[11] White cells also contain a procoagulant factor similar or identical with thromboplastin which appears when white cells are activated.[12] Thus during cardiopulmonary bypass, coagulation can be initiated by activation of factor XII, platelets, and probably white cells; whether synthetic surfaces can directly activate other coagulation factors is unknown.

HEPARIN

Heparin is a prerequisite for extracorporeal perfusion and usually 3 mm (300 IU)/kg body weight is given before starting bypass. An addi-

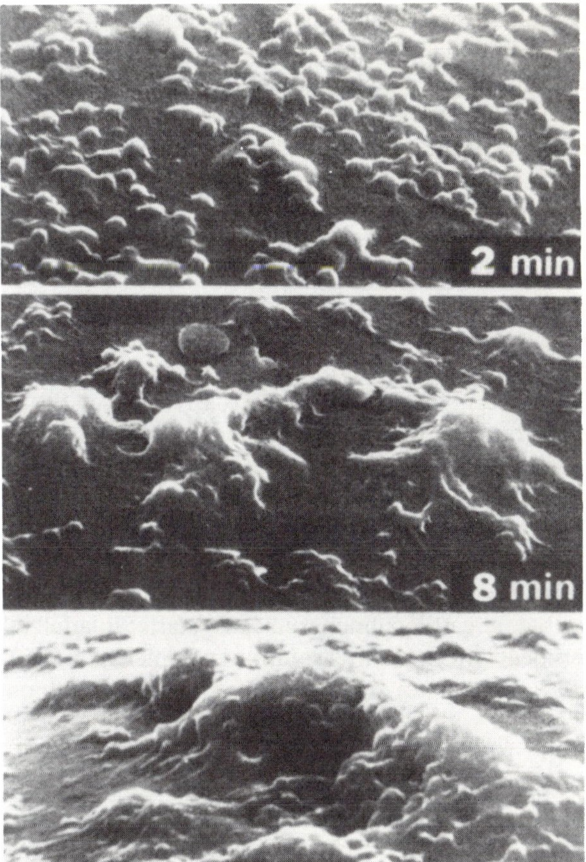

Figure 18-3 Sequential photographs of platelet adhesion onto pyrolytic carbon beads from citrated blood. (Reproduced with permission from Salzman EW, Landon J, Brier D.[9])

tional 1 mg/kg is given after each hour of bypass. Since threshold sensitivities and rates of heparin metabolism vary between individuals, heparin administration is monitored by activated clotting time measurements which should remain over 400 seconds during the period of bypass.[13] Even with clinically adequate heparin doses, partial coagulation as evidenced by measurements of fibrinopeptide A may occur in some patients.[14] At the end of bypass heparin is neutralized by administration of 1.3 mg protamine sulfate for each milligram of heparin given. This should return the activated clotting time to the normal range of 80 to 120 seconds.

Commercial heparin is extracted from beef lung or porcine gut and purified to a highly sulfated mucopolysaccharide. Within commercial heparin preparations two fractions with very high anticoagulant activity and relatively low molecular weights can be separated from the bulk material that has high molecular weight and much less anticoagulant activity.[15] Low molecular weight, highly active heparin preparations are not yet available for widespread clinical use.

Heparin greatly accelerates the active of antithrombin III.[15] Antithrombin III is a serine protease inhibitor which normally slows the reactions of serine proteases in the coagulation cascade. In the presence of heparin the action of antithrombin III accelerates so that these reactions are essentially inhibited. The heparin-antithrombin III complex inhibits factors XIIa, XIa, Xa, and IXa and conversion of fibrinogen to fibrin by thrombin.[15] Thus heparin inhibits coagulation at several points in the coagulation cascade but does not inhibit activation of factor XII nor activation of platelets. In fact heparin actually reduces the threshold of platelets to aggregating agents. Heparin does not prolong bleeding time.

DILUTION AND DEPLETION OF COAGULATION FACTORS

The heart-lung machine requires one to 2.5 liters of fluid to prime the machine before cardiopulmonary bypass starts. In adults the machine is usually primed with crystalloid solutions to which albumin may or may not be added. Thus when bypass starts, the patient's blood volume is thoroughly mixed with the nonblood priming volume. This causes the concentration of all blood constituents to decrease to 40% to 70% of their prebypass values.[16]

As mentioned, blood contact causes adsorption of plasma proteins to the synthetic surface of the heart-lung machine. Coagulation proteins are not selectively adsorbed, but dilution and some adsorption routinely decrease factors II, V, VII, VIII, IX, and X to 20% to 60% of prebypass concentrations.[16] Within 20 minutes after bypass the concentration of coagulation proteins is restored to 45% or higher of prebypass levels; these levels are sufficient to restore hemostasis.[16] Dilution and depletion of soluble coagulation factors during bypass almost never cause a deficiency in coagulation.

Surface contact activates complement, specifically C_2 and C_5 which can enhance leukocyte adhesion and aggregation.[17] Perfusions lasting more than two hours slightly reduce concentrations of IgA, IgG, IgM, C_3, and C_4 proteins beyond that expected by dilution.

Platelets are the most important hemostasis element affected by cardiopulmonary bypass and are the cause of prolonged bleeding times that occur during the first few hours after cardiopulmonary bypass. In vitro studies using fresh heparinized human blood recirculated through membrane or bubble oxygenator extracorporeal perfusion systems show a loss of circulating platelets to 20% to 50% of prebypass counts (Figure 18-4),

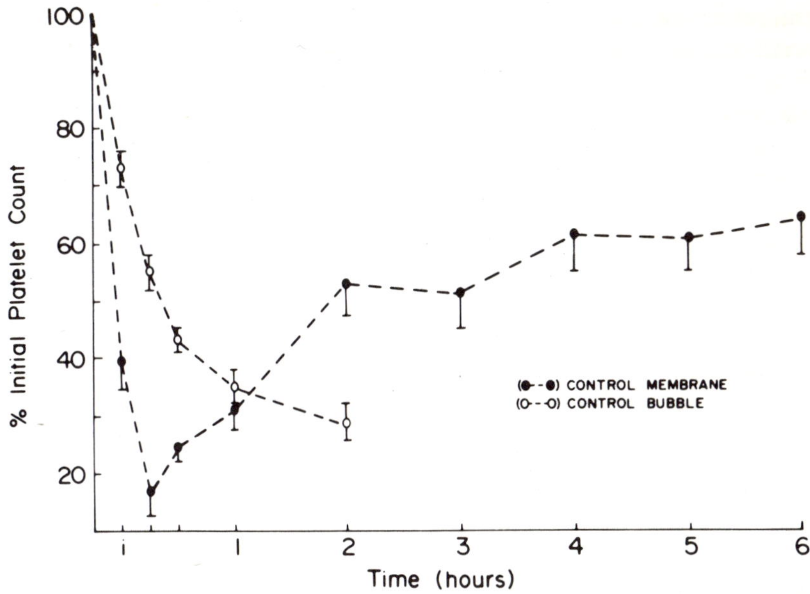

Figure 18-4 Change in platelet count during in vitro recirculation of fresh heparinized human blood in membrane and bubble oxygenator extracorporeal perfusion circuits. In membrane oxygenator circuits platelet counts decrease rapidly to 20% of control counts during initial blood-surface contact. Decrease of platelet counts is less rapid but progressive in bubble oxygenator systems.

loss of sensitivity to aggregating agents, and progressive release of low affinity platelet factor 4 and acid phosphatase, a lysosomal enzyme.[18] Thromboxane B_2, the stable metabolite of thromboxane A_2, which is synthesized by activated platelets appears and increases progressively.[18] Scanning electron micrographs show individual and groups of platelets attached to synthetic surfaces and filter studies have demonstrated platelet aggregates in circulating blood.[10] Although transmission electron micrographs show large numbers of circulating platelets that have not released granule contents, these platelets do not function in response to aggregating agents. Recent evidence suggests that platelet membrane receptors, specifically epinephrine receptors, may be altered during extracorporeal perfusion.

In patients undergoing open heart surgery actual platelet counts decrease during cardiopulmonary bypass, but little or no decrease occurs when counts are corrected for dilution.[19] Low-affinity platelet factor 4, a platelet-specific protein found in alpha granules, progressively increases. Postoperative bleeding times are prolonged, presumably until new platelets enter the circulation in numbers.

White cells are activated during cardiopulmonary bypass and, like platelets, are initially reduced in number by dilution. However as bypass

384

progresses, the number of white cells increases. During and after bypass white cells have reduced opsonification, metabolism, and phagocytosis.

TRAUMA TO BLOOD ELEMENTS

Extracorporeal perfusion injures blood elements. In addition to surface adsorption, proteins and lipoproteins are denatured during extracorporeal perfusion. Blood viscosity increases, plasma may become turbid, and serum has reduced bacteriostatic activity.[1]

Bypass hemolyzes red cells particularly in areas of cavitation, turbulence, and high shear stress. Red cells release ADP and free hemoglobin which circulates bound to haptoglobulin and hemapexin until these plasma proteins become saturated. The cardiotomy sucker system, oxygenator, and roller or centrifugal pump are the major sources of hemolysis within extracorporeal perfusion systems.

As bypass continues beyond three to four hours with bubble oxygenators, progressive hemolysis, denaturation of plasma proteins, and lipoproteins, formation of platelet aggregate emboli and probably cytolysis of platelets and white cells result in progressively deteriorating organ function and impairment of microcirculation of various organs. Cardiotomy suction return systems and vent catheters also traumatize blood. Membrane oxygenators with larger solid surface areas cause similar injury to formed and unformed blood elements initially, but as bypass continues beyond three to four hours, further blood damage is minimal. Since the membrane surface in contact with blood does not change, nearly all of the blood injury occurs in the first few moments after blood contact. In contrast, new blood-gas surfaces in the form of bubbles are constantly produced in bubble oxygenator systems. This results in progressive and continuing alteration of both formed and unformed blood elements.

MICROEMBOLI

Extracorporeal perfusion systems produce vast numbers of microemboli that may obstruct the circulation to the microvasculature.[20] The majority of microemboli are foreign gaseous or solid particles, but significant numbers are derived from blood elements. Efficient filters, placed within the cardiotomy suction return system, and in arterial perfusion lines significantly reduce the numbers of emboli larger than 35 to 40 μm diameter. The emboli have been causally related to some of the complications of cardiopulmonary bypass. Undoubtedly vast numbers of microemboli less than 35 μm are produced during cardiopulmonary bypass, but these have not been conclusively shown to cause organ damage.

The major sources of gaseous emboli are the cardiotomy sucker return system and bubble oxygenators.[20] Foreign materials such as fat, fibrin, calcium, talc, and cellular debris may enter the circulation through the cardiotomy sucker system if blood is not filtered. Other sources of foreign material include spallation of tubing compressed by roller pumps, antifoam compounds, inorganic debris in crystalloid solutions, and debris left within sterile components of the heart-lung machine. Stored blood contains platelet and leukocyte aggregates, bits of fibrin, lipid precipitates, and red cell debris that may become microemboli if blood is not filtered before introduction into the perfusion system.

Emboli also develop from the formed and unformed elements of circulating blood. Fibrin may form in areas of stagnant flow, on rough surfaces, and in areas of turbulence and cavitation within bypass circuits. Fibrin deposits are prone to develop at connections within oxygenators and in arterial line filters. Bubble oxygenators tend to form more fibrin emboli than membrane oxygenators.

There are no conclusive data that denatured proteins form aggregates and microemboli.

Denaturation of proteins and lipoproteins causes fat to come out of solution during extracorporeal perfusion.[20] Bubble oxygenators cause more denaturation of soluble blood elements than membrane oxygenators. The emboli produced are aggregates of chylomicrons or free fat and contain principally triglycerides and cholesterol. Size varies between 4 and 200 μm. Hemodilution reduces generation of imiscible fat during bypass, but there are no means to completely prevent formation of fat emboli during bypass.

Contact between blood and synthetic surfaces activates platelets and causes the formation of platelet aggregates. Most platelet aggregates probably disaggregate in the microcirculation; however, some platelet aggregate emboli have been observed in the central nervous system of patients who have died after open heart surgery.[21] Experimentally, aggregated leukocytes have been found in the lungs of dogs following cardiopulmonary bypass.[22] Leukocyte aggregates may release lysosomal enzymes which in turn cause extravasation of plasma into surrounding tissues. Pharmacologic inhibitors of platelets such as alprostadil or epoprostenol can largely prevent the formation of platelet aggregates during cardiopulmonary bypass, but because of vasodilatory properties cannot be used routinely. At present there are no means to prevent leukocyte aggregation during bypass; however, aside from the lung, organ damage due to leukocyte aggregation has not been demonstrated.

Cardiopulmonary bypass reduces the ability of red cells to change shape during passage through the microcirculation. Although hypothermia and hypotension may cause stagnant flow and red cell sludging

386

in the capillary circulation, altered red cells have not been shown to permanently obstruct capillaries during cardiopulmonary bypass.

In current cardiopulmonary bypass systems blood returning from the cardiotomy suction return system is always filtered and bubble oxygenator systems always employ an arterial line filter. An arterial line filter is optional with membrane oxygenator systems. Stringent measures are used to reduce the number of microemboli that enter the patient. Nevertheless psychomotor test scores are temporarily reduced and psychiatric disturbances occur in a few patients after open heart surgery. Whether or not these temporary complications are due to microemboli that develop from blood elements during the period of bypass is not known.

ACTIVE SUBSTANCES RELEASED FROM BLOOD ELEMENTS

Platelets and leukocytes release active substances during bypass either in response to activation or from cytolysis.[18] The effects of these released substances on the patient is somewhat obscured by the patient's endocrine response to anesthesia, operation, and bypass. Operations utilizing cardiopulmonary bypass increase blood levels of epinephrine and norepinephrine and vasopressin.[1] Total plasma cortisol decreases at the beginning of bypass, but free cortisol increases during bypass to reach normal concentrations. ACTH concentrations decrease during bypass. Free thyroxin and serum amylase concentrations increase. Glucose and free fatty acid concentrations increase markedly up to three- to fourfold during bypass, and insulin levels decrease.

Thromboxane B_2 and 6 keto-$PGF_{1\alpha}$, the stable metabolites of thromboxane A_2 and prostacyclin, increase during cardiopulmonary bypass. In addition, platelets release serotonin, catecholamines, acid hydrolases, a vascular permeability factor, a chemotactic factor, and various coagulation factors.

Hemolyzed red cells release ADP, but the significance of this during bypass is not known. White cells are activated and occasionally destroyed during bypass. Biopsies of many tissues before and immediately after bypass reveal increased numbers of white cells, particularly granulocytes, in most tissues. Activated white cells release a variety of proteases, peroxidases, a tissue thromboplastin procoagulant, and lysosomal enzymes including several hydrolases.

Even in the presence of heparin, plasminogen is activated to plasmin during cardiopulmonary bypass.[23] Presumably kininogen is activated to bradykinin also. Heparin does not inhibit activation of factor XII although it does inhibit activated factor XII.[15] The amount of plasmin generated may produce measurable amounts of fibrin breakdown products,[14] but the amounts are small, and except in very rare circumstances fibrinolysis does not cause bleeding problems after open heart surgery.[23]

Extracorporeal perfusion has been considered a cause of disseminated intravascular coagulation. However, as noted above, in the presence of adequate heparin only small amounts of plasmin are generated[23] and only small concentrations of fibrinopeptide A can be detected in *some* patients. In the absence of sepsis diffuse intravascular coagulopathy probably does not occur in patients after open heart surgery. However this serious and frequently fatal disease occurs occasionally in patients with low cardiac output who require prolonged intravascular monitoring catheters and inotropic drugs to enhance cardiac output.[24] These patients are at increased risks for septicemia, which is probably the initiating cause of disseminated intrasvascular coagulopathy. Appropriate antibiotics and systemic heparin are required to avert death or limb loss in these very uncommon patients.

CONSEQUENCES OF BLOOD-SURFACE INTERACTION DURING BYPASS

With adequate heparin, careful priming of clean, sterile equipment and filters for stored blood, cardiotomy suction return, and the arterial line, short-term cardiopulmonary bypass for up to three hours causes little morbidity in infants, children, and most adults. Operation and bypass are less well tolerated in underweight neonates and elderly patients with compromised function of multiple organ systems. Aside from the accumulation of extravascular fluid during the period of bypass, morbidity due to short-term extracorporeal perfusion cannot be separated from that due to the operation.

Cardiopulmonary bypass activates and inhibits platelets. Other coagulation factors do not change sufficiently to impair coagulation. However the reduced numbers of platelets and the functional impairment of those remaining cause prolonged bleeding times for one to four hours after bypass stops and heparin is neutralized.[16] The mechanism by which circulating platelets are inhibited is not known.[19] There is evidence to suggest that in vivo platelet activation leads to an acquired platelet storage pool deficiency state.

Approximately 1% to 2% of patients who have open heart surgery require subsequent reoperation for operative site bleeding. When excessive postoperative bleeding occurs after cardiopulmonary bypass, a platelet count, prothrombin time, partial thromboplastin time, and fibrinogen concentration should be measured. The activated clotting time should also be measured and protamine given if the activated clotting time is prolonged over 120 seconds. Usually fresh frozen plasma is also given to augment concentrations of some of the soluble coagulation proteins. Platelet transfusions are helpful if counts are less than 80,000 and if the template bleeding time is prolonged. Other measures include the use of positive end expiratory airway pressure and pharmacologic

388

controlled hypotension if the patient can tolerate these measures. Nevertheless 1% to 2% of patients require re-exploration of the mediastinum. Usually surgical bleeding sources are found; less often no explanation is found, but bleeding stops after the incision is closed.

Prolonged bypass (more than 4 hours) with systemic heparin is associated with increased postoperative bleeding problems. Even when partial bypass is used for prolonged respiratory or circulatory support, bleeding from small groin or axillary wounds can become major sources of blood loss. In these patients replacement therapy is all that is available; sometimes bypass must be stopped because of bleeding.

Several studies have reported the use of prostaglandin E_1 or prostacyclin to temporarily inhibit platelets during extracorporeal perfusion.[25,26] Although these short-acting platelet inhibitors prevent platelet activation and postoperative increases in bleeding times, in monkeys and baboons[16,27] (Figure 18-5) doses sufficient to inhibit platelet activation in patients also cause severe vasodilatation and unacceptably low mean blood pressures during bypass.[25] Furthermore, postoperative

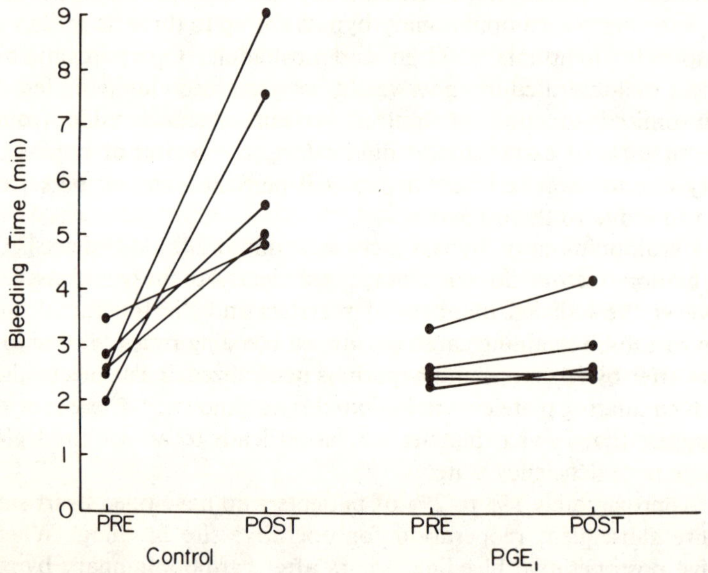

Figure 18-5 Template bleeding times before and after one hour of cardiopulmonary bypass in rhesus monkeys. Heparin was neutralized with protamine after bypass in each group. The experimental group of animals received a constant infusion of prostaglandin E_1 up to 5 μg/kg/min during the period of bypass. (Reproduced with permission from Addonizio VP Jr, Strauss J, Macarak EJ, et al: Preservation of platelet number and function with prostaglandin E_1 during total cardiopulmonary bypass in rhesus monkeys. *Surgery* 1978;83: 619–625.)

bleeding does not decrease.[26] A satisfactory means to preserve platelets and numbers during cardiopulmonary bypass is not yet available.

Prostacyclin has been used to inhibit platelets in patients undergoing hemodialysis.[27] Prostacyclin is not an anticoagulant; therefore the drug should be used with some concentration of heparin to prevent activation of the coagulation cascade. Experimental work suggests that prostacyclin in combination with surface-bound heparin can prevent coagulation during partial left heart bypass with an extracorporeal perfusion system.[28]

CONCLUSION

Blood reacts to synthetic surfaces in complex ways that are just beginning to be addressed. For short-term cardiopulmonary bypass with systemic heparin the interaction between blood and extracorporeal surfaces does not cause serious morbidity; however, if platelets could be preserved, some of the blood loss and bleeding problems associated with open heart surgery could be reduced. Other consequences of bypass such as effects of chemicals secreted from activated platelets and white cells on organs and vessels need to be more carefully studied and defined.

The interaction between blood and synthetic surfaces greatly limits the potential use of extracorporeal perfusion systems to partially or completely substitute for the circulation to the whole body or individual organs. Without nonthrombogenic surfaces, mechanical and chemical devices cannot be developed to substitute for diseased internal organs. Moreover, temporary but nonetheless long-term (days or weeks) use of extracorporeal circulatory, respiratory, renal, or hepatic assist devices is curtailed by the need for systemic heparin and the adverse effects of synthetic surfaces on blood. Since blood reacts with every known surface except the endothelial cell, means to control the adverse effects of this interaction are a necessary prerequisite for the development of long-term paracorporeal assist devices as well as artificial organs.

REFERENCES

1. Edmunds LH Jr, Stephenson LW: Cardiopulmonary Bypass for Open Heart Surgery, in Glenn WWL, Baue AE, Lindskog BS (eds): *Thoracic and Cardiovascular Surgery*, New York, Appleton-Century-Crofts, 1982, pp 1091–1106.
2. Edmunds LH Jr: Pulseless cardiopulmonary bypass. *J Thorac Cardiovasc Surg* 1982;84:800–804.
3. Colman RW: Deficiencies of Factor XII, prekallikrein and high molecular weight kininogen, in Colman RW, Hirsh J, Marder VJ, Salzman EW (eds): *Hemostasis and Thrombosis: Basic Principles and Clinical Practice*, Philadelphia, JP Lippincott Co, 1982, pp 3–17.
4. Baier RE, Dutton RC: Initial events in interactions of blood with a foreign surface. *J Biomed Mater Res* 1969;3:191–205,1969.
5. Kim SW, Wisniewski S, Lee ES, et al: Role of proteins and fatty acid

absorption on platelet adhesion and aggregation at the blood-polymer interface. *J Biomed Mater Res (Symposium 8)* 1977;11:23–31.

6. Vroman L, Adams AL, Klings M, et al: Fibrinogen, globulin, albumin and plasma at interfaces. *Adv Chem* 1975;145:255–289.

7. Vroman L, Adams AL, Fischer GC, et al: Interaction of high molecular weight kininogen Factor XII and fibrinogen in plasma at interfaces. *Blood* 1980;55:156–159.

8. Packhan MA, Evans G, Glynn MF, et al: The effect of plasma proteins on the interaction of platelets with glass surfaces. *J Lab Clin Med* 1969;73:686–697.

9. Salzman EW, Landon J, Brier D: Surface-induced platelet adhesion, aggregation and release, in Vroman L, Leonard EF (eds): *The Behavior of Blood and Its Components at Interfaces*. New York, New York Academy of Science 1977, pp 114–127.

10. Dutton RC, Edmunds LH Jr, Hutchinson JC, et al: Platelet aggregate emboli produced in patients during cardiopulmonary bypass with membrane and bubble oxygenators and blood filters. *J Thorac Cardiovasc Surg* 1974;67:258–265.

11. Walsh PN: Platelet-coagulant protein interactions, in Colman RW, Hirsh J, Marder VJ, et al (eds): *Hemostasis and Thrombosis: Basic Principles and Clinical Practice*, Philadelphia, JB Lippincott Co, 1982, pp 404–420.

12. Needleman SW, Hook JC: Platelets and leukocytes, in Colman RW, Hirsh J, Marder VJ, et al (eds): *Hemostasis and Thrombosis: Basic Principles and Clinical Practice*, Philadelphia, JB Lippincott Co, 1982, pp 716–725.

13. Bull BS, Huse WM, Brauer FS, et al: Heparin therapy during extracorporeal circulation: The use of a drug response curve to individualize heparin and protamine dosage. *J Thorac Cardiovasc Surg* 1975;69:685–689.

14. Davies GC, Sobel M, Salzman EW: Elevated fibrinopeptide A and thromboxane A_2 levels during cardiopulmonary bypass. *Circulation* 1980;61:808–814.

15. Rosenberg RD: Heparin-antithrombin system, in Colman RW, Hirsh J, Marder VJ, et al (eds): *Hemostasis and Thrombosis: Basic Principles and Clinical Practice*, Philadelphia, JB Lippincott Co, 1982, pp 962–985.

16. Harker LA, Malpass TW, Branson AG, et al: Mechanism of abnormal bleeding in patients undergoing cardiopulmonary bypass: Acquired transient platelet dysfunction associated with selective granule release. *Blood* 1980;56:824–834.

17. Chenoweth DE, Cooper SW, Hugli TE, et al: Complement activation during cardiopulmonary bypass: Evidence for generation of C3a and C5a anaphylatoxins. *N Engl J Med* 1981;304:497–503.

18. Edmunds LH Jr, Addonizio VP Jr: Platelet physiology during cardiopulmonary bypass, in Utley JR (ed): *Pathophysiology and Techniques of Cardiopulmonary Bypass*, Baltimore, Williams & Wilkins, 1981, pp 106–119.

19. Edmunds LH Jr, Ellison N, Colman RW, et al: Platelet function during open heart surgery: Comparison of membrane and bubble oxygenators. *J Thorac Cardiovasc Surg* 1982;83:805–812.

20. Edmunds LH Jr, Williams W: Microemboli and the use of filters during cardiopulmonary bypass, in Utley, JR (ed): *Pathophysiology and Techniques of Cardiopulmonary Bypass*, vol 2. Baltimore, Williams & Wilkins, 1983, pp 110–114.

21. Hill JD, Aguilar MJ, Baranco A, et al: Neuropathological manifestations of cardiac surgery. *Ann Thorac Surg* 1969;7:409–419.

22. Ratliff NB, Young WG Jr, Hackel DB, et al: Pulmonary injuries secondary to extracorporeal circulation. *J Thorac Cardiovasc Surg* 1973;65:425–432.

23. Ekert H, Montgomery D, Aberdeen E: Fibrinolysis during extracorporeal circulation. *Circ Res* 1971;28:512–517.
24. Colman RW, Robboy SJ: Postoperative disseminated intravascular coagulation and fibrinolysis. *Urol Clin North Am* 1976;3:379–392.
25. Radegran K, Aren C, Teger-Nilsson AC: Prostacyclin infusion during extracorporeal circulation for coronary bypass. *J Throac Cardiovasc Surg* 1982;84:601–608.
26. Faichney A, Davidson KG, Wheatley DJ, et al: Prostacyclin in cardiopulmonary bypass operations. *J Thorac Cardiovasc Surg* 1982;84:601–608.
27. Turney JH, Fewel MR, Williams LC, et al: Platelet protection and heparin sparing with prostacyclin during regular dialysis therapy. *Lancet* 1980;2:219–222.
28. Palatianos GM, Edmunds LH Jr, Cohen DJ, et al: Extracorporeal left ventricular assistance with prostacyclin and heparinized centrifugal pump. *Ann Thor Surg* 1983;35:504–515.

19 *Thromboembolism in Hemodialysis*

Michael J. Weston

Hemodialysis is by far the most widely used extracorporeal circuit today and it has revolutionized the treatment of both acute and chronic renal failure. Clinical hemodialysis was developed by Kolff in occupied Holland during World War II and a major factor in its success was the availability of heparin to prevent clotting of blood upon contact with the foreign surfaces of the dialysis circuit. Experimental hemodialysis had been demonstrated in dogs much earlier in the twentieth century by Abel, Rowntree, and Turner but anticoagulation had been difficult and expensive, depending upon the hirudin obtained from freshly ground leeches; as with the grape harvest, the first "pressing" gave the best quality material! Hemodialysis had been much refined since those early days and in recent years the problems associated with the use of heparin, not least of which is still its expense even today, have received attention.

ANTICOAGULATION FOR HEMODIALYSIS

The rapid action of heparin which, together with antithrombin III, an α_2 globulin, inhibits the conversion by thrombin of fibrinogen to fibrin and the action of activated factors X, XII, and IX, makes it an apparently ideal anticoagulant for hemodialysis. There is little doubt that in the majority of cases this is so if success is judged by the prevention of massive clotting in the dialysis circuit. This unfortunate event does not usually result in clinically significant embolization of clot to the patient but it causes loss of blood in the dialyzer and tubing, delays the patient's treatment while the circuit is changed, and increases the expense of the procedure because fresh disposable components are needed. It is customary to administer heparin either as a bolus at the start of dialysis or as a bolus followed by an infusion into the circuit, the amounts given ranging from 5,000 to 30,000 IU depending upon the requirements of the patient. A bolus of 30 IU/kg body weight followed by 30 IU/kg intravenously per hour is sufficient to prolong activated whole blood clotting times (vide infra) by 60 seconds in most patients, but often adjustments are made on pragmatic lines by the nursing staff. For example, clotting of a dialyzer circuit might result in doubling of the dose but troublesome bleeding after removal of needles from the fistula used for access may necessitate a reduction in dosage, particularly during the last hour of

394

dialysis. Heparin might be increased to improve the "wash back" of blood from the dialyzer and when done properly this seldom leaves more than a milliliter or two of blood in the circuit. Along these lines most patients achieve satisfactory hemodialysis for long periods.

Thus, the laboratory's help in controlling heparin administration for hemodialysis is seldom needed, and indeed it is not known which test of clotting and by how much it should be prolonged, would be the most appropriate. Whole blood clotting times in clean glass tubes at body temperature (Lee White clotting time) may be done at the bedside, but are time-consuming and it is probable that decline of heparin activity in vivo may proceed at a different pace than in the aliquot in the test tube; there is little point in quantifying further a Lee White clotting time of more than 20 minutes and a result of only a minute or two longer than the baseline value at the start of dialysis would indicate the need for a further dose of heparin. Prothrombin times, kaolin-cephalin clotting times, and thrombin clotting times all have their applications, particularly in a research capacity, but require an experienced laboratory scientist for their measurement. Another method is to titrate the heparin in aliquots of blood from the circuit against protamine sulfate or hexadimethrine bromide and to try to maintain levels of 0.3 to 0.7 IU/ml. More recently automated systems measuring activated whole blood clotting times (eg, the Hemochron system) in matters of seconds rather than minutes have been used by the bedside and have improved the control of heparin anticoagulation. How much prolongation of the activated whole blood clotting time is decided by the clinician, and monitoring is frequently required in a patient who is bleeding or at risk of doing so during dialysis. In these circumstances it may be wise to avoid prolonging the activated whole blood clotting time by more than 60 seconds over base line.

Problems Associated with the Use of Heparin

Heparin is a heterogeneous substance composed of a number of molecular weight fractions possessing different potential for inhibiting thrombin and activated factors X, XI, IX (Figure 19-1). Its sources include lung and mucosa from beef and pork and it is therefore not surprising that there is variability between commercial sources and even between batches from the same commercial source. Attempts are usually made to standardize the product but this is difficult because of lack of knowledge of which property of heparin is most important for use in extracorporeal circulations. Application of the clotting tests alluded to above not only show different responses to a given dose of heparin from one batch in different patients but also variability from day to day in the same patient. In this latter respect, intercurrent febrile illnesses, myocardial infarction, and cancer, all of which may alter acute phase proteins, often seem to increase heparin requirements for dialysis, but thrombocytopenia and liver dysfunction reduce them. In view of the release of heparin-neutralizing activity from platelets during aggregation and the central role of the liver in the synthesis of clotting factors, this is not unexpected.

Osteoporosis and alopecia   Use of heparin after myocardial infarction has been sometimes associated with the development of osteoporosis although the mechanisms are unknown. Many patients on maintenance hemodialysis suffer from renal osteodystrophy but the contribution to this of heparin used for routine hemodialysis is unclear. Nevertheless, it seems reasonable to try to reduce the heparin to a minimum required to prevent clotting during dialysis in view of this complication. Means by which this may be achieved are discussed below. Occasionally delayed-onset alopecia may be attributed to heparin therapy during dialysis.

Thrombocytopenia   This may be a transitory phenomenon after administration of heparin resulting from the production of platelet aggregates and their sequestration in the reticuloendothelial systems. More serious however, is the immune thrombocytopenia induced by heparin thought to be mediated by IgG antibodies which promote platelet aggregation and a number of thromboembolic complications. It is worth trying heparin from different sources in these circumstances but the patient may need to use a different form of anticoagulation in the form of vitamin K analogues (warfarin), antiplatelet agents, etc.

White thrombus formation and microembolization   The clot which blocks the dialysis circuit completely if insufficient heparin is used is a large classical red one composed mostly of red cells and fibrin. Use of heparin in sufficient quantities to prevent this does not stop deposition on

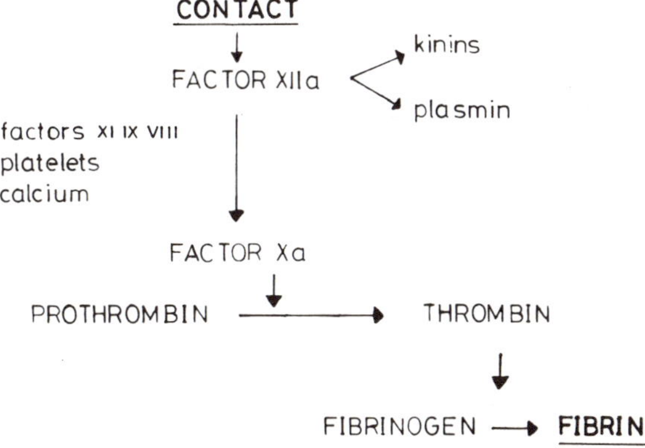

Figure 19-1   Simplified version of the intrinsic coagulation pathway which is activated by contact with the dialyzer surface. The sub-set a indicates an activated clotting factor. The main actions of heparin are to combine with antithrombin III to inhibit activated factor X and to inhibit thrombin-mediated conversion of fibrinogen to fibrin.

the foreign surfaces of the circuit of "white thrombus." Found in the areas of high shear stress in the circuit (eg, within the dialyzer at the points of blood entry and exit), it is composed mainly of platelets, leukocytes, and fibrin. The fibrin may derive from the intraplatelet stores of fibrinogen, deposition of which is not stopped by heparin unless concentrations of 50 IU/ml or more are achieved, which are unacceptably high for clinical use. On the contrary, by promoting platelet aggregation, heparin might actually promote the formation of white thrombus. White thrombus is undesirable, particularly in hollow-fiber dialyzers, the efficacy of which may be reduced by occlusion of capillary pathways. Since the main component of white thrombus is platelets, it is not surprising that drugs with antiplatelet actions reduce this phenomenon. This has been shown with aspirin, dipyridamole, and sulfinpyrazone, all of which have been given to the patient orally prior to dialysis. A potential disadvantage of aspirin therapy, however, is its predisposition to gastrointestinal blood loss which, even in its occult form, may increase four- to five-fold.

The place of the potent antiplatelet agent prostacyclin in hemodialysis is discussed below.

Dialysis and hypoxia Heparin does not prevent the deposition on the foreign surfaces of the dialyzer of proteins, leukocytes, or platelets. The complement, kinin, and fibrinolytic systems are all activated to varying degrees but precoating of the surface with albumin renders it more biocompatible. One of the readily demonstrable effects of hemodialysis using Cuprophane membranes is the production of arterial hypoxia during the first hour of dialysis. Microembolization to the lungs from white thrombus or platelet aggregates formed within the dialyzer may contribute to this hypoxia and although incorporation of particle filters within the circuit between the dialyzer and venous side of the circulation may reduce it, the filters themselves may give rise to thromboembolism. One mechanism for induction of hypoxia during dialysis appears to be complement activation by the foreign surface of the dialyzer promoting leukocyte aggregation within the lungs. Complement activation and leukocyte sequestration within the lungs is not readily preventable by pharmacologic means and more promising in this respect has been the development of membranes for dialysis which do not activate complement. The hypoxia is of little importance to otherwise healthy patients but may be troublesome to those with heart or lung disease.

Bleeding During Dialysis

Use of anticoagulation during hemodialysis to prevent thromboembolism and clotting may aggravate bleeding. This chapter would be incomplete without some consideration of this problem since it is so frequently encountered in dialysis practice. The postoperative patient or one with a bleeding peptic ulcer are obvious examples, but bleeding into the pericardium or the pleura and the development of subdural hematomas and retroperitoneal bleeding are equally serious and life-threatening problems. Thus, prevention of thromboembolism may be the major requirement of anticoagulants during dialysis but it is equally important that bleeding risks must be minimized. There is little doubt that if blood flow rates are high enough, hemodialysis may be carried out without heparin or other anticoagulation in certain patients. Regular flushing of the dialyzer with saline has been used to reduce clotting. It seems very likely, however, that contact between the blood and the foreign surface will result in activation of clotting factors and exhaustion of platelets. The high flow rates may prevent gross clotting but a form of disseminated coagulation may develop and actually aggravate hemostatic problems. The studies reported of this technic have not documented platelet function before or after, or fibrinogen degradation products, for example, and most renal units have not adopted this procedure.

Regional heparinization is a technic employing neutralization of heparin in the blood returning to the patient from the dialyzer by protamine infusion. In skilled hands this may be effective but the large number of clotting tests required both on the patient's blood and the blood in the dialyzer, the delay in response to altered infusion rates of heparin and protamine, and the predisposition of the latter agent to inhibit platelets and activated factor XI and thus to cause rebound anticoagulation make the technic difficult to use and therefore unpopular. The administration of small doses of heparin with measurement of activated whole blood clotting times or Lee White clotting times, known as "tight heparinization" is probably as effective a method as any in minimizing bleeding during dialysis.

Alternatives to Heparin

Vitamin K analogues   The long duration of action of these agents, slow reversibility, and the need for laboratory control preclude the routine use of vitamin K analogues as anticoagulants for hemodialysis. However, they may be useful in patients who have displayed sensitivity to heparin.

Prostacyclin   The involvement of platelets in white thrombus formation despite heparin therapy and the predisposition of heparin to increase platelet reactivity make the use of an antiplatelet agent during hemodialysis desirable. The isolation of the potent antiplatelet agent prostacyclin, a product of arachidonic acid metabolism in vascular endothelium, has permitted an evaluation of platelet activation in hemodialysis as well as other extracorporeal circulations including charcoal hemoperfusion and cardiopulmonary bypass. Charcoal hemoperfusion

398

employed to treat liver failure had dramatic effects on platelet reactivity inducing platelet aggregate formation in blood flowing over the charcoal column, a problem which was not solved by manipulation of the heparin regimen or by use of dipyridamole or sulfinpyrazone. Prostacyclin is thought to be a major mechanism for the protection of healthy vascular endothelium from platelet adhesion and subsequent aggregation (Figure 19-2). The foreign surfaces of dialyzers or charcoal columns or cardiopulmonary bypass circuits are not protected since they are not covered by endothelium (Figure 19-3) and thus the scene is set for platelets to adhere to foreign surfaces and then to aggregate and perhaps break free as microemboli, a process predisposed to by the enhancement of platelet aggregation induced by heparin infusion (Figure 19-4). Infusion of prostacyclin during use of extracorporeal circulation into the blood line leading into the device, whether it be charcoal column, dialyzer or cardiopulmo-

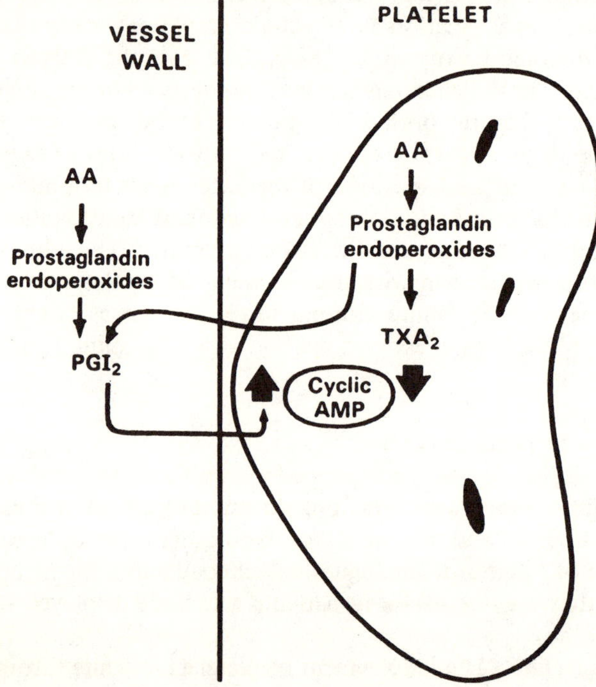

Figure 19-2 Postulated mechanism by which platelet adhesion to healthy endothelium is prevented by the synthesis of prostacyclin (PG1$_2$) in the endothelium from prostaglandin endoperoxides formed within the platelet from arachidonic acid (AA). Thromboxane A$_2$ (TXA$_2$), the other main product of AA metabolism, causes platelet aggregation. (Reproduced with permission from Moncada S, Vane JR: Unstable metabolites of arachidonic acid and their role in haemostasis and thrombosis. *Br Med Bull* 1978;34:129–135.)

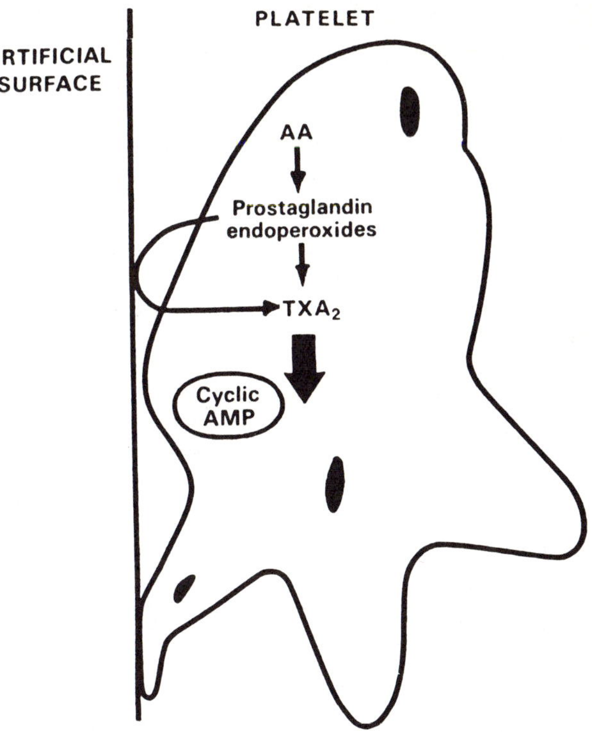

Figure 19-3 Platelet adhesion occurring on a foreign surface which cannot be prevented because there is no enzymatic pathway within the foreign surface to form prostacyclin. Thromboxane generation proceeds from arachidonic acid unopposed. (Reproduced with permission from Moncada S, Vane JR: Unstable metabolites or arachidonic acid and their role in haemostasis and thrombosis. *Br Med Bull* 1978;34:129–135.)

nary bypass circuit, has been carried out both experimentally and in humans and the results of these studies may be summarized as follows:

1. Falls in platelet count are minimized.
2. Platelet aggregate formation is eliminated.
3. The biologic activity of heparin is enhanced (Figure 19-5).
4. Dialysis may be carried out without any heparin at all although this is not possible for charcoal hemoperfusion.
5. During hemodialysis the patient's vascular endothelium is protected from the results of infusion of activated platelets and clotting factors from the dialyzer.

The potency and short duration of action of prostacyclin make it an ideal agent for temporary platelet removal during use of extracorporeal

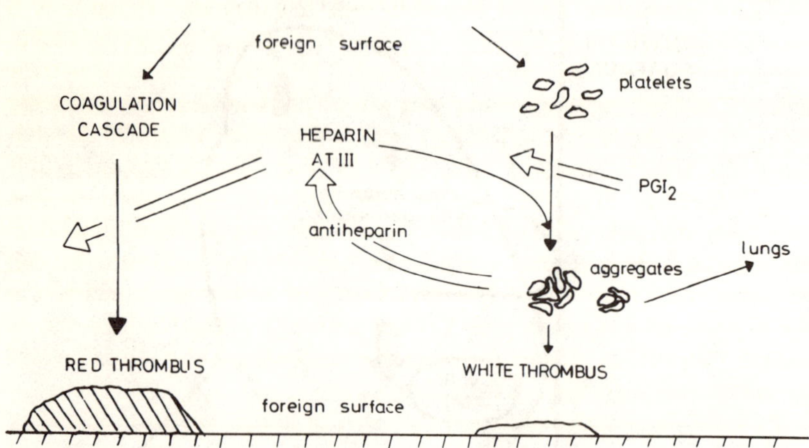

Figure 19-4 Relationship between the coagulation cascade, heparin, antithrombin III (AT-III), platelet activation, and prostacyclin (PGI$_2$) when whole blood comes into contact with a foreign surface. Although heparin is needed to prevent activation of the coagulation cascade, many preparations of heparin promote platelet activation and aggregation and it therefore seems advisable to include in the anticoagulation regimen a potent inhibitor of platelet activation such as prostacyclin.

circulation. By preserving platelets from being exhausted and depleted by the foreign surfaces of the circuit and reducing or eliminating the need for heparin, hemostasis is preserved. Drawbacks to the routine use of prostacyclin during extracorporeal circulation in conscious patients (ie, the majority of patients on hemodialysis but not charcoal hemoperfusion for liver coma or cardiopulmonary bypass during which the patient is anesthetized) include facial flushing, nausea, and sometimes abdominal cramps. Blood pressure needs careful monitoring as does heart rate. More experience with its use is still required but apart from permitting safe dialysis in the patient at risk of bleeding it raises the possibility that its long-term use (or that of a stable analogue) during hemodialysis may reduce the morbidity that such patients suffer from arteriosclerosis. The evidence for this is indirect and derives from the fact that hemodialysis with heparin alone results in elevation of factor VIII–related antigen produced by normal healthy endothelium and also antithrombin III levels. Addition of prostacyclin to the anticoagulation regime prevents such changes, presumably by preventing the release of these two factors from the patient's endothelium. If derangements of factor VIII and antithrombin metabolism reflect damage to endothelium, which may predispose to atherosclerosis, then use of prostacyclin routinely during dialysis may prevent this process.

Low molecular weight heparins and heparinoids Heparin is a heterogeneous mixture of polysaccharide chains which vary in their affinity for the naturally occurring antithrombin III complex and thus in their potency as anticoagulants. Fractionation of heparin has shown that the higher molecular weight substance (average molecular weight 20,000 daltons) has greater reactivity with platelets than that of low molecular weight (average molecular weight 7000 daltons). Evaluation of low molecular weight heparin with sufficient affinity for antithrombin III during hemodialysis is needed, but it seems unlikely that such heparins can be introduced into routine clinical use without an inevitable increase in the expense of this procedure. Various naturally occurring heparinoids such as Org 10172, isolated from porcine mucosa, are also under investigation as anticoagulants in hemodialysis.

Ideally, any anticoagulation regimen for hemodialysis or any other extracorporeal circuit should be cheap, short-acting, and capable of

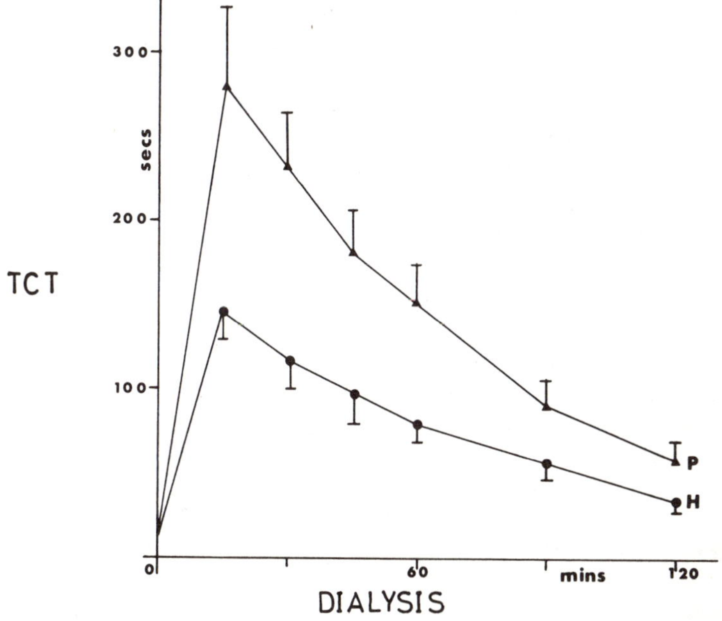

Figure 19-5 The biologic activity of heparin as assessed by thrombin clotting times (TCT), during hemodialysis in humans with uremia with heparin alone (H), or heparin plus prostacyclin (P). This shows obvious enhancement of the biologic activity of heparin in the presence of prostacyclin and that this was maximal at the start of dialysis reflects the fact that the heparin in this investigation was given as a bolus at the start of dialysis. (Reproduced with permission from Turney JH, Williams LC, Fewell MR, et al: Platelet protection and heparin sparing with prostacyclin during regular dialysis therapy. *Lancet* 1980;2:219.)

402

inhibiting the serine proteases of the soluble coagulation cascade as well as inhibiting platelet activity. This is a tall order for any one drug and it seems likely that a combination of heparin and antiplatelet agents may meet these requirements.

SUMMARY

1. For the majority of patients on hemodialysis, heparin is a satisfactory anticoagulant and easy to use although expensive.
2. Individual patient requirements for heparin are often worked out empirically.
3. Closer monitoring of heparin is desirable in the patients at risk of hemorrhage and the most simple regimen is to administer sufficient heparin to maintain a prolongation of the base-line activated whole blood clotting time by 60 seconds.
4. Heparin does not prevent platelet activation during use of extracorporeal circulation and may indeed promote it.
5. Such activation of platelets may contribute to heparin neutralization and to hemostatic defect in the short term. In the longer term platelet activation may damage the patient's endothelium.
6. The addition of a potent antiplatelet agent such as prostacyclin can prevent such platelet activation and by inhibiting release of heparin neutralizing material reduce heparin requirements.
7. Use of prostacyclin thus may render hemodialysis safer in the patient at risk of hemorrhage and in the longer term reduce the incidence of arteriosclerosis.
8. Further evaluation of prostacyclin and other alternatives of heparin is needed, but to gain acceptance for hemodialysis and to prevent a realistic alternative to heparin, must be considerably cheaper.

FURTHER READING

1. Kakkar VV, Thromas DP (eds): *Heparin—Chemistry and Clinical Use*. New York, Academic Press, 1976.
2. Mann RG, Chuang HYk, Mohammad SV, et al: Extracorporeal thrombogenesis and anticoagulation, in Drukker W, Parsons, F, Maher JF (eds): *Replacement of Renal Function by Dialysis*. Martinus Nijhoff, 1979, p 199.
3. Weston MJ: Prostacyclin and extracorporeal circulation. *Br Med Bull*, to be published.

Index